HIV/AIDS FINANCING AND SPENDING IN EASTERN AND SOUTHERN AFRICA

EDITED BY VAILET MUKOTSANJERA

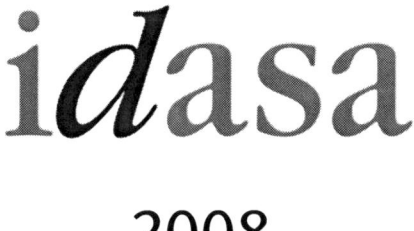

2008

Published by Idasa, 357 Visagie Street, Pretoria 0001

© Idasa 2008
ISBN 978-1-920118-69-3

First published 2008

Edited by Lois Henderson
Cover by Marco Franzoso
Layout by Bronwen Müller
Production by Idasa Publishing

Bound and printed by ABC Press, Cape Town

ACKNOWLEDGEMENTS

The publication of *HIV/AIDS Financing and Spending in Eastern and Southern Africa* would not have been possible without the consistent and invaluable contribution of various individuals and organisations. Considering the many challenges involved, we thank all those who contributed either directly or indirectly to the completion of the project. First and foremost, Idasa–GAP wishes to thank the Swedish International Development Agency (SIDA) for their financial support to the three-year multicountry study. Secondly, we extend our thanks to United Nations Programme on AIDS (UNAIDS) for the technical support rendered during both the formative and intermediate phases of the project. Without the participation of representatives from government, civil society, AIDS Councils, People Living with HIV/AIDS and donor agencies, this work would not have emerged as it has.

Finally, our gratitude to our country partners and their in-country stakeholders who made the collection, analysis of the data and documentation possible:

MALAWI

We thank the following Malawian in-country stakeholders:
- Malawi Economic Justice Network (MEJN);
- Action Aid International Malawi;
- Malawi National AIDS Commission; and
- UNAIDS Malawi.

The Malawi Economic Justice Network (MEJN) also wishes to thank the following organisations for their financial and technical support of the current study:
- The MoH (most notably for the permission to produce the HIV/AIDS section of the main NHA report);
- The US Agency for International Development (USAID)/Malawi;
- WHO/Malawi;
- Action Aid International Malawi;
- Idasa;
- SIDA;
- UNAIDS/Malawi;
- NAC;
- The MEJN:
- Actionaid Malawi; and
- USAID, through the Partners for Health Reformplus (PHRplus) Project based in Bethesda, Maryland, USA.

ETHIOPIA

We thank the following Ethiopian in-country stakeholders:
- The Institute for Development Research (IDR), Addis Ababa University;

- The HIV/AIDS Prevention Control Programme (HAPCO), the Ministry of Health (MoH);
- The Ministry of Finance and Economic Development (MoFED); and
- ActionAid.

ZAMBIA

We thank the following Zambian in-country stakeholders:
- The INESOR, University of Zambia (UNZA); and
- The Zambian National AIDS Council (NAC).

TANZANIA

We thank the following Tanzanian in-country stakeholders:
- The Economic and Social Research Foundation (ESRF);
- Youth Action Volunteers (YAV);
- The Tanzanian Commission for AIDS (TACAIDS);
- The Zanzibar AIDS Commission (ZAC); and
- The Ministry of Finance (MoF).

KENYA

We thank the following Kenyan in-country stakeholders:
- The University of Nairobi Enterprises and Services (UNES);
- The Department of Economics, University of Nairobi;
- The Kenyan Treatment Access Movement (KTAM);
- The MoF; and
- The National AIDS Control Council (NACC).

The project encountered many challenges, including the departure of the original research team from Idasa at a critical phase of the study, which served to slow the pace and minimise the impact of the experience gained from previous related Idasa interventions. However, Teresa Guthrie, one of the initiators of the project, made herself available to assist with the external review; the reorientation of the new team, led by Vailet Mukostanjera; and technical edits. We are most grateful for her commitment and contribution in this regard. Similarly, Elesani Njobvu, a senior economist who served with the UNAIDS intercountry team during the course of the study, pinpointed shortcomings and provided guidance during the initial stages of the project. Several members of GAP, including the former Unit Manager of the AIDS Budget Unit, Nhlanhla Ndhlovu; the researcher Rabelani Daswa and the administrator Vasanthie Naicker, worked on the project.

ZANZIBAR

The Zanzibar AIDS Commission (ZAC) also wishes to thank those individuals who shared their knowledge in their areas of expertise, providing the requisite data. Researchers were mainly drawn from:

- The Zanzibar AIDS Control Programme (ZACP);
- The Ministry of Finance and Economic Affairs (MoFEA);
- The Zanzibar HIV/AIDS NGO Cluster (ZANGOC);
- The Zanzibar Association of People Living with HIV/AIDS (ZAPHA+); and
- Action Aid Tanzania.

In particular, we wish to thank Ms Asha Abdullah (ZAC); Ms Amina Makame (ZAC); Mr Ameir Khamis (ZACP); and Ms Asha Ahmed (ZANGOC).

ZAC also wishes to express gratitude to the Office of the Chief Government Statistician (OCGS) for providing requisite data for this study. The technical support provided by Dr Flora Kessy, Dr Oswald Mashindano and Mr Samwel Kessy of the ESRF is also highly appreciated. ZAC is also grateful to Idasa for the financial support to undertake this important study.

The final phases of the project benefited from the editing skills of the GAP staff, Kondwani Chirambo, Marietjie Myburg and Christele Diwouta. Finally, we take the opportunity to thank Etienne Yemek, an economist from Idasa's Economic Governance Programme, who provided further technical support and the internal review, as well as Idasa's Publishing Unit for the final editing and design of the publication.

Vailet M. Mukotsanjera, Regional Coordinator, AIDS Budget Unit

The opinions, conclusions and recommendations in this publication do not necessarily reflect the donors' opinion.

CONTENTS

TABLES   PAGE

FIGURES   PAGE

Acronyms and Abbreviations

ABC	Abstinence, Being faithful, and Condom
ABCZ	AIDS Business Coalition in Zanzibar
ABU	AIDS Budget Unit
ACU	AIDS Control Unit
AGO	Accountant-General's Office
AIA	Appropriation in Aid
AIDS	Acquired Immuno-Deficiency Syndrome
ApUIy	Appropriation Utilisation Index
ASC	AIDS Spending Categories
AUIy	Allotment Utilisation Index
BCC	Behaviour Change Communication
BLM	Banja la Mtsogdo
BoFED	Bureau of Finance and Economic Development (regional)
BoP	Balance of Payments
BoT	Bank of Tanzania
BP	Beneficiary segments of population
BPIy	Budget Programming Index
BSC	Budget Steering Committee
BSD	Budgetary Supplies Department
BSS	Behaviour Surveillance Survey
CACC	Constituency AIDS Control Committee
CAG	Controller and Auditor-General
CARF	Community AIDS Response Fund AIDS or Action
CBO	community-based organisation
CBS	Central Bureau of Statistics
CCJDP	Catholic Commission of Justice and Development
CCM	Chama cha Mapinduzi
CDC	Centre for Disease Control
CFS	Consolidated Fund Services
CH	Child Health
CHAI	Clinton Foundation against HIV/AIDS
CHAM	Christian Health Association of Malawi
CHF	Community Health Fund
CIDA	Canadian International Development Agency
CMAC	Council Multisectoral AIDS Committee
CMO	Chief Minister's Office
CO	Clinical Officer
CPU	Central Planning Unit
CRDA	Catholic Relief and Development Agency
CSA	Central Statistics Authority
CSD	Constitutional Statutory and Debt Servicing

CSO	CIVIL SOCIETY ORGANISATION
CSW	COMMERCIAL SEX WORKER
DAC	DEVELOPMENT ASSISTANCE COMMITTEE
DACCOMs	DISTRICT AIDS COORDINATING COMMITTEES
DATF	DISTRICT AIDS TASK FORCE
DBCC	DEPARTMENT OF BUDGET COORDINATION COMMITTEE
DBM	DEPARTMENT OF BUDGET AND MANAGEMENT
DBS	DIRECT BUDGET SUPPORT
DFID	DEPARTMENT FOR INTERNATIONAL DEVELOPMENT
DHS	DEMOGRAPHIC AND HEALTH SURVEY
DOH	DEPARTMENT OF HEALTH
DRI	DISTRICT RESPONSE INITIATIVE PROGRAM
EMSAP	ETHIOPIAN MULTISECTORAL HIV/AIDS PROGRAMME
ERD	EXTERNAL RESOURCE DEPARTMENT
ESRF	ECONOMIC AND SOCIAL RESEARCH FOUNDATION
EU	EUROPEAN UNION
FA	FINANCING AGENT
FBO	FAITH-BASED ORGANISATION
FDRE	FEDERAL DEMOCRATIC REPUBLIC OF ETHIOPIA
FHAPCO	FEDERAL HIV/AIDS PREVENTION AND CONTROL OFFICE
FHI	FAMILY HEALTH INTERNATIONAL
FMA	FINANCIAL MANAGEMENT AGENCY
FS	FINANCING SOURCES
FY	FINANCIAL YEAR
GAA	GOVERNMENT APPROPRIATIONS ACT
GDP	GROSS DOMESTIC PRODUCT
G8	GROUP OF EIGHT (INDUSTRIALISED COUNTRIES)
GER	GROSS ENROLMENT RATIO
GFATM	GLOBAL FUND TO FIGHT AIDS, TUBERCULOSIS AND MALARIA
GFCCM	GLOBAL FUND COUNTRY COORDINATING MECHANISM
GFS	GOVERNMENT FINANCE STATISTICS
GNI	GROSS NATIONAL INCOME
GOK	GOVERNMENT OF KENYA
HAPCO	HIV/AIDS PREVENTION CONTROL PROGRAMME
HBS	HOUSEHOLD BUDGET SURVEY
HDI	HUMAN DEVELOPMENT INDEX
HQ	HEADQUARTERS
HSDP	HEALTH SECTOR DEVELOPMENT PROGRAM
HSSP	HEALTH SERVICES AND SYSTEMS PROJECT
ICASA	INTERNATIONAL CONFERENCE ON AIDS AND STDs IN AFRICA
IDR	INSTITUTE FOR DEVELOPMENT RESEARCH
IDU	INJECTING DRUG USER
IEC	INFORMATION, EDUCATION AND COMMUNICATION

IFMS	INTEGRATED FINANCIAL MANAGEMENT SYSTEM
IHRDC	IFAKARA HEALTH RESEARCH AND DEVELOPMENT CENTRE
ILO	INTERNATIONAL LABOR ORGANIZATION
IMF	INTERNATIONAL MONETARY FUND
IMG	INDEPENDENT MONITORING GROUP
IMR	INFANT MORTALITY RATE
IMTC	INTERMINISTERIAL TECHNICAL COMMITTEE
INESOR	INSTITUTE FOR ECONOMIC AND SOCIAL RESEARCH
IPAR	INSTITUTE OF POLICY ANALYSIS AND RESEARCH
JAPR	JOINT AIDS PROGRAMME REVIEW
JAS	JOINT ASSISTANCE STRATEGY
JFA	JOINT FINANCING AGREEMENT
KCMC	KILIMANJARO CHRISTIAN MEDICAL CENTRE
KDHS	KENYA DEMOGRAPHIC HEALTH SURVEY
KHADREP	KENYA HIV/AIDS DISASTER RESPONSE PROJECT
KNASP	KENYA NATIONAL AIDS STRATEGIC PLAN
KTAM	KENYAN TREATMENT ACCESS MOVEMENT
M&E	MONITORING AND EVALUATION
MAP	MULTICOUNTRY HIV/AIDS PROGRAMME
MARP	MOST-AT-RISK-POPULATIONS
MCH	MATERNAL AND CHILD HEALTH
MDAs	MINISTRIES, DEPARTMENTS AND AGENCIES
MDG	MILLENNIUM DEVELOPMENT GOAL
MDHS	MALAWI DEMOGRAPHIC AND HEALTH SURVEY
MEDaC	MINISTRY OF ECONOMIC DEVELOPMENT AND COOPERATION
MEFF	MACROECONOMIC AND FISCAL FRAMEWORK
MEJN	MALAWI ECONOMIC JUSTICE NETWORK
MK	MALAWI KWACHA
MMR	MATERNAL MORTALITY RATIO
MOALE	MINISTRY OF AGRICULTURE, LIVESTOCK AND ENVIRONMENT
MoE	MINISTRY OF EDUCATION
MoF	MINISTRY OF FINANCE
MoFEA	MINISTRY OF FINANCE AND ECONOMIC AFFAIRS
MoFED	MINISTRY OF FINANCE AND ECONOMIC DEVELOPMENT
MoFNP	MINISTRY OF FINANCING AND NATIONAL PLANNING
MoH	MINISTRY OF HEALTH (AND POPULATION)
MoHSW	MINISTRY OF HEALTH AND SOCIAL WELFARE
MoPND	MINISTRY OF PLANNING AND NATIONAL DEVELOPMENT
MOTTI	MINISTRY OF TRADE, TOURISM AND INVESTMENT
MP	MEMBER OF PARLIAMENT
MPAC	MULTISECTORAL POLICY ADVISORY COMMITTEE
MPER	MINISTERIAL PUBLIC EXPENDITURE REVIEW
MSH	MANAGEMENT SCIENCES FOR HEALTH

MSM	Men who have sex with other men
MTEF	Medium-term Expenditure Framework
MTP	Medium-term Plan
NAA	National AIDS Account
NAC	National AIDS Commission; National AIDS Council
NACC	National AIDS Control Council
NACP	National AIDS Control Programme
NASA	National AIDS Spending Assessment
NASCOP	National HIV/AIDS and STI Control Programme
NBPC	National Budget and Planning Committee
NBS	National Bureau of Statistics
NER	Net Enrolment Ratio
NGO	Non-governmental Organisation
NHA	National Health Accounts
NHIF	National Health Insurance Fund
NMSF	National Multisectoral Strategic Framework
NRB	National Review Board
NRE	National Resource Envelope
NSF	National Strategic Framework
NSGRP	National Strategy for Growth and Reduction of Poverty
NSP	National strategic plan
NZP+	Network of Zambians Living with HIV/AIDS
OACIy	Overall Absorptive Capacity Index
OCGS	Office of the Chief Government Statistician
OI	Opportunistic infection
OOPE	Out-of-pocket expenditure
OP	Office of the President
OPC	Office of the President and Cabinet
ORID	Other related infectious diseases
OSY	Out-of-school youth
OUNHC	Office of the United Nations High Commission
OVC	Orphans and vulnerable children
OVP	Office of the Vice-President
PAF	Policy Assessment Framework
PAPs	Programmes, activities and projects
PASDEP	Plan for Accelerated and Sustained Development to End Poverty
PATF	Provincial AIDS Task Force
PDCC	Provincial Development Coordinating Committee
PEP	Post-exposure prophylaxis
PEPFAR	Presidential Emergency Plan for AIDS Relief
PER	Public Expenditure Reviews
PF	Production factors
PFMRP	Public Financial Management Reform Program
PHC (C)	Primary Health Care (Center)

PHF	Primary Health Facility
PHRplus	Partners for Health Reformplus
PLWHA	People Living with HIV/AIDS
PMO	Prime Minister's Office
PMTCT	Prevention of Mother-to-Child Transmission
PoW	Programme of Work
PPP	Purchasing Power Parity
PRBS	Poverty Reduction Budget Support
PRS	Poverty Reduction Strategy
PRSC	Poverty Reduction Support Credit
PS	Permanent Secretary
PSI	Population Services International
PTR	Pupil teacher ratio
RAB	Regional Advisory Board
RALG	Regional Administration and Local Government
RAPIDS	Reaching HIV/AIDS-Affected People with Integrated Development and Support
RAS	Regional Administrative Secretary
RBB	Results-based budgeting
RC	Regional Committee
RFE	Rapid Fund Envelope
RGoZ	Revolutionary Government of Zanzibar
RH	Reproductive Health
RHAPCO	Regional HIV/AIDS Prevention and Control Office
RTS	Resource Tracking Software
SADC	Southern African Development Community
SAP	Structural Adjustment Programme
SARPN	Southern African Regional Poverty Network
SER	Special Exchequer Requisitions
SFH	Society for Family Health
SHACCOM	Shehia AIDS Coordinating Committee
SHARE	Support to the HIV/AIDS Response in Zambia
SIDA	Swedish International Development Agency
SNA	Systems of Health Accounts
SOE	Statement of Expenditure
SSA	Sub-Saharan Africa
STI	Sexually transmitted infection
SU	Substance user
SWAp	Sector-wide Approach
SWG	Sector Working Group
TAC	Technical AIDS Committees
TACAIDS	Tanzania Commission for AIDS
TAS	Tanzania Assistance Strategy
TB	Tuberculosis

TFHAE	Total Foreign HIV/AIDS Expenditure
THAE	Total HIV/AIDS Expenditure
THE	Total Health Expenditure
THIS	Tanzania HIV/AIDS Indicator Survey
TMAP	Tanzania Multi-Sectoral AIDS Project
TPE	Total Public Expenditure
TPHAE	Total Public HIV/AIDS Expenditure
TPHE	Total Public Health Expenditure
TPHME	Total Public HIV/AIDS Expenditure
TRA	Tanzania Revenue Authority
UN	United Nations
UNAIDS	United Nations Programme on AIDS
UNDP	United Nations Development Programme
UNGASS	United Nations General Assembly Special Session on HIV/AIDS
UNHCR	United Nations High Commissioner for Refugees
UNICEF	United Nations Children's Fund
UNIP	United National Independence Party
UNZA	University of Zambia
UPE	Universal Primary Education
URT	United Republic of Tanzania
USAID	United States Agency for International Development
US$	United States dollar
VAT	Value-added tax
VCT	Voluntary counselling and testing
VMAC	Village Multisectoral AIDS Committee
WB	World Bank
WFP	World Food Programme
WHO	World Health Organization
WMAC	Ward Multisectoral AIDS Committee
YAV	Youth Action Volunteers
ZAC	Zanzibar AIDS Commission
ZACP	Zanzibar AIDS Control Program
ZAIADA	Zanzibar against AIDS Infection and Drug Abuse
ZANARA	Zambia National Response to AIDS
ZANGOC	Zanzibar NGO Cluster for HIV/AIDS Prevention
ZAPHA+	Zanzibar Association of People Living with HIV/AIDS
ZIADA	Zanzibar Association of Interfaith on AIDS and Development
ZNAN	Zambia National AIDS Network
ZNSP	Zanzibar National Strategic Plan
ZPCT	Zambian Prevention, Control and Treatment
ZPRP	Zanzibar Poverty Reduction Plan
ZRB	Zanzibar Revenue Board
ZWRCN	Zimbabwe Women's Resource Centre and Network

GLOSSARY OF ECONOMIC TERMS

ABSORPTIVE CAPACITY: THE ABILITY OF SERVICE PROVIDERS TO SPEND ALL THE RESOURCES THAT HAVE BEEN ALLOCATED TO THEM

ALLOCATION: THE FUNDS SET ASIDE FOR A PARTICULAR PURPOSE

BALANCED BUDGET: EQUALITY BETWEEN REVENUES AND EXPENDITURES THAT CONSTITUTE A BUDGET

BALANCE OF PAYMENTS: THE DIFFERENCE BETWEEN THE FUNDS RECEIVED BY A COUNTRY AND THOSE PAID OUT BY A COUNTRY FOR ALL INTERNATIONAL TRANSACTIONS

BUDGET: A STATEMENT OF THE FINANCIAL POSITION OF AN ENTITY – ESPECIALLY A HOUSEHOLD, BUSINESS, OR GOVERNMENT – BASED ON ESTIMATES OF ANTICIPATED REVENUE AND EXPENDITURE

BUDGET DEFICIT: AN EXCESS OF BUDGETARY EXPENDITURE OVER REVENUE

BUDGET SURPLUS: AN EXCESS OF BUDGETARY REVENUE OVER EXPENDITURE

CONSUMER PRICE INDEX: AN INDEX OF THE PRICES OF GOODS, SUCH AS FOOD AND CLOTHING, AND SERVICES, SUCH AS HEALTH AND TRANSPORT, TYPICALLY PURCHASED BY THE URBAN CONSUMER

ECONOMIC DEVELOPMENT: THE PROCESS OF IMPROVING THE ECONOMY'S ABILITY TO SATISFY CONSUMER WANTS AND NEEDS

ECONOMIC GROWTH: LONG-TERM EXPANSION OF THE ABILITY OF AN ECONOMY TO PRODUCE OUTPUT

EFFICIENCY: THE CAPACITY TO OBTAIN THE MOST SATISFACTION POSSIBLE FROM A GIVEN AMOUNT OF RESOURCES

EMPIRICAL: BASED ON, OR RELATING TO, REAL-WORLD DATA OR ANALYSIS; OTHER THAN THEORETICAL

EQUITY: THE FAIRNESS OF INCOME OR WEALTH DISTRIBUTION

EXCHANGE RATE: THE PRICE OF ONE NATION'S CURRENCY IN TERMS OF ANOTHER NATION'S CURRENCY, WITH THE EXCHANGE RATE BEING SPECIFIED AS THE AMOUNT OF ONE CURRENCY THAT CAN BE TRADED IN TERMS OF UNIT OF THE OTHER

EXPENDITURE: THE AMOUNT OF MONEY SPENT

FISCAL: THE 12-MONTH PERIOD THAT GOVERNMENT USES FOR COLLECTING TAXES, APPROPRIATING SPENDING, AND OTHERWISE TABULATING ITS BUDGET

GDP DEFLATOR: A PRICE INDEX BASED ON THE CALCULATION OF THE REAL GROSS DOMESTIC PRODUCT THAT IS USED AS AN INDICATOR OF AVERAGE PRICES IN THE ECONOMY

GDP PRICE DEFLATOR: A PRICE INDEX CALCULATED AS THE RATIO NOMINAL GROSS DOMESTIC PRODUCT TO REAL GROSS DOMESTIC PRODUCT

GOVERNMENT BORROWING: THE DEMAND FOR LOANS OBTAINED THROUGH THE FINANCIAL MARKETS BY THE GOVERNMENT SECTOR TO FINANCE GOVERNMENT PURCHASES OVER AND ABOVE TAXES

GOVERNMENT EXPENDITURE: SPENDING BY THE GOVERNMENT SECTOR, INCLUDING BOTH THE PURCHASE OF FINAL GOODS AND SERVICES, OR THE GROSS DOMESTIC PRODUCT, AND TRANSFER PAYMENTS; USED BY THE GOVERNMENT SECTOR TO UNDERTAKE KEY FUNCTIONS; FINANCED WITH A COMBINATION OF TAXES AND BORROWING

GROSS DOMESTIC PRODUCT (GDP): THE TOTAL MARKET VALUE OF ALL GOODS AND SERVICES PRODUCED WITHIN THE POLITICAL BOUNDARIES OF AN ECONOMY DURING A GIVEN PERIOD OF TIME, USUALLY ONE YEAR

GROWTH RATE: THE PERCENTAGE CHANGE IN A VARIABLE FROM ONE YEAR TO THE NEXT; A MEASURE OF HOW MUCH THE VARIABLE IS GROWING OVER TIME

HUMAN CAPITAL: THE SUM TOTAL OF A PERSON'S PRODUCTIVE KNOWLEDGE, EXPERIENCE, AND TRAINING; THE GREATER THE ACQUISITION OF HUMAN CAPITAL, THE MORE PRODUCTIVE THE PERSON

INFLATION: A PERSISTENT INCREASE IN THE AVERAGE PRICE LEVEL IN THE ECONOMY; OCCURS WHEN THE AVERAGE PRICE LEVEL (THAT IS, PRICES IN GENERAL) INCREASES OVER TIME; NEITHER MEANING THAT ALL PRICES INCREASE BY THE SAME AMOUNT, NOR THAT ALL PRICES NECESSARILY INCREASE

NOMINAL: THE ACTUAL DOLLAR PRICE OF ITEMS WHEN THEY ARE BOUGHT OR SOLD; AS OPPOSED TO TERM "REAL", WHICH IS ACTUAL VALUE ADJUSTED IN ACCORDANCE WITH PRICE CHANGES OR INFLATION

NOMINAL GDP: THE TOTAL MARKET VALUE, MEASURED IN CURRENT PRICES, OF ALL GOODS AND SERVICES PRODUCED WITHIN THE POLITICAL BOUNDARIES OF A CERTAIN ECONOMY DURING A GIVEN PERIOD OF TIME, USUALLY ONE YEAR

OFF-BUDGET EXPENDITURE: ALLOCATIONS MADE TO A GOVERNMENT MINISTRY OR DEPARTMENT, WHICH ARE NEITHER ALLOCATED THROUGH THE NATIONAL BUDGET, NOR ACCOUNTED FOR BY THE GOVERNMENT

ON-BUDGET EXPENDITURE: ALLOCATIONS MADE THROUGH THE BUDGET, WHICH ARE ACCOUNTED FOR BY THE GOVERNMENT

REAL: THE VALUE OF GOODS AND SERVICES AFTER ADJUSTMENTS FOR INFLATION

REAL GDP: THE TOTAL MARKET VALUE, MEASURED IN PRICES, OF ALL GOODS AND SERVICES PRODUCED WITHIN THE POLITICAL BOUNDARIES OF AN ECONOMY DURING A GIVEN PERIOD OF TIME, USUALLY ONE YEAR

RESOURCE ALLOCATION: THE DIVIDING UP AND DISTRIBUTION OF AVAILABLE, LIMITED RESOURCES TO COMPETING, ALTERNATIVE USES THAT SATISFY UNLIMITED WANTS AND NEEDS

REVENUE: THE MONEY COLLECTED IN THE FORM OF TAXES, FEES, FINES, FEDERAL GRANTS, BOND SALES AND OTHER SOURCES DEPOSITED IN THE STATE TREASURY, WHICH SERVES AS A SOURCE OF FUNDING FOR THE GOVERNMENT

NATIONAL AIDS SPENDING ASSESSMENT TERMINOLOGY

(BASED ON THE UN PROGRAMME ON AIDS DEFINITIONS)

AIDS SPENDING CATEGORIES (ASCs) COMPRISE HIV/AIDS-RELATED INTERVENTIONS AND ACTIVITIES, SUCH AS HUMAN RESOURCE INCENTIVES AND RESEARCH.

BENEFICIARY SEGMENTS OF POPULATION (BPs) ARE THOSE SECTORS OF THE POPULATION, SUCH AS PLWHAs, SEX WORKERS, MSM AND IDUs, BENEFITING FROM A CERTAIN PROVISION.

FINANCING AGENTS (FAs) ARE ENTITIES, SUCH AS GOVERNMENT MINISTRIES AND DEPARTMENTS, LOCAL AUTHORITIES AND CSOs, THAT POOL THEIR FINANCIAL RESOURCES TO FINANCE THE PROGRAMMES OF SERVICE PROVIDERS.

FINANCING SOURCES (FSs) ARE ENTITIES, SUCH AS THE GOVERNMENT AND BILATERAL AND MULTILATERAL INSTITUTIONS, THAT FINANCE THE PROVISION OF HIV/AIDS-RELATED SERVICES BY THE AGENTS CONCERNED.

PRODUCTION FACTORS (PFs) / RESOURCE COSTS ARE INPUTS, SUCH AS LABOUR, CAPITAL, NATURAL RESOURCES, ENTREPRENEURIAL RESOURCES AND DISTRIBUTION COSTS.

PROVIDERS (PSs) ARE ENTITIES, SUCH AS HOSPITALS AND CSOs, THAT PRODUCE, PROVIDE AND DELIVER HIV/AIDS-RELATED SERVICES.

ABOUT THE AUTHORS

EDITOR

Vailet Mukotsanjera holds both an MSc in Economics and a BSc Hons in Economics from the University of Zimbabwe. Vailet is currently the Regional Coordinator of the AIDS Budget Unit (ABU) of Idasa's Governance and AIDS Programme. As such, she is responsible for the coordination of the ABU's multicountry research on HIV/AIDS financing and spending in Africa. Her unit also undertakes capacity-building targeted at both state and nonstate actors in Africa.

Prior to joining Idasa, Vailet worked with the Zimbabwe Women's Resource Centre and Network (ZWRCN) as a gender budgeting specialist, defining, designing, implementing and monitoring a gender budgeting action strategy for the organisation. She was also involved in the development of research frameworks and training tools aimed at building gender budget literacy. Before joining the ZWRCN, she worked for MoFED in Zimbabwe as an economist. Her job involved carrying out research and developing economic models that enhance the relevance and utility of fiscal measures, developing and maintaining a database on different economic variables and making recommendations for economic policy formulation. Prior to joining the MoF, as an assistant researcher for the Department of International Development (DfiD) (United Kingdom), she helped to conduct a labour survey entitled *"Where has all the education gone in Zimbabwe?"*.

TANZANIA

Flora Lucas Kessy, a Senior Social Scientist at the Ifakara Health Research and Development Centre (IHRDC), holds a PhD in Agricultural and Consumer Economics, with a major in Family and Consumer Economics and a minor in Women and Gender in Global Perspective from the University of Illinois in Urbana Champaign, USA. She has researched and published material relating to poverty, gender and development, and reproductive health (RH), in particular family planning and HIV/AIDS. Kessy has also published articles in the Tanzania Journal of Development Studies, the American Behavioural Scientist Journal, Uongozi Journal, the Tanzania Journal of Population Studies and Development, and the Journal of Biosocial Science. Before joining IHRDC, Dr Kessy was a Senior Research Fellow at the ESRF (2002–2006), and a lecturer in the Development Studies Institute at Sokoine University of Agriculture (1992–2001). Her email addresses are fkessy@gmail.com and fkessy@ihrdc.or.tz.

Oswald Mashindano is a Senior Research Fellow with the ESRF and the Coordinator of Research and Monitoring at the Foundation. For the past 20 years, Dr Mashindano has been involved with research and teaching at the University of Dar es Salaam, Tanzania. He teaches Microeconomics, Agricultural Economics and Rural Development, and Natural Resources and Environmental Economics. Mashindano has also taught Quantitative Methods and Research Methodology.

Irenei Kiria is an Executive Director for YAV, a health policy and governance-related non-governmental organisation (NGO) based in Dar es Salaam, Tanzania. He has ten years of NGO leadership experience, with a first degree in Sociology, majoring in medical sociology. Kiria is active in the Tanzanian health sector policy and with budget analysis and advocacy aimed at improving the participation of youth in their communities, as well as the equity and quality of health services for youth and the poor. As founder of YAV, he is also involved in mobilising youth volunteers to demand quality health service delivery. Since 2005, YAV, through Irenei, has played an active role in the Health Equity Group, emphasising equitable access to quality health services, in particular as regards reproductive and child health (CH).

ETHIOPIA

Getnet Alemu, a senior researcher and lecturer, currently heads the Macroeconomic and Policy Studies Division at the Institute of Development Research at Addis Ababa University. He obtained a BA degree in Economics from Addis Ababa University in 1987 and both an MA degree in Economic Policy and Planning, in 1992, and a PhD in Development Studies, in 2002, from the Institute of Social Studies in The Hague in the Netherlands in 1992. Until joining Addis Ababa University, he worked for the Ethiopian Government from September 1987 onwards. After filling the role of graduate assistant at the Jimma Health Science Institute (now Jimma University) and of senior economic researcher at the National Urban Planning Institute, he served as a senior investment policy expert for the Ethiopian Investment Authority (currently the Ethiopian Investment Commission).

Abdulhamid Bedri, a senior researcher and lecturer, currently heads the Social and Poverty Studies Division at the Institute of Development Research at Addis Ababa University. After obtaining both his BA and MA degrees in Economics from Addis Ababa University, he successfully defended his PhD in Economics at the University of Kweele in 1992. Since earning his BA degree, he has worked for the Institute of Development Research, serving as Acting Director of the Institute of Development Research from 1993 to 1995.

Yimer Hassen has, since June 2007, worked as an Implementation Support Officer for UNDP. Prior to joining UNDP, he served as the Finance Manager of the Multi-country HIV/AIDS Programme (MAP) (consisting of the World Bank (WB), the United Nations Children's Fund (UNICEF), UNDP, IRISH AID, ActionAid and other donors) in the Federal HIV/AIDS Prevention and Control Office (FHAPCO). He obtained his BA degree in Accounting from the University of Addis Ababa in 1984. At the time of going to press, he is working towards becoming a professional-level Chartered Certified Accountant via distance education in ACCA.

Nigussie Tefera is currently an internal auditor for MoFED. Since obtaining his BA degree in Accounting from Addis Ababa University, he has worked in the Ministry of Finance and Economic Development.

KENYA

Paul Odundo is a specialist in planning, administration and impact evaluation, holding a PhD in planning and administration, and both an MA and a BED in education. He has participated in extensive health-related research at both the national and regional level, including health care financing, the preparation of modules for health management teams, social health insurance and the evaluation of the socio-economic impact of HIV/AIDS. At the time of going to press, he is a lecturer in the School of Education at the University of Nairobi. His main interests are advocacy work and HIV/AIDS resource tracking.

Enos Njeru is an Associate Professor of Sociology and Anthropology in the Department of Sociology at the University of Nairobi. He holds a PhD in Cultural Anthropology from the University of California and both a BA and MA in Sociology from the University of Nairobi. He is a Medical Anthropologist and Fellow in Social Medicine at the Harvard Medical School in Boston, with many years of research and teaching experience in the above fields. Currently on consultancy, Professor Njeru is widely experienced in both consultancy and research work in areas and projects to do with water projects; health and sanitation; poverty analysis and reduction; gender mainstreaming; HIV/AIDS; governance and organisational approaches and project design.

Urbanus Kioko is a Health Economist and lecturer in the School of Economics at the University of Nairobi. He is a holder of an MPhil in Health Economics, an MA in economics and a BED in Economics and Business Studies. He has substantial experience in the field of health and social science research at both an academic level and as a consultant. His main areas of focus are HIV/AIDS; economic evaluation; efficiency analysis; health care financing; and the costing of health interventions. His participation in numerous research activities at both the national and international level include his involvement with the costing of the Kenya National AIDS Strategic Plan (KNASP) (2005/2006–2009/2010), the health sector strategic plan ((2005/2006–2009/2010), the Kenyan post-rape care services and the strategic plan relating to orphans and vulnerable children. He is currently a research associate at the Institute of Policy Analysis and Research (IPAR).

Julius Kipkemoi Korir is an economist and lecturer in the Department of Economics at Kenyatta University, holding both an BA and an MA in Economics. He was also due to complete his doctoral studies by the end of 2007. He has considerable experience in costing health interventions, being involved in the costing of the KNASP from 2005 to 2010, the health sector strategic plan from 2005/2006 to 2009/2010, the Kenyan post-rape care services, and the integrated HIV/AIDS and RH services, as well as with the analysis of the effect of user fees on antenatal and delivery care services in the public health sector in Kenya, and the decentralisation of health services and management capacities at district level in Kenya. He has previously worked with the IPAR as a researcher.

Zambia

Jolly Kamwanga holds degrees in both Demography and Economics and has many years' experience of research into development and health economics and policy issues. He works as a Research Fellow at the INESOR at UNZA, and as a part-time Associate in the Frontiers Development and Research Group. He has worked with public sector institutions, such as the Ministries of Health, Education and Agriculture, as well as with the Cabinet Office. He has also undertaken much consultancy and commissioned work for a variety of bilateral and multilateral organisations.

Paul Chitenge holds degrees in Biochemical Science and Public Health. He is currently employed as a Monitoring/Evaluation and Researcher Officer with the NAC of Zambia, for which body he oversees the collation and analysis of HIV/AIDS-related data from district level through to the NAC level. He has extensive knowledge of the HIV/AIDS programmes in the health sector and a wide working knowledge of a variety of data collection and analysis methodologies.

Emmanual Mali holds a degree in Economics and currently works as a Programme Officer at the Catholic Commission for Justice and Development (CCJDP) in Lusaka, Zambia. As a Programme Officer, he has been charged with the responsibility of overseeing the Commission's work on the national budget process. Due to his extensive advocacy and lobbying skills on budget issues, he has continuing contact with the National Assembly in carrying out the CCJDP's advocacy work.

Malawi

James Brown Gwaza is a Project and Resource Management Specialist, with more than fifteen years experience of business, technical, financial and economic appraisal and development. He is a specialist in fiduciary risk (the compliance monitoring of public finance and procurement), budget tracking and economic analysis in all sectors of the economy. Currently, he is part of the consultation team representing civil society in the development of the Malawi Development Assistance Strategy. Having worked with all the major multilateral donors, he understands their respective modus operandi.He has an in-depth knowledge of HIV/AIDS-related issues, such as advocacy, mainstreaming, capacity-building, and monitoring, evaluation and research, as well as of the development of HIV/AIDS workplace policies and programmes.

Gloria Chisala Hamela holds a Master of Science Degree in Comparative Social Work obtained in 2005 from Bodo University in Norway. She also holds a Bachelor of Social Science Degree with a major in Sociology, which she obtained in 1999 from Chancellor College in Zomba. As Regional Coordinator for the MEJN she is responsible for coordinating the implementation of MEJN programmes on budget tracking, trade justice and budget monitoring at regional level. Previously, she worked as an Acting Budget Monitoring Officer for the same organisation. She also formerly worked for the Ministry of Women and Child Welfare as Gender Programme Officer and Social

Welfare Officer. Currently, she works for the University of North Carolina Project in Lilongwe as a social behavioural scientist who is responsible for the implementation of Truvada Sociobehavioural Research. Her main areas of work experience include budget tracking, budget analysis, participatory research, social research, HIV/AIDS, gender mainstreaming and advocacy.

EXTERNAL REVIEWERS

TERESA GUTHRIE

Teresa Guthrie joined Idasa's AIDS Budget Unit as a Regional Coordinator in May 2003. She holds a Bsc (Hons) in Social Work from the University of Zimbabwe and is undertaking an MPhil on critical issues in HIV/AIDS at the University of Cape Town. She has been involved in health and development projects in various countries for several years. She is the founder and Executive Director of the Centre for Economic Governance and AIDS in Africa (CEGAA).

ELESANI DICKSON NJOBVU

Elesani Dickson Njobvu holds a BA (Economics) degree from the University of Zambia (1979) and an MPA in Macro-economic Policy in Developing Countries from the Kennedy School of Government, Harvard University (1993). He has spent most of his working life serving the Government of the Republic of Zambia. He also worked with UNAIDS Regional Support Team for East & Southern Africa (RST-ESA) as a Programme Advisor – Resource Mobilisation. He is currently serving as Counsellor (Economic) at the Zambian Embassy in Brussels, Belgium, a mission accredited to the Economic Commission (EC) and the ACP, and the Benelux countries.

INTRODUCTION

VAILET MUKOTSANJERA

The occurrence of HIV/AIDS is relatively severe in countries and territories, as well as among population groups that are socially, economically or politically impoverished (Farmer, 1999; Mann, 1996). The related effects tend to be catastrophic for all sectors of the economy, leading to HIV/AIDS being declared a national disaster in many African countries, including Malawi, Lesotho, Swaziland and Kenya.[1] Many national HIV/AIDS policies and strategic plans have, accordingly, been put in place.

To date, many financial and human resources of multilateral and bilateral donors, governments, civil society organisations and the private sector have been committed to, and disbursed for purposes of funding, HIV/AIDS responses in Africa. However, according to the Joint United Nations Programme on HIV/AIDS (UNAIDS) (2007a), more resources still must be mobilised in order to meet global HIV/AIDS resource requirements.

The assessment and establishment of the nature of HIV/AIDS resources is critical to using them efficiently, equitably and effectively. Evaluating whether such resources are being used for their intended purpose and are truly benefiting the targeted groups is also very important. Issues of absorptive capacity (meaning the ability of the different service providers to spend the disbursed funds), especially at the country level, are also of critical importance.

HIV/AIDS Financing and Spending in Eastern and Southern Africa is therefore an attempt to assess the financial response to the pandemic. In assessing the financing of, and expenditure on, AIDS-related efforts, this study also discusses, at length, the implications for the selected countries regarding their international commitments, which set benchmarks for success. In line with such coverage, we therefore consider related issues, including the progress made towards the Abuja Declaration of 2001,[2] which stipulates that African countries should allocate at least 15% of their national resources towards the health sector, the "three ones", and the Paris Declaration, which recommends the adoption of collaborative approaches to managing the pandemic among all stakeholders, including governments, donors, civil societies and the private sector.

For the different nonstate actors in the health and HIV/AIDS sector, the Abuja target facilitates holding governments accountable and ensuring the adequate funding of health sectors (including those concerned with HIV/AIDS). *HIV/AIDS Financing and Spending in Eastern and Southern Africa* focuses on, and distinguishes between, the relevant pledges, allocations, disbursements and actual spending.

The current study examines the encapsulation of the essence of citizen participation during the policy formulation process and budget cycle. Spending is also assessed from the democratic governance perspective.

OBJECTIVES OF THE STUDY

The objective of this study was to provide participating countries, as well as Africa as a whole, with evidence of some of the pertinent issues surrounding HIV/AIDS financing and spending in Africa. The aim was to enable appropriate recommendations to be made to the relevant stakeholders.

The specific objectives of the multicountry HIV/AIDS resource-tracking project were:

- To track HIV/AIDS financing and spending resources, and to analyse the budget from an HIV/AIDS perspective;
- To analyse the adequacy of HIV/AIDS funds and to assess their use by different stakeholders;
- To make recommendations to national-level policy makers on the effectiveness and efficiency of budgeting and funding mechanisms supportive of the government response to HIV/AIDS;
- To train civil society and research organisations in the participating countries to undertake HIV/AIDS budget analyses by means of the National AIDS

Spending Assessment (NASA);
- To establish an African regional network of non-governmental organisations (NGOs) involved with HIV/AIDS budget analysis to enable the sharing of research methodologies and research results;
- To work with NGO research partners to develop a common framework for tracking HIV/AIDS-targeted expenditure as deployed in terms of the country budget, using a rights-based framework; and
- To improve public knowledge of the fiscal obligations and responses of individual governments to the HIV/AIDS epidemic.

METHODOLOGY

The current study employed both primary and secondary data-collection methods. The responses provided by donors, government ministries and HIV/AIDS service providers to the UNAIDS-structured questionnaires provided primary data. Related government, donor and service provider documentation was also subjected to a desk review.

This study employs a combination of conventional budget analysis and resource-tracking tools, namely the National Health Accounts (NHA), the National AIDS Accounts (NAA) and the recently developed NASAs. It was a first attempt to use NASA as a methodology, and challenges and limitations encountered by this initial attempt are explained.

EXISTING RESOURCE TRACKING AND BUDGET ANALYSIS FRAMEWORKS

The numerous resource tracking and budget analysis frameworks developed since the early 1990s include the System of Health Accounts (SHA), the NHA, the NAA and the recently developed NASA, which complement one another. A brief description of each of the resource-tracking methods used in this study follows.

National Health Accounts (NHA) is, according to the United States Agency for International Development (USAID) (2007), well recognised internationally as an important tool for informing financial policy. UNAIDS (2007), defines NHA as a framework that provides for the systematic, comprehensive and consistent monitoring of resource flows through a country's health system. NHA identifies and quantifies parameters, while focusing on describing the different components of the health system. Standard methodologies have been developed for ensuring that complete and consistent datasets are collected and comparable among countries. The NHA framework also collects nonfinancial data, such as details of the personnel, the numbers of facilities provided and the activities (such as outpatient visits and hospital in-patient days) performed.

Financial data relating to the sources of health-care funding, the financing intermediaries through which such funds flow and the uses to which the funds are put (amounting to the expenditure patterns) can be collected. Expenditure patterns may be expressed in one of two ways: either in terms of type of input, such as personnel, drugs and capital expenditure, or in terms of type of provider, such as facility or health programmes on which the expenditure took place (UNAIDS, 2007a). Linking NHA and NAA makes the information, on which relevant decisions pertaining to the broader health-system context are made, more readily accessible and harmonises national demographics by monitoring all health-system expenditure (UNAIDS, 2007a).

NASA, a tool developed by UNAIDS[3] for tracking resource allocations and expenditures, encompasses all countrywide HIV/AIDS resource-tracking activities. According to UNAIDS (2007a), NASA is based on other globally standardised and internationally accepted and recognised tools, such as the System of National Accounts (SNA), the National AIDS Accounts (NAA), the NHA and budget analysis. NASA analyses national HIV/AIDS expenditure in order to obtain a comprehensive description of the flow of resources from their sources to the beneficiaries. NASA helps to determine the flow and utilisation of HIV/AIDS resources from the financing sources (FSs), the financing agents (FAs) and the service providers, as well as to determine how such resources are dispersed among different activities, objects of expenditure, and beneficiaries (UNAIDS, 2007a). The assessment tool also helps to identify the level and determinants of expenditure on HIV/AIDS and so measure the national response to HIV/AIDS.

Easily adaptable to different country scenarios, NASA tracks all HIV/AIDS expenditure from all public, private and international (foreign aid) sources. NASA not only captures what was actually spent, as opposed to what was allocated or committed, but also identifies any discrepancies, together with their contributing factors (Guthrie, 2006). Institutionalising NASA greatly enhances a country's monitoring and evaluation (M&E), allowing for cross-country comparisons due to its standardised categories and classifications.

Most of the countries involved in the current survey collected their primary data using the UNAIDS-structured NASA questionnaire to map the flow of resources, budgetary allocations and expenditures for FY 2004/2005. The responses obtained allowed for the compilation of details relating to HIV/AIDS-related resource allocation/transfer and actual expenditure by following the path of the funding from the source to the beneficiary. The use of NASA enabled the collection of data on HIV/AIDS-related financial flows and expenditures according to sources, agents, service providers, objects of expenditure, functions and beneficiaries. However, not all of the countries involved in the study were able to provide all of the necessary details due to the many challenges that they encountered.

Even in cases where alternate methodologies were employed, the outcomes within the said limitations provide sufficient basis for reasoned action by both state and nonstate actors seeking to achieve accountable governance. Malawi, for instance, used the NHA's assessment methodology, which is yet another internationally recognised approach for tracking resources and assessing expenditure. Though different methodologies were used by some of the participants in this study, some aspects are, nevertheless, comparable and hence provide a reasonably sound basis for more general recommendations.

Based on the outcome of the questionnaire, interviews were also conducted with donor representatives and key informants in both government ministries and departments. The information on total government allocations and public-sector health allocations used in this study was drawn from the public documents of the governments concerned. Zanzibar, Tanzania and Kenya all relied heavily on their Public Expenditure Review (PER) as a source of their data. Detailed estimates of HIV/AIDS-related expenditures were obtained from the source FAs in terms of both service provider and function (including the prevention, treatment and mitigation of the impact of AIDS). In cases where information was missing, incomplete or inconsistent, experts and previous studies were consulted to verify or complete the findings.

Though the study lasted from 2000/01 to 2004/05, the report focuses on 2004/05, which was the only common year of analysis for all the countries concerned. To improve the cross-country comparability of the study, all allocations and expenditures were converted to US$ using the annual average exchange rates for the year specified for each country.

NASA CHALLENGES ENCOUNTERED IN THE COURSE OF THIS STUDY

The current research is the first attempt made by Idasa and its partners to apply the NASA methodology. Though the lack of technical expertise held by the implementing partners and Idasa hampered the successful implementation of such methodology, and difficulties were encountered by the researchers with the NASA Resource Tracking Software (NASA RTS), as the product was still in its development stages, overall the study was a success. In most cases, a solid effort was made to collect the data using the NASA guidelines available.

The solution to the abovementioned difficulties was a compromise consisting of a budget analysis and an NHA exercise using the NASA concepts, with Tanzania being the only country that successfully managed to pilot NASA in a few selected districts. The report does, however, not fulfil all the requirements of a complete NASA study, though this does not compromise the original intention to track resources.

The researchers encountered the following challenges while executing the NASA framework:
1. The data, especially that provided by the various governments concerned, was not disaggregated on the basis of the NASA categories of expenditure.
2. The researchers' technical capacity in the execution of NASA was inadequate.
3. The NASA RTS was difficult to use, as it was still in development stage at the time of the study and the final version was not ready in time for the analysis.
4. As the HIV/AIDS spending categories of the countries concerned employed different definitions to those of NASA, they were unable to present their find-

5

ings in the UNAIDS-recommended format, as it was difficult to harmonise the two.

5. Accessing adequate data proved challenging – in some cases, the FSs and service providers were reluctant to disclose private and confidential information on financing and spending.

6. NASA requires a comprehensive tracking of all HIV/AIDS-related expenditure, including that of all donors and both public and private contributions, down to district level. Such tracking proved very challenging, especially for the larger countries of Ethiopia and Tanzania, given the financial and human capacity constraints.

7. Weak or absent financial M&E systems, especially within government departments, resulted in the absence of actual expenditure information.

8. Some inconsistencies in terms of the funds allocated occurred due to the underreporting of received funds by service providers, resulting from the fact that not all of the countries in the study had a centralised database providing comprehensive information on HIV/AIDS financing and expenditure.

9. Certain key experienced and trained AIDS Budget Unit (ABU) staff resigned during the implementation of the project, compromising the technical backstopping. As a result, the continuity of the project was threatened by country partners facing a high staff turnover.

Such challenges can, in future, be overcome by more rigorous training of partners and the ensuring of more consistent support by NASA experts at all levels of research, including during data collection, analysis, documentation and the dissemination of findings. Despite the limitation, the findings, in our view, remain useful to the broader policy environment, particularly in light of the expenditure on AIDS becoming increasingly a key measure of political commitment by African governments.

THE SCOPE AND PROCESS OF THE PROJECT

The current study, which was coordinated by the ABU of GAP, follows the first phase of a Swedish International Development Cooperation Agency (SIDA)-funded project, *Funding the Fight, Budgeting for HIV/AIDS in Developing Countries*, which studied five Latin American countries (Argentina, Chile, Ecuador, Mexico and Nicaragua) and four African countries (Kenya, Namibia, Mozambique and South Africa). One of the main achievements of the first phase of the current project is that it has helped to empower civil society to engage governments on AIDS-related resource issues. Phase 2 has built on these experiences by including Ethiopia and Tanzania in the existing sample of countries.

A key lesson learnt from the first phase was that the development of a partnership between researchers and civil society is crucial for advocacy purposes, enabling skills transfer in both directions. Such collaboration existed in all participating countries. Phase 2 involved building a strong network of civil society organisations (CSOs) with experience in resource tracking, and supporting their capacity alongside that of the research partners in each country. The choice of country and CSO participants in the project was based on, though not limited to, the following factors:

- Previous experience of resource tracking or general HIV/AIDS research;
- The viability of organisations in terms of capacity, a good track record, availability, interest and legal existence;
- Continuation from Phase 1 (e.g. Kenya);
- Stakeholder (government, CSO, donor and academic institution) interest in the project;
- The receipt of Global Fund to Fight AIDS, Tuberculosis and Malaria (GFATM) or Presidential Emergency Plan for AIDS Relief (PEPFAR) funds by the country concerned;
- The nature of the country's budgeting systems (the use of the Medium-term Expenditure Framework (MTEF));
- The availability of two experienced researchers (or one from both the research agency and the CSO) who could be assigned to the project for its duration; and
- The potential for regional collaboration and overlap with GAP's electoral project countries.

The research teams in each country consisted of a research agency with health economic professionals, an advocacy group and a representative of the National AIDS Commission or Council (NAC).

A number of exploratory visits, the identifying of potential partners and the holding of stakeholder meetings were performed in 2005 in Tanzania and Zanzibar, Kenya, Zambia, Ethiopia, Malawi and South Africa. During these visits, both individual and stakeholder meetings were held with as many stakeholders as possible across the board, representing government, CSOs (especially associations of People Living With HIV/AIDS (PLWHAs)), donors and research institutions, who then formed the reference group in each country studied.

In June 2005, the ABU and UNAIDS held consultations during which ABU's budget tracking[4] and the UNAIDS' NASA methodologies were assessed and evaluated, allowing for Idasa methodology to be enriched by means of recourse to NASA methods. The latter made provision for highly disaggregated information, while also focusing on HIV/AIDS fund allocations and expenditure in the selected countries.

In July 2005, the countries concerned embarked on initial training in budget analysis, expenditure monitoring and basic resource-tracking methods. In October 2005, they underwent further in-depth training in the NASA methodology, which was facilitated by a UNAIDS NASA consultant. To maximise the benefits gained from the study, comparable terms of reference were agreed upon, setting out the basic principles aimed at guiding the investigation.

UNAIDS then offered to provide the necessary technical expertise and to build the capacity of Idasa staff and researchers. The country research teams subsequently began developing their own research methodologies and plans, together with the training of their research assistants. The difficulties that some countries experienced with gaining authorisation from their respective NACs and Ministries of Health (MoHs) prevented them from undertaking a complete NASA study.

In February 2006, the ABU undertook site visits to each country participant in order to monitor their progress and to provide technical assistance. Later in the same year, the country research teams (consisting of three representatives from each country) attended an "interim meeting" in Zanzibar to present their preliminary findings, to share challenges and good practices, and to begin developing key advocacy themes and strategies. As, at that point, the country data presentations showed weaknesses in terms of data collection and analysis, the technical support of Idasa and UNAIDS was elicited to master the NASA methodology involved. However, due to certain key members of the original research team leaving Idasa during this period, as well as during the transitional phases, the country partners were unable to benefit fully from the arrangement.

STRUCTURE OF THE BOOK

After presenting an overview of the HIV/AIDS financing and spending, the individual case studies are covered in the following alphabetical order: Ethiopia, Kenya, Malawi, Tanzania (and Zanzibar), and Zambia. The overview also includes recommendations based on the findings from the different selected countries.

BACKGROUND

In 2006, 63% of all persons infected with HIV lived in Sub-Saharan Africa (SSA). Therefore, since the discovery of the first HIV cases in the early 1980s, HIV has increasingly become a major developmental issue in Africa, posing an unprecedented threat to human welfare and socioeconomic development. According to UNAIDS (2005), AIDS deaths in SSA represented 72% of the global AIDS deaths in the year under review.

In East Africa (including Kenya, Tanzania and Ethiopia), the HIV prevalence rate has either decreased or remained stable over the past few years. East Africa continues to provide the most hopeful indications that serious AIDS epidemics can be reversed, as declines in prevalence have been recorded in both Kenya and Uganda. The decline in prevalence in Kenya from 10% in the late 1990s to about 6% in 2005 has been attributed to the delay in sexual débuts, increased condom use and fewer sexual partners (UNAIDS, 2006a). The relatively low prevalence rates in Tanzania, Kenya and Uganda are also partly due to the traditional male circumcision practice, which is common in such countries. The studies conducted by the Center for Disease Control (CDC) in Uganda and Kenya in 2007 showed that male circumcision had reduced the chances of men contracting HIV from women by 51% and 53% respectively.

According to UNAIDS (2006a), Southern Africa (including Malawi and Zambia) remains the most affected region in the world, with approximately 30% of the world's PLWHAs living in this subregion. About 43% of all HIV+ children under the age of 15 live in Southern Africa, as do approximately 52% of all HIV+ women older than 15.

Several factors contribute to the spread of the HI virus in Southern Africa:

1. Much stigma is still associated with PLWHAs, discouraging people from getting tested and leading to their nondisclosure of status.

2. Denialism that HIV causes AIDS is fostered by those who believe that they will only develop AIDS if they are bewitched.

3. Condom use is also very low, and, according to the prevailing culture, men may have multiple sexual partners (MRC, 2008). With the exception of Zimbabwe, Southern African countries show little evidence of a decline in the epidemic.

That Southern African countries are the hardest hit is confirmed by the prevalence rates shown in the following graph, with the rates for the former being higher than those for the East African countries. While Zambia was shown to have had the highest prevalence rate (16%) in 2005, Zanzibar was reported as having had the lowest (0.9%).

Figure 1.1: Prevalence rates for selected countries for 2005

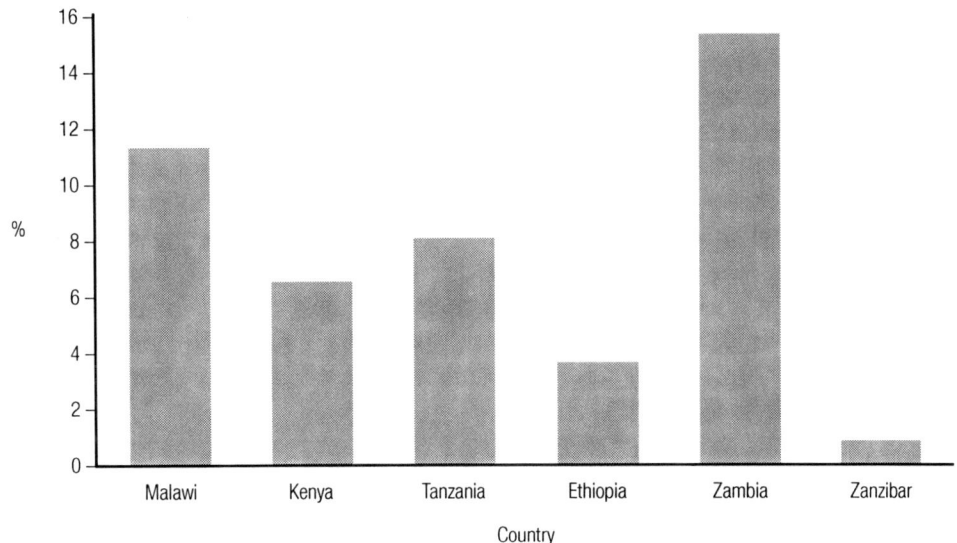

Source: UNAIDS, 2005

GENDER AND GEOGRAPHICAL DIMENSIONS OF HIV/AIDS

The epidemic is becoming increasingly feminised, with women not only being more likely to become infected with HIV than men, but also being the primary care-givers to the sick. The feminisation of the epidemic reflects the different physiological, economic, sociocultural and legal factors that contribute to the susceptibility of women to HIV infection. According to UNAIDS (2005), women and girls make up 57% of PLWHAs in SSA.

Former UN Secretary-General Kofi Annan described the vicious cycle in 2004:

> *As AIDS forces girls to drop out of school, whether they are forced to take care of a sick relative, run the household, or help support the family, they fall deeper into poverty. Their children, in turn, are less likely to attend school and more*

likely to become infected. Thus society pays many times over the deadly price of the impact on women of AIDS. – Kofi Annan statement on International Women's Day, 2004. www.un.org/news/press/docs/2004/sgsm9177.doc.htm

Evidence has shown that African women are at greater risk of becoming infected at an earlier age than men.[5] According to UNFPA (2005), the proportion of infected women has risen over the years from 35% in 1990, to 41% in 1997 and 48% in 2004. The scenario is even more pronounced among the youth (15–24 years). A review compared the ratio of young women to young men living with HIV, which ranged from 20 women for every 10 men in South Africa to 45 women for every 10 men in Kenya and Mali (UNAIDS/UNDP, 2004). Such discrepancies have been explained by the gender-related constraints caused by a patriarchal ideology and culture, which gives men disproportionate power and ownership over resources. They are also explained by a combination of biological, social, legal, economic and cultural factors, which include widow inheritance, female genital mutilation, polygamy, domestic violence and the inability of women to negotiate safer sex (Langen, 2005). In African cultures, men are the decision-makers, meaning that they also make decisions about when and how sex should take place.

In all the countries studied, the HIV prevalence rates were found to be higher among women than among men. In Zanzibar, women show infection rates that are four to six times higher that those of their male counterparts. The gender disparities go far deeper than mere sexual relations. African women cannot own property and lack access to financial resources, resulting in their having to depend on the men in their lives (their husbands, fathers, brothers and sons) for support. The femininity of poverty also reduces women to a state of economic dependency, which also makes them more vulnerable to HIV/AIDS.

In Southern Africa, many older men choose to have sex with young women and adolescent girls in return for their providing them with school fees, food or highly sought-after consumer goods (Hallman, 2004). Women who are beaten or dominated by their partners are more vulnerable to contracting HIV. Without resources, women tend to be susceptible to abuse.

Though, on average, more than 80% of the population have been found to live in the rural areas, HIV prevalence is higher among the urban population. A study conducted in Tanzania (URT, 2005b) showed that HIV/AIDS prevalence is higher in urban areas (12% for women and 9.6% for men) compared with that in rural areas (5.8% for women and 4.8% for men). The urban areas tend to be densely populated. The growth of poor and informal communities, which are generally excluded from basic services and subjected to high densities and the disintegration of social fabric, aid the rapid spread of the epidemic. According to a report by UN Habitat (2002), the close proximity and frequency of interaction among diverse groups of people leads to relatively high and more rapid rates of infection and transmission.

MODES OF TRANSMISSION

According to UNAIDS (2004), unsafe sexual practices are responsible for the majority of HIV infections in SSA. In the African countries studied, the predominant mode of

HIV transmission was found to have remained heterosexual intercourse, accounting for an average of more than 70% of the HIV transmissions. In Kenya, heterosexual intercourse was found to account for 98% of all transmissions. Mother-to-child transmission and blood transfusion are also common modes of transmission. In Tanzania, heterosexual intercourse, blood transfusion and mother-to-child transmission was found to account for 83% of transmission, while 17% of modes were unstated. Gear (2005) affirmed in her study of sexual violence in prisons that, though most African countries, apart from South Africa, do not recognise homosexuality, the practice is nevertheless common, especially in prisons, and therefore such a phenomenon requires attention. There is growing concern that HIV may be spreading undetected among prison inmates, due to failure to report the phenomenon for fear of disclosure, since the victims of sexual assault tend to be victimised further as a result of the stigma and discrimination practised against them.

SOCIOECONOMIC ENVIRONMENT

The HIV/AIDS pandemic affects not only the health sector, but also forms of governance, the way in which states manage their political, economic and social affairs (Poku NK *et al*, 2007), which demands an assessment of the socioeconomic environment within which each country operates.

The Human Development Index (HDI) is a composite index that measures the average achievement in a country in terms of three basic dimensions of human development:

- A long and healthy life, as measured in terms of life expectancy at birth;
- Knowledge, as measured by the adult literacy rate and the combined Gross Enrolment Ratio (GER) for primary, secondary and tertiary schools; and
- A decent standard of living, as measured by the Gross Domestic Product (GDP) per capita in Purchasing Power Parity (PPP) in terms of US$.

More than 60% of the populace of the countries reviewed for the purpose of this study were reported to be living in rural areas. In SSA, of the nearly 80% of the population living in rural areas, 70% are estimated to depend on farming or livestock keeping for their livelihood. According to a report by Practical Action/ PELUM (2005), small-scale farming provides most of the food produced in Africa, as well as employment for 60% of the employed. Agriculture, which is the backbone of most economies, remains the key to achieving the Millennium Development Goals (MDGs) in Africa, as it is one of the leading sources of foreign currency and the main generator of savings and revenue. Zambia has been found to have 75.8% of the population living on less than US$1 per day, exhibiting dire poverty levels.

Cohen (1993) identified the bicausal relationship between poverty and HIV, showing that poverty accentuates people's vulnerability to HIV/AIDS by increasing their exposure to unsafe sexual practices. AIDS also compounds poverty by impoverishing households, requiring funding of the sick and the payment of funeral expenses (Booysen and Buchmann, 2002). Booysen and Buchmann (2002) found that, in South Africa's Free State province, the adult equivalent per capita income in HIV/

AIDS-affected households represented only between 50% and 60% of the level of income earned in nonaffected households, with household income clearly falling if household members lose their jobs due to illness.

Those living in rural areas also have poor access to communication systems, such as radios, newspapers, televisions and the Internet, which are all important technologies for the dissemination of anti-AIDS messages. The paucity of health-care facilities in rural areas demands that sick people walk long distances to the nearest health care facility. According to a report by the World Bank (WB) (2005), poverty in Africa is predominantly rural, with the rural population tending to be poorly organised and often isolated, beyond the reach of special safety nets and poverty programmes.

Table 1.1: Cross-country demographics for countries under review

Country	Malawi	Kenya	Tanzania	Ethiopia	Zambia
Indicators					
Population (million), 2005, (UN Population Division)	10.1	27.4	29.9	60.3	9.3
HIV prevalence rate (%)	12	7.3	8.9	4.4	16
Exchange rates (2005) local currency per US$	108.9	76.74	1 076	8.66	4 200
Inflation - year on year (%)	15.5	10.3	13.6	18.4	16.8
GDP 2005 (US$ million) (World Bank, 2005)	2 000	19 100	12 400	11 300	6 800
GDP per capita US$ (Idasa calculations)	198	697	414.7	187.4	731
Population density (people per square kilometre) (World Bank, 2006)	138.33	60.97	42.26	66.78	15.53
Human Development Index (HDI) (UNDP, 2004)	0.400	0.491	0.430	0.371	0.407
Percentage of population living in rural areas	86.7	81	79.5	86.1	62.9
Human Development Rank (UNDP, 2004)	166	152	162	170	165
Life expectancy (years) (UNDP, 2004)	39.8	47.5	45.5	47.8	37.7
Adult literacy (%) (UNDP, 2004)	64.1	73.6	69.4	41	68.0
Human Poverty Index (HPI) (%) (UNDP, 2006)	43.0	35.5	36.3	53.3	68.0
Population living on less than $1 per day (%) (UNDP, 2006)	41.7	22.8	57.8	23.0	75.8
Maternal mortality (per 100 000) (UNDP, 2004)	1 800	1 000	1 500	850	750
Infant mortality (per 1 000 live births) (UNFPA, 2005)	115.9	68	90.4	104.6	105.4
Under-five mortality rate (per 1 000 live births) (UNFPA, 2005)	185	110	153	179	181

Sources: UNFPA (2005) State of World Population, 2005. UNDP (2005) Human Development Report, 2005. UNDP (2006) Human Development Report, 2006. World Bank, 2006

Table 1.1 summarises the socioeconomic variables for the countries under study. A strong relationship exists between HIV/AIDS and the socioeconomic situation in any country. The table shows that countries with the highest prevalence (Malawi and Zambia) are characterised by high Infant Mortality Rates (IMRs); more people living below US$1 per day; a low population rate; a low life expectancy, and the lowest economic growth, as reflected by the low GDP. Malawi and Zambia were found to have the highest infant and under-five mortality rates, while Kenya had the lowest. Adetunji (2000) showed that under-five mortality rates increased in most countries with high adult HIV prevalence rates, but decreased in countries with low prevalence, showing that HIV/AIDS contributes to infant mortality. In the 11 African countries with prevalence rates above 13%, the average life expectancy is 47.7 years, which is 11 years less than might have been expected in the absence of HIV/AIDS.

IMPACT OF HIV ON DIFFERENT SECTORS OF THE ECONOMY

The disease (HIV/AIDS), moving like a ravaging Tsunami wave, is attacking productive sectors such as agriculture (thus threatening food security in the region) and other key sectors that are crucial to economic recovery. The disease … threatens to decimate entire populations, cripple national economies and reverse developmental gains so far recorded. It has overstretched national budgets by gobbling resources meant for investments that are essential to economic growth and development… (SARPN, 2006)

Until recently, HIV/AIDS was mainly considered a health issue. However, a paradigm shift has now taken place, with HIV becoming widely viewed as a development crisis (Barnett and Whiteside, 1999). The adverse effects of HIV/AIDS on development institution programmes in Africa have forced both health and nonhealth development agencies to approach the problem from an entirely different, more critical perspective. The HIV epidemic is now being considered as an important cross-sectoral developmental issue, due to its having far-reaching implications for both the policies and programming of governments and international development agencies.

The negative effects of HIV/AIDS have been felt at the micro (individual, household, and community), meso (institution) and macro (national) levels of the economy. According to the International Labour Organization (ILO) (2004), estimates of HIV/AIDS indicate that the epidemic would reduce the average annual GDP growth rate by 0.5–4% per annum in the most affected countries of the African region.

Cohen (1993) relates labour productivity and efficiency to poverty reduction. Sichone (2004) showed that economic productivity fell and economic costs associated with loss of labour due to increased mortality accounted for a decline of 3% in the GDP. HIV/AIDS has also been shown to reduce the labour force and life expectancy among the economically active population (Guiness and Alban, 2000; Theodore, 2001).

Table 1.2: The impact of HIV/AIDS on different economic sectors	
Sector	Impact
Agriculture	• An inadequate labour supply; • Absenteeism of seasonal workers; • Low productivity, low output; • Low foreign currency inflows; • Food insecurity for households, communities and the nation as a whole; • Reduction in the amount of area under cultivation; • Distortion of the supply chain; and • Low economic growth.
Health	• Overstretched medical care facilities: • High doctor–patient ratios, leading to low staff morale; • High staff recruitment and training costs; and • High HIV/AIDS-related bed occupancy rates of 50% in Tanzania and 30% in Kenya.
Education	• High recruitment and training costs; • High absenteeism resulting from infected and affected teachers, with the learning process consequently affected; • High teacher–pupil ratios; • Low completion rates; and • A high school dropout rate, with especially girls becoming care-givers.
Households/ community	• Low household incomes, with increased levels of poverty; • Increased medical, funeral and transport expenses; • Low savings and high borrowing rates; • Loss of household assets due to labour losses and loss of employment; • The erosion of intergenerational dependency structures; • An increase in elder- and child-headed households; and • Lower productivity, with a decrease in the availability of food leading to malnutrition.
Business	• A high rate of absenteeism, leading to low productivity and declining profits; • High medical insurance bills; • High costs of recruitment and training; and • High funeral insurance costs.
Sources: Arndt, 2000; Barnett and Whiteside, 1999a; Cohen, 2000; Guiness and Alban, 2000; Theodore, 2001	

Some under-resourced governments have relied on large contributions from foreign donors to sustain wide-ranging response mechanisms focused on mitigating the impact of the HIV/AIDS pandemic. With a restive civil society, exemplified by such movements as the Treatment Action Campaign (TAC) in South Africa, in some countries beginning to organise across boundaries, the international commitments signed by political leaders have attracted closer scrutiny.

INTERNATIONAL AND REGIONAL COMMITMENT TO CURB THE EFFECTS OF HIV/AIDS

As all the leaders of the countries under review in this study[6] are signatories to numerous global and regional declarations and commitments aimed at fighting HIV/AIDS, such declarations and commitments require analysis. However, the signing of such documentation is a necessary but insufficient condition for upholding their principles in practice. As such commitments are not legally binding, the governments concerned cannot be held accountable for not complying with them (UNAIDS, 2001). State parties require continual prodding to implement dedicated instruments for the general public good, making civil society's role critical in this regard.

The countries under review are all signatories to the following global and regional commitments.

GLOBAL COMMITMENTS

- *United Nations' MDGs – 2000.* World leaders from 189 countries adopted the UN's MDGs in 2000. The goals include the eradication of extreme poverty, the promotion of gender equality, the empowerment of women, and the countering of HIV/AIDS, malaria and other ravaging diseases.
- *UNGASS Declaration of Commitment on HIV/AIDS – 2001.* During the United Nations General Assembly Special Session (UNGASS) on HIV/AIDS held in 2001, themed "Global crisis requiring global action", the heads of states agreed that the AIDS pandemic had caused untold suffering and death worldwide. However, they also agreed that, with sufficient will and resources, communities and countries could positively intervene in the crisis. The resultant declaration remains a powerful tool that is helping to guide and secure action, commitment, support and resources in support of the AIDS response.
- *The G8 Communiqué – 2005.* The leaders of the Group of Eight (G8) industrialised countries agreed to take concrete actions to tackle HIV/AIDS in terms of this communiqué, which includes the following statement:

With the aim of an AIDS-free generation in Africa, [we will work to] significantly reduce HIV infections and, working with WHO, UNAIDS and other international bodies to develop and implement a package for HIV prevention, treatment and care, with the aim of as close as possible to universal access to treatment for all those who need it by 2010.

The G8 pledge was broadened at the 2005 United Nations (UN) General Assembly World Summit, at which the member states committed themselves to:
- Developing and implementing a package for HIV prevention, treatment and care, aimed at attaining near-universal access to treatment by 2010, including the allocation of more resources, and working towards the elimination of stigma and discrimination, the enhancement of access to affordable medicines and the reduction of the vulnerability of those, especially orphans and vulnerable children and older persons affected by HIV/AIDS and other health issues; and
- Working actively to implement the "Three Ones" principles in all countries.
- *Paris Declaration on Aid Effectiveness – 2005.* The Paris Declaration was adopted by the senior ministers from donor and host countries, as well as by the heads of bilateral and multilateral institutions (UNAIDS, 2006b). The Declaration

offers a holistic approach towards aid effectiveness, with targets set for both the donors and the recipients to achieve. They resolved to "scale up for more effective aid" by:

- Strengthening the host countries' capacity to develop and deliver results-driven national development strategies;
- Defining performance standards and measures for the host countries' financial management systems and other systems;
- Reforming and simplifying donor policies and procedures to make them as cost-effective as possible, in order to reduce unnecessary duplication and the bureaucratic burden on countries;
- Achieving progressive alignment with the host countries' policies and procedures, providing more predictable, multiyear aid flows consistent with the sustainable development needs of host countries;
- Improving the integration of global initiatives in areas such as HIV/AIDS management into the host countries' broader development agendas; and
- Enhancing both donor and host countries' accountability to their citizens and parliaments by increasing the transparency of their policies, procedures and activities.

In terms of the Declaration, the country partners are expected:

- To exercise leadership in developing and implementing their national development strategies through broad consultative processes;
- To translate the national development strategies into prioritised results-oriented operational programmes, as expressed in Medium Term Expenditure Frameworks (MTEF) and annual budgets; and
- To take the lead in coordinating aid at all levels, in conjunction with other development resources, in dialogue with donors and through encouraging the participation of civil society and the private sector.

REGIONAL COMMITMENTS

- *Abuja Declaration – 2001*. In April 2001, African heads of state and government adopted the Abuja Declaration and Plan of Action on HIV/AIDS, Tuberculosis (TB) and Other Related Infectious Diseases (ORIDs). The primary goal of the Declaration was to arrest and reverse the accelerating rate of HIV infection, TB and ORID. During the summit, due to the prevalence of AIDS throughout the continent, a state of emergency was declared in Africa. The African signatories to the Declaration, accordingly, committed themselves to allocating at least 15% of the national budget to the health sector.
- *The Maputo Resolution on Acceleration of HIV Prevention in Africa – 2005*. The World Health Organization (WHO) and the AFRO Regional Committee adopted the Maputo Resolution, which called on member states to declare 2006 the year for accelerating HIV prevention.
- In November 2005, WHO/AFRO spearheaded an initiative involving UNAIDS, United Nations Development Programme (UNDP), United Nations Population Fund (UNFPA), United Nations Development Fund for Women (UNIFEM),

United Nations Educational, Scientific and Cultural Organisation (UNESCO) and the United Nations Children's Fund (UNICEF). The initiative was intended to support countries in the region to accelerate HIV prevention. The seven UN agencies, accordingly, signed a declaration agreeing to ensure synergy in implementing a joint regional plan to support the acceleration of HIV prevention, including key milestones for 2006 and mechanisms for monitoring implementation.

- *The Maseru (Lesotho) Declaration on HIV and AIDS in the Southern African Development Community (SADC) Region – 2003.* The Declaration reaffirms the commitment of heads of state and government to combating the HIV/AIDS epidemic in all its manifestations, which is regarded as a matter of urgency, by way of the multisectoral strategic initiatives contained in the new SADC HIV/AIDS Strategic Framework and Programme of Action 2003–2007. The Declaration also urges the continuation of efforts aimed at allocating at least 15% of the signatory countries' national budgets to the cause – an intention that is consistent with the Abuja Declaration.
- *The Gaborone Declaration on Universal Access to Prevention, Treatment, Care and Support – 2005.* The African Union countries committed themselves to the achievement of universal access to treatment and care through the Gaborone Summit Declaration, which recommends an integrated AIDS, TB and malaria health-care delivery system based on an essential health package (EHP). The Declaration also calls for the allocation of at least 15% of each country's national budget to health, as was resolved in the Abuja Declaration.
- *Brazzaville Commitment on Scaling up Towards Universal Access to HIV and AIDS Prevention,Ttreatment, Care and Support in Africa by 2010 – 2006.* Utilising the outcomes of the country consultations on scaling up towards universal access to HIV prevention, treatment, care and support by 2010, an African continental consultation was held in Brazzaville in 2006. The consultation resulted in a set of recommendations contained in the Brazzaville Commitment (AU, 2006).

THE "THREE ONES" PRINCIPLES

In April 2004, UNAIDS and other major bilateral and multilateral donors, as well as their country partners, endorsed a framework of principles aimed at improving efficiency in the global struggle to combat the spread and impact of HIV/AIDS at a national level. According to UNAIDS (2005), the principles, referred to as the "Three Ones", are as follows:

1. One agreed HIV/AIDS action framework, containing a budget and a work plan, should provide the basis for coordinating the work of all partners.
2. One national, legally recognised AIDS coordinating authority with broad-based multisectoral mandate should have full technical capacity for coordination, M&E, resource mobilisation, financial tracking and strategic information management.
3. One agreed country-level M&E system should be integrated into the HIV/AIDS framework in accordance with a set of standardised indicators.

RATIONALE FOR TRACKING HIV/AIDS RESOURCES

According to UNAIDS (2005), the annual funding for HIV/AIDS responses in low- and middle-income countries increased 28-fold since UNAIDS' inception in 1996 to US$8.3 billion in 2005. The total amount of resources estimated to be available for HIV/AIDS initiatives by the end of 2007 was US$10 billion, against an estimated need of US$18.1 billion by the end of the same year – revealing a funding gap of US$8.1 billion (UNAIDS, 2007a). However, the rate of increase of the existing pledges and commitments is declining, with the available funds being unlikely to meet the estimated resource needs for HIV/AIDS responses by 2015 (UNAIDS, 2007b). The funding gap for 2005 was estimated to stand at US$2.8 billion, with the estimated funding gap for the period 2005–2007 standing at US$16.9 billion.

Figure 1.2: Total annual resources available for HIV/AIDS, 1986–2007

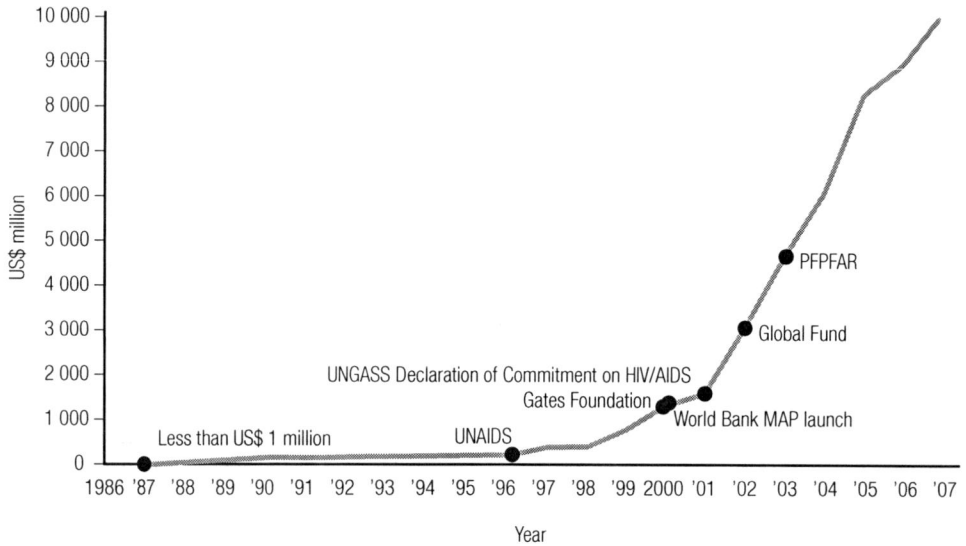

Source: Graph adapted from UNAIDS, 2007a

Though both low- and middle-income countries are still experiencing HIV/AIDS financing gaps, appreciating the role that different FSs[7] have played in reducing the impact of HIV/AIDS in Africa is important. Multilateral agencies, developed country governments and private institutions mobilised significant resources to assist developing countries in their quest to provide quality health care services. Households have also played a significant role, though sometimes unknowingly, in out-of-pocket expenditure (OOPE).[8] OOPE takes the form of cost sharing (in the payment of user fees), self-medication and other expenditure paid directly by private households for health care.

African countries are faced with the daunting task of having to prioritise scarce resources for various sectors of their economies. Other socioeconomic challenges include high levels of poverty;[9] weak health-care systems; unemployment; and low, or sometimes negative, economic growth. Such challenges have been compounded by the HIV/AIDS pandemic, as they exert more pressure on already ailing health care systems, diminishing the attention that can be paid to patients with other ailments (Buve, 1997). In most of the countries under review, more than 45% of the hospital bed occupancy is estimated to be HIV/AIDS-related (Buve, 1997). Buve found that, not only was 53% and 46% of bed occupancy in Kinshasa and Zambia respectively due to HIV/AIDS, but that the increase in hospital bed capacity was not keeping up with demand as a result of the HIV/AIDS pandemic.

Such a scenario seriously impacts on the availability and redistribution of the already scarce resources made available through the national budget. Redistributing national resources is problematised by the multiplicity of wants and the scarcity of resources, especially due to the presence of HIV/AIDS. Nevertheless, governments are expected to allocate adequate resources to all sectors. While being expected to inject more funds into the productive sectors of the economy, which directly contribute to economic growth (such as agriculture, manufacturing, mining and tourism), they are also expected to ensure that the nation is healthy and has access to affordable and accessible health services, including HIV/AIDS services.

Though the challenges posed by HIV/AIDS must not only be understood in economic and social terms, but also from a human development perspective (UNDP/SADC/SAPES 2000), the current study focuses only on financing and expenditure.

General Overview of Findings

Vailet Mukotsanjera

O ur overview of the key findings from Kenya, Zambia, Tanzania, Zanzibar, Malawi and Ethiopia is divided into two sections, the first of which deals with the appraisal of the five countries in respect of their adherence to the "Three Ones", which provide a sense of how their overall response mechanism is shaped. Each country has been affected to different degrees by the HIV/AIDS pandemic and therefore employs different HIV/AIDS financing and spending strategies.

BUDGETING

After assessing UNAIDS' appraisal of the national response mechanisms, we explain in detail the health allocations and expenditure of each country studied, comparing and contrasting the varying degrees to which the governments commit themselves to reversing the negative trends generated by HIV/AIDS. After defining the roles, composition and components of the budgets, the transparency, timeliness and accessibility of the budget processes in the selected countries are discussed, ending with a financing and expenditure analysis.

BUDGETS AND THEIR ROLE

A budget is a list of all planned expenses and revenues, which is stated in monetary terms and serves as an annual statement of government priorities.[10] A government budget summarises the intended revenues and expenditures of that government, reflecting both the amount that will need to be spent to achieve planned activities (expenditure) and the amount that will need to be generated to cover the costs of getting the envisaged work done (income). National budgets assist in the planning and control of the socioeconomic activities of a country. CSOs can use national budgets to monitor government's commitments and levels of accountability in terms of HIV/AIDS allocations. Ideally, a national budget "…reflects the values of a country – who it values, whose work it values and who it rewards… and who and what and whose work it does not…" (Govender, 1996).

BUDGET COMPOSITION

The Development Initiatives Network (1996) elucidates revenues and expenditures. The main components of revenue are:
- Statutory allocations, as provided for under the Constitution;
- Internally-generated revenue from taxes, fines, fees, licenses, rent on government properties and other earnings from investments; and
- Capital receipts, which are derived from loans, grants and the share of value-added tax (VAT).

The main components of expenditure are:
- Recurrent (routine) costs, such as personnel and overhead costs; and
- The capital costs of infrastructure development.

If the revenue estimates exceed expenditure this represents a budget surplus, and if the expenditure exceeds the revenue, the budget is said to be in deficit. Any government experiencing a budget deficit is compelled to borrow money to make up the shortfall, with the deficit being financed by printing money,[11] selling government assets, or issuing government bonds.

Approaches to Budgeting

The *incremental (or traditional) budget*[12] has two identifying characteristics:
1. Funds are first allocated to departments or organisational units, of which the managers allocate funds to activities.
2. An incremental budget, which is easier to coordinate and simpler to operate, then develops out of the previous budget.

Each period's budget uses that of the preceding period as a reference point, with only incremental changes in the budget request being reviewed by top management (Hayes, 2001). Identifying inefficiencies in the allocation and spending of resources is, however, difficult under the incremental budget. Typically, allocations are not reduced for the subsequent financial year (FY). Unit managers add a percentage for inflation and requests for envisaged new or expanded activities to the funds allocated for the preceding period.

According to Abraszewski et al (1999), *results-based budgeting (RBB)* aligns resources with results. RBB is a results-driven budget process, in terms of which programme formulation and resources justification involve a set of predefined objectives, expected results, outputs, inputs and performance indicators. Expected results justify resource requirements, which are derived from, and linked to, outputs to be delivered. RBB is also linked to actual performance in achieving results, as measured in terms of predefined performance indicators.

The *Medium-term Expenditure Framework (MTEF)* is a recent innovation for economic policy-making and government budget processes. According to the World Bank,[13] the MTEF aims to promote order and a disciplined approach to economic planning and budget processes, ensuring the efficient use of public resources. The framework requires that governments should prepare fiscal and monetary programmes, and estimates of revenue and expenditure, for a three-year rolling period. Consequently, the budget for a given FY must link proposed expenditure with the government's medium-term planning priorities. Such linkage helps government departments to document and plan how and where to spend the resources.

The multicountry research project has shown that all the countries studied have implemented budget reforms, using the three-year rolling MTEF for their budget, though, in Ethiopia, the MTEF is referred to as the Macroeconomic and Fiscal Framework (MEFF). The MTEF/MEFF provides three-year forecasts of economic growth, inflation, GDP, government revenue and expenditure. The MTEF clarifies policy objectives and enhances predictability in budget allocation, the comprehensiveness of coverage, and renders more efficient and transparent the use of resources.

The MTEF enables:
- The linkage of policies to budgets;
- The maintenance of aggregate *fiscal discipline* (restraint in spending by the government);
- The improvement of inter- and intrasectoral resource allocation-based projects and programme priorities; and
- Increased effectiveness and efficiency of public expenditure.

On both the Tanzanian mainland and Zanzibar, the MTEF is linked to the Poverty

Reduction Strategy (PRS), which is dubbed "Mkukuta" in Tanzania and "Mkukuza" in Zanzibar. However, for an MTEF to work well, a country must have sound macro-economic policies with which the budgets are transparently aligned.

THE BUDGET PROCESS

The countries' budget process/cycles, which bear close similarity to one another,[14] consist of four stages according to McIntyre et al (1999):
- Budget preparation (the drafting/design process);
- Budget approval and appropriation (the legislative process);
- Budget execution (the implementation process); and
- Budget control (performance monitoring – the audit and evaluation process).

In East Africa (Kenya, Uganda and Tanzania), the *formulation/preparation* stage involves a consultative session among the three East African Community Governments, allowing them to compare notes on their budgetary frameworks. As the budget is perceived as a "technocrat's project", CSO participation in its formulation is limited. Whether the budget is responsive to the needs of the population in its resource allocation is debatable.

After preparing their budgets for the FY, before they receive the expenditure ceilings from the treasury, ministries are expected to budget downwards in order to be in line with the ceiling, which is usually lower than what they had anticipated.

The *legislative* part of the budget involves its tabling before Parliament for approval. Constitutionally, the Parliament has to review, amend and approve the budget (Lee et al, 2007). Based on their mandates, Parliament is expected:
- To examine government revenue and expenditure proposals;
- To authorise revenue collection and expenditures through the passing and enactment of the Finance and Appropriation Acts; and
- To authorise supplementary revenue collection and supplementary expenditures by passing and enacting supplementary Finance and Appropriation Acts.

While Parliament is responsible for approving the budgetary allocations, its role in the budget process is relatively limited, mostly participating *after* the budget presentation in Parliament. As Parliamentarians have limited time and capacity to critically examine or assess the budget during the enactment stage, the assessment of whether Parliament is fulfilling its mandate is critical.

Generally, all the countries under review have M&E mechanisms in place. The ministries have to submit quarterly and annual reports to Parliament, detailing the utilisation rates of the resources allocated. The Office of the Auditor-General presents the findings of its audits of government departments in the form of reports to Parliament. Often, such reports are not produced on time and are not user friendly, being overly detailed and technical. In Ethiopia, though federal and regional budget laws and allocations appear in the *Negarit Gazetta*, the official law gazette of the government, the publication is not accessible to all citizens. Implementation of the budget is inadequately monitored, with little or no link between allocations, targets and actual spending. Very little is done to monitor the budget in terms of its effectiveness, efficiency and equity.

The CSOs are mostly involved in the post-budget processes, monitoring budget implementation by way of the Public Expenditure Reviews (PERs), which serve to evaluate the budgetary performance of the various ministries in the preceding FY and to analyse the budget after its presentation in Parliament.

HIV/AIDS Financial Sources, Flows and Reporting

According to the UNAIDS NASA classifications (2007), an FS assigns resources solely in response to the national response in the country. As such, FSs provide resources to the FAs for pooling and distribution, with the major sources of HIV/AIDS funds being government, donors and the private sector. *Government funds* are allocated to the government ministries and departments by way of the Treasury/Ministry of Finance (MoF). The funds consist of government revenue primarily from taxes, including funds that originate from the central authorities, provincial authorities, local authorities, social security fund, government employee insurance schemes and parastatal organisations.

The Tanzanian government is trying to ensure that HIV/AIDS activities are well funded within the different government departments. Each MDA (ministries/departments/agencies) is expected to have an HIV/AIDS objective aimed at ensuring that HIV/AIDS activities are adequately funded in terms of a "Z" code implemented between 2003 and 2005. In Malawi, 2% of any ministry's budget is allocated to HIV/AIDS activities. Though governments try to ensure that HIV/AIDS activities are well funded, assessing the types of activities on which the different ministries are to embark is important. Evaluating the *quality* of the spending would help to prevent misspending of the funds.

Donor funds, which originate outside a country, can be allocated to:
- The government through the Treasury (in the form of *on-budget allocations*);
- Specific government ministries or departments for specified projects (*off-budget allocations*); and
- International and local CSOs.

Table 1.3 shows the different foreign donors for the selected countries.

Table 1.3: Foreign donors supporting countries under review	
Country	Foreign donors supporting country
Ethiopia	Global Fund to Fight AIDS, Tuberculosis and Malaria; World Bank
Kenya	Department for International Development; European Union; Finland; Global Fund to Fight AIDS, Tuberculosis and Malaria; Japan; Sweden; UN; USAID; World Bank
Malawi	Canada; Department for International Development; Global Fund to Fight AIDS, Tuberculosis and Malaria; Japan International Cooperation Agency; Norway; UN; USAID; World Bank
Tanzania	Belgium; Canada; Clinton Foundation against HIV/AIDS; Department for International Development; European Union; Finland; Germany; Global Fund to Fight AIDS, Tuberculosis and Malaria; Ireland; Japan; the Netherlands; Norway; Sweden; Switzerland; UN; USAID; World Bank
Zanzibar	Clinton Foundation against HIV/AIDS; Global Fund to Fight AIDS, Tuberculosis and Malaria; UN; USAID; World Bank
Zambia	Canada; Department for International Development; European Union; Global Fund to Fight AIDS, Tuberculosis and Malaria; Japan; Sweden; the Netherlands; Norway; UN; USAID; World Bank

The financial support, which all the specified countries receive from the GFTAM, WB, UN and USAID, also funds HIV/AIDS initiatives in all of the countries except Ethiopia, with countries with more donors having a higher proportion of HIV/AIDS donor financing. No clear relationship exists between the number of donors in any country and the HIV prevalence rate.

Private sector funds include the contributions of employers, households, not-for-profit institutions, for-profit institutions, private nonparastatal organisations, parastatal households in the form of OOPE, and company health insurance policies for employees.

The FAs concentrate financing resources from different sources, transferring them to finance a programme or as payment for goods and services, such as health treatment and prevention activities (UNAIDS, 2007c). FAs decide on the use of the resources they receive from the FSs. According to Hanlon (2005), donors prefer channeling funds through off-budget mechanisms or the other CSOs, with, in most countries, 60% of aid being off-budget. However, such a financing method is inefficient and lacking in transparency, due to its unclear accounting mechanisms. The government has little control over such resources, often lacking knowledge of funding and its intended purpose. The departments that receive the funds report directly to the donor, excluding government involvement.

Reporting mechanisms mainly consider the source of funding and the FA. Donor organisations usually have complicated procedures and guidelines that are time-consuming and involve much paperwork. The lack of expertise of the implementing agencies has led to slow and low utilisation rates of the disbursed funds, making it difficult to achieve the intended objectives. Generally, government and donors have varying accountability and reporting requirements. To ensure accountability in the transfer and utilisation of funds, the donors engage a local fund agency to manage the disbursement of, and accounting for, funds transferred to government and local CSOs. All funded organisations are required to implement their activities according to their approved workplans and budgets, and to report on resource utilisation within a specified time period after receiving such funds.

Progress on the "Three Ones"

Assessment of the progress made by the different countries towards achieving the "Three Ones" principles shows how governments commit themselves to improving country-level responses to HIV/AIDS.

One Agreed National HIV/AIDS Action Framework

At the end of 2004, a UNAIDS Secretariat survey found that, of the 66 countries covered by the survey, 82% had up-to-date national HIV/AIDS action frameworks in place. The survey, as well as other more detailed country assessments, however, identified few multisectoral agreements. Many key stakeholders are not consulted during the developing, reviewing and updating of frameworks. Of the countries surveyed, 9% had no participation by women and only 5% had full participation by women.

All the countries under review have clearly laid-out HIV/AIDS policies with objectives and priorities, with the latter revolving around issues of prevention, treatment and care, social mitigation and research. In Ethiopia, emphasis was placed on the importance of women and youth empowerment, perhaps due to their being the most economically disadvantaged, and therefore more vulnerable to HIV infection. Ethiopia and Tanzania have a framework in place that safeguards the rights of PLWHAs, underscoring the importance of research in the fight against HIV/AIDS. Zanzibar also aims to enhance the institutional capacity of the key implementers of HIV/AIDS initiatives (UNAIDS, 2005).

As many of the existing frameworks have not been translated into workplans and budgets, donors have difficulty identifying the countries' national priorities, making it difficult for them to identify the most beneficial interventions. Of all the countries surveyed, 23% have no system either for aligning their budgets with their objectives or of tracking expenditures to see that they are meeting objectives (UNAIDS, 2005).

Since UNAIDS recommended that strategic plans should be costed, this study had to assess whether the countries had costed strategic plans in place and whether their policy objectives and priorities were being matched by adequate resource allocation. According to UNAIDS (2005), unless the national HIV/AIDS policy outlines firm commitments to objectives and milestones that need to be achieved, they merely serve as a statement of intent. UNAIDS has thus recommended that HIV/AIDS strategic plans be prioritised and costed in order to determine the future financial resources needs for HIV/AIDS activities. A comprehensive and costed multisectoral response is most likely to yield results where there is a strong alignment of national development plans/instruments, such as Poverty Reduction Strategies, MTEFs and the national HIV/AIDS policies.

Though many countries have national HIV/AIDS policies and strategic plans in place, most are not costed, so it is difficult to know the amount of resources required to achieve the set objectives. Kenya provides some useful insights in this regard.

KENYA'S COSTED STRATEGIC PLAN

In Kenya, the National AIDS Control Council (NACC) and a broad range of partners have been committed to applying the "Three Ones", leading to their developing the Kenya National HIV/AIDS Strategic Plan for 2006–2010. The plan contains a detailed workplan, with a budget as illustrated in Table 1.4.

Table 1.4: Estimated financing requirements for Kenya National HIV/AIDS Strategic Plan, 2005/06-2009/10						
Activity	2005/06	2006/07	2007/08	2008/09	2009/10	Total
	KES, million					
Prevention	5 740	7 765	8 661	9 788	11 173	43 127
Improving quality of life	7 229	8 832	10 898	12 041	13 155	52 155
Mitigation of socioeconomic impact	7 252	9 221	10 865	12 126	14 441	53 905
Overall total	20 221	25 818	30 424	33 955	38 769	149 187
Source: Kenya National HIV/AIDS Strategic Plan, 2005/06–2009/10; National AIDS Control Council, 2005						

The strategic plan discussed above clearly shows that the key priority for Kenyans from 2005/2006 to 2009/2010 is the mitigation of the socioeconomic impact of HIV/AIDS, with a total of KES53 905 million for the five years. Its main objectives are to adopt existing programmes and to develop innovative responses to reduce the impact of the epidemic on communities, socioeconomic services and economic productivity. Prevention has the least budget over the strategic period, with only KES43 127 million suggesting changing priorities.

Figure 1.3 illustrates the HIV/AIDS resource requirements for Zanzibar, based on the Zanzibar National Strategic Plan (ZNSP). An HIV/AIDS resource requirement exercise would involve estimating the resource requirements based on the projections of key variables that determine expenditure on each HIV/AIDS activity. The graph shows the large financing gap (the difference between what is needed and what is available). The available resources that are needed for the HIV/AIDS response are far less than the resources that are needed to achieve the objectives of the national HIV/AIDS policy. The projection of required resources is a necessary but insufficient condition for the achievement of the national HIV/AIDS goals. Making realistic resource projections for the domestic and international community during the costing stage is possible. However, governments need to translate such commitments into action by allocating adequate resources to the HIV/AIDS initiatives.

Figure 1.3: HIV/AIDS resource requirements for Zanzibar

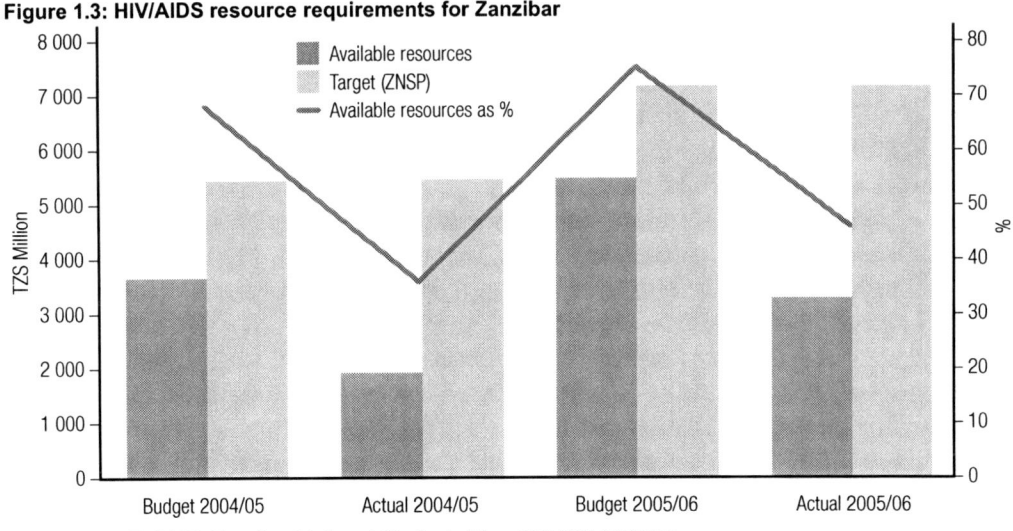

Source: RGoZ, 2007; Zanzibar National Strategic Plan, 2004/05-2008/09

27

Figure 1.4 shows the resources required for the different HIV/AIDS-related activities in Zanzibar, based on the costed strategic plans. The findings show that very few resources are being allocated to prevention, treatment and care compared with what is required, while institutional strengthening is the only activity that was allocated more than required.

Figure 1.4: Required versus actual resources allocated for HIV/AIDS-related efforts in Zanzibar, 2004/05

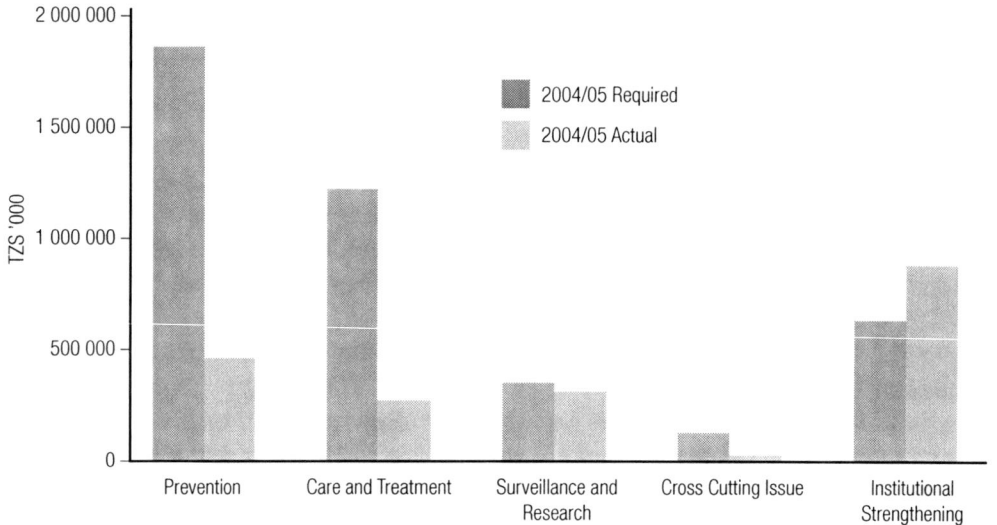

Source: RGoZ, 2007

Though Kenya and Zanzibar have costed strategic plans, this is a necessary but insufficient condition for the success of HIV/AIDS interventions. There is the need to ensure that resources are *adequately* (meaning that the projected cost is equal to the allocated amount), *efficiently* and *equitably* distributed.

ONE AGREED NATIONAL HIV/AIDS AUTHORITY

Two models of NACA have been developed over the last 15 years: One treats NACA as a stand-alone institution (independent of a government ministry) and the other treats NACA as a unit within a given ministry. In Kenya and Malawi, the national AIDS coordinating body falls under the Office of the President (OP). In Ethiopia and Tanzania,[15] the body falls under the Prime Minister's Office (PMO), while, in Zanzibar, it is located in the Chief Minister's Office (CMO). This has been in line with the principle agreed upon by AU and endorsed by UNGASS, that NACAs should be positioned under the highest political offices (OP or the OPM). This is aimed at giving NACAs greater authority and independence from other government departments so that they can carry out their mandate well. In Kenya, the NACA is a state corporation and has an enabling legal environment to take a strategic and influencing role in the national response. Assessing whether NACAs are more successful and effective under the MoH or under a high political office, such as the OP, is key.

ROLES AND FUNCTIONS OF A NACA: COORDINATING AND FACILITATING THE NATIONAL RESPONSE TO HIV/AIDS

The roles and functions of a NACA, according to Dickson (2006), entail:
- Facilitating HIV/AIDS policy development, adoption, dissemination, and periodic review;
- Spearheading advocacy and social mobilisation on HIV/AIDS in all sectors at all levels;
- Building partnerships among all stakeholders in the countries, with regional and international linkages;
- Leading resource mobilisation allocation and the tracking of effective utilisation;
- Guiding the development of HIV/AIDS national strategic frameworks (NSFs) and strategic plans;
- Facilitating and supporting the development of strategic frameworks and plans throughout all sectors and decentralised units;
- Developing strategies for the mainstreaming of HIV/AIDS in all sectors at all levels;
- Promoting the principle of greater involvement of people living with HIV/AIDS Greater Involvement of People Living With HIV/AIDS (GIPA) through capacity strengthening, active participation in all decision- and policy-making forums, and the support and facilitation of PLWHA organisations;
- Developing a national HIV/AIDS M&E system;
- Managing knowledge through documentation and exchange of experiences, approaches and practices, and promotion of best practices;
- Mapping out initiatives, indicating the geographical coverage and the scope of initiatives and actors throughout a country;
- Facilitating and supporting the development of human capacities for responding to HIV/AIDS at all levels; and
- Identifying research priorities and use of findings for policy development.

Evidence has, however, shown that NACA roles and functions are both too ambitious and very difficult to execute. The absence of direct lines of accountability between NACAs and other government departments also makes it difficult for NACAs to be influential in the design and implementation of sector AIDS action plans. Increased donor funding is also changing the role of NACAs to one of resource management and implementation. As alluded to in the UNAIDS (2005) report on the progress on the "Three Ones" most NACAs lack enough human and financial resources to be able to fulfil their mandate. In Malawi, the establishment of the NACA led to the migration of staff from the MoH, leading to the crippling of the ministry in service delivery (Putzel, 2004).

The UNAIDS Secretariat's survey found that, of the 66 countries covered by the survey, 95% had national HIV/AIDS authorities, including all those countries with national frameworks. However, many of the authorities lacked strong mandates and support from the highest levels of government, broadening out to cover all sectors at all levels from national to local. The national HIV/AIDS authorities sometimes also had insufficient accountability, authority, legitimacy and overall leadership of the national response. They were found to have sometimes been excluded from participating in critical processes involved in planning and coordinating the national HIV/AIDS response. The national authorities were also dogged by the absence of human resource capacity and/or management and institutional authority.

Few national HIV/AIDS authorities had all the capacity they needed to perform the functions of planning, resource mobilisation, coordination, information management and M&E. The low salaries paid by the public sector made it difficult to attract qualified people, and the lack of in-country vocational and professional training was even more dire. While only one of the 66 countries covered by the survey was found to have all of the human resource capacity necessary, only 9% had sufficient capacity for coordination.

ONE NATIONAL M&E SYSTEM

By the end of 2004, UNAIDS (2005) found that, of the 66 countries covered by the survey, 79% had begun to work on the development of M&E systems, with there still being a long way to go before the systems were in place. Only 60% had developed plans to the point of being endorsed by all partners, with only 35% having budgets and only 26% having national databases. They also lacked human resource capacity. Only 25% of the countries had trained personnel to develop and manage national databases, and only 5% had all the human resources they needed to do M&E.

A MULTISECTORAL APPROACH TO THE HIV/AIDS RESPONSE

Efforts to encourage a multisectoral response to HIV/AIDS depended on increased knowledge of the pandemic in all areas of the community, increased political commitment, and improved delivery of primary health care (PHC) in general and of HIV/AIDS/STD services specifically (Bates and Altanchimeg, 1998).

There is general consensus that the success of a national HIV/AIDS response to the epidemic depends on a strong, effective strategic partnership between national and international stakeholders, government, civil society and the private sector. In Tanzania, the *central government*, through both the Ministry of Health and Social Welfare (MoHSW), its departments and agencies, and NACA are responsible for service delivery in prevention and care initiatives, including patient care, blood safety and Voluntary Counselling and Testing (VCT), the procurement and distribution of condoms and learning materials and research. Other ministries are also responsible for formulating and implementing HIV/AIDS plans, policies and activities in their respective sectors (URT, 2003e). In Kenya, each government ministry has an AIDS Control Unit for undertaking the mainstreaming of HIV in all core functions of the planning process. In addition to mainstreaming HIV/AIDS in core activities, the

ACUs are expected to mainstream HIV/AIDS into constituency development activities. Constituency AIDS Control Committees (CACCs) are the foci for spearheading the fight against the epidemic at grassroots level through the CBOs and individual organisations.

In Kenya, the regional administrative secretary (RAS), as well as the regional technical entities, play an intermediate role in planning, implementation and monitoring activities at the *regional level*. Local government councils are responsible for bringing together and coordinating all actors working on HIV/AIDS in the respective districts. They serve as the foci for involving and coordinating the public and private sector, NGOs and faith-based organisations (FBOs) in planning and implementing HIV/AIDS initiatives through the council, ward and village multisectoral committees (the council multisectoral AIDS committees (CMACs), the ward multisectoral AIDS committees (WMACs) and the village multisectoral AIDS committees (VMACs)), respectively. They also have the responsibility of ensuring that the councils mainstream HIV/AIDS into plans and budgets through the hamlet, village, ward and council levels. Thus, the local government, from the council to the village level, is responsible for policy making, the budget, decision making and service delivery.

HEALTH FINANCING – ATTAINMENT OF THE ABUJA DECLARATION[16]

As stated earlier, the African leaders met in Abuja in 2001, where they declared that "AIDS is a state of emergency in the continent", committing themselves to place the HIV/AIDS response at the forefront as the highest priority issue in development plans. African countries declared that they would ensure that the needed resources for HIV/AIDS initiatives would be made available from all sources, and that they would be efficiently and effectively utilised. They also pledged to set a target of allocating at least 15% of their annual budgets to improving the health sector.[17]

According to a report by the AU (2006), only 33% of the 53 AU countries had allocated 10% or more of their national resources to the health sector by the end of 2004. For FY 2004/2005, none of the countries under review had managed to reach the set target. Figure 1.5 shows that Ethiopia had the least proportion of resources allocated to health (4.9%), while Zambia and Malawi had the highest (9.3%). Though knowing the amount of resources that the government allocates to the health sector is important, even more critical is assessing whether the resources are being used effectively and efficiently, and ascertaining whether the health ministry has adequate absorptive capacity.

Figure 1.5: Attainment of the Abuja Declaration by countries under review, 2004/05

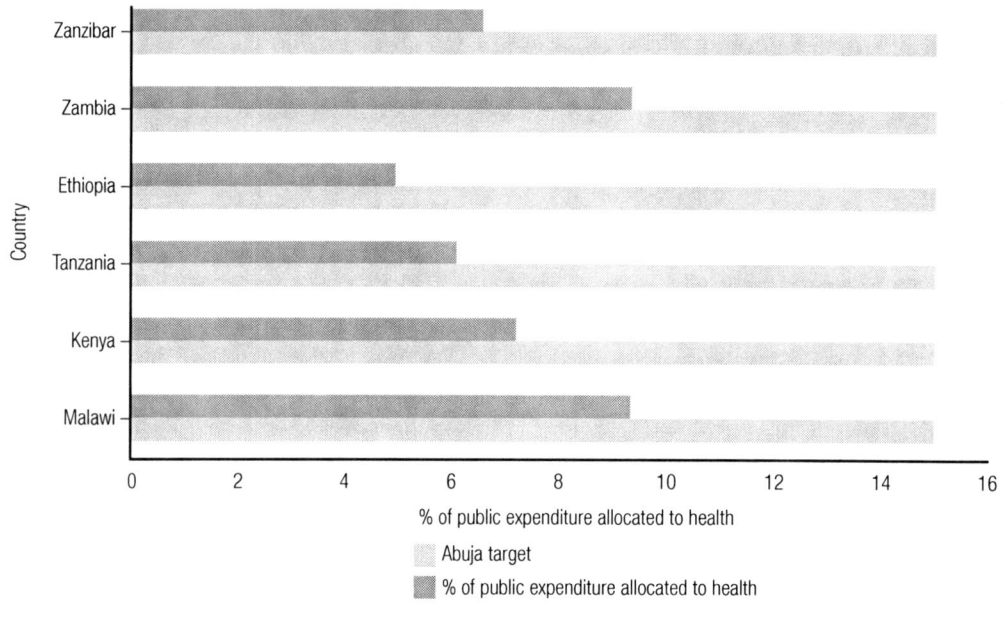

Sources: *Kenya, Malawi NHA report, 2006; MoFED, (Ethiopia) various years, 1997–2005; MoFNP, various years, 2002–2006; MoH, PER various years (Tanzania); RGoZ (Zanzibar) various years, 2004–2007. Calculations by author.*

Effect of the Structural Adjustment Programmes on Health Financing

The failure of governments to meet the Abuja target has largely been blamed on the Structural Adjustment Programmes (SAPs) initiated in Africa by the Bretton Woods institutions (the International Monetary Fund (IMF) and the WB) in the early 1980s. Under SAPs, African governments were encouraged to dramatically reduce government expenditure on the social sectors (including health and education) in line with cost recovery programmes, and to abolish food and agricultural subsidies in order to reduce the government deficit. SAPs were built on fundamental objectives including:

- The promotion of the free movement of capital;
- The opening of national markets to international competition;
- The privatisation of public services and companies;
- The deregulation of labour relations;
- The cutting of social safety nets; and
- The improving of competitiveness (Toissant and Comanne, 1995:14).

SAPS made an effort to reduce government expenditure and to concentrate more on increasing economic growth through investing in the major productive sectors, such as manufacturing, agriculture and mining. The SAPs had far more disastrous effects on those countries which had adopted them (Colgan, 2002), which are characterised by high unemployment rates, increased poverty and very high interest rates.

Zambia took the most dramatic steps to fully implement Economic Structural Adjustment Programmes (ESAPs), and local industries disappeared as measures to protect local industries were dropped, leading to worker retrenchments and high levels of unemployment. According to Goncalves (1996), external debts in Zambia were very high and between 1990 and 1993 the Zambian government spent 35 times more funds on debt repayment than on primary school education. SAPs prevented the achievement of any sustainable economic development that might have enabled the meeting of national priorities. Chossudovsky (1995: 66) pointed out that the "...IMF–WB reform package constitutes a coherent programme for economic and social collapse...They destroy the entire fabric of the domestic economy."

Though SAPs are well documented as not achieving their intended objectives in Africa, whether the failure by governments to achieve the Abuja target can be entirely attributed to them is debatable. While such a matter falls beyond the immediate goal of the current project, the need to understand government limitations in this regard is paramount.

HIV/AIDS FINANCING

THE AMOUNT OF HEALTH CAKE ALLOCATED TO HIV/AIDS

Though it has been established that most of the HIV/AIDS responses are the responsibility of NACA, the health ministry remains an important actor in the HIV/AIDS response, implementing a wide range of HIV/AIDS activities aimed primarily at treatment (including antiretroviral provision and treatment of opportunistic infections (OIs)). The share of HIV/AIDS funds allocated in the health sector budget will be critically assessed in this section.

The health ministries need to balance their resource allocation among the different diseases and other priorities. Overexpenditure on HIV/AIDS alone may lead to the overburdening of the health system, making the achievement of HIV/AIDS targets even more difficult.

UNGASS emphasised the need for an urgent, coordinated and sustained response to the HIV/AIDS epidemic, acknowledging that the HIV/AIDS challenge could not be met without new, additional and sustained resources. An increase in national budgetary allocations for HIV/AIDS initiatives is also a prerequisite for successful HIV/AIDS initiatives, though care should be taken that other diseases are not neglected.

Figure 1.6 shows the share of intended resources allocated by the MoH for HIV/AIDS activities, but does not take into consideration the resources allocated to other ministries that also implement HIV/AIDS activities.

Figure 1.6: The proportion of total public health resources allocated for HIV/AIDS, 2004/05

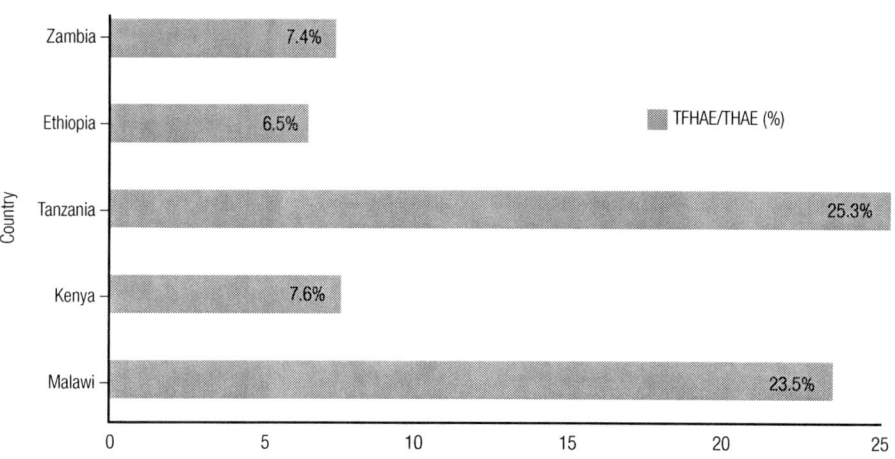

Sources: Kenya, Malawi NHA report, 2006; Malawi NHA report, 2006; MoFED (Ethiopia) (various years, 1997–2005; MoFNP various years, 2002–2006; MoH PER various years (Tanzania); RGoZ (Zanzibar) various years, 2004–2007. Calculations by author.

Figure 1.6 shows that Tanzania had the highest allocation of public resources for HIV/AIDS (25.3%), followed by Malawi (23.5%). Ethiopia had the least allocation of 6.5%, followed by Zambia with 7.4%. It is interesting to note that, despite Zambia having the highest HIV prevalence rate among the countries reviewed in this study, it allocates only 7.4% of its public health resources towards HIV/AIDS. Although Tanzania has one of the lowest prevalence rates, it acknowledges that HIV/AIDS is a health issue and therefore allocates 25.3% of its public health resources towards HIV/AIDS. Although this study is not exhaustive, it would be critical to analyse how governments allocate HIV/AIDS resources to other government departments. A small allocation of funds from the health budget may not necessarily mean that governments are not doing enough to curb the effects of HIV/AIDS. It is however important that governments allocate enough resources for HIV/AIDS from their public funds in order to complement donor efforts and sustain the programmes.

DONOR DEPENDENCY

For many decades, the key feature of African relations with the developed world has been the donor dependency relationship (Riddell, 1999). Donor dependency involves the receipt of more financial resources from external financiers than those contributed by the domestic sources of any particular activity, entailing overreliance on foreign aid to achieve the required HIV/AIDS response. Such a phenomenon is partly due to the lack of government resources, requiring donors to complement government efforts.

Donors have prioritised using aid resources to help solve Africa's HIV/AIDS and poverty challenges. However, the sustainability of donor aid has often been questioned (Games), as foreign funders can withdraw at short notice for political and economic reasons.[18] According to Bulir and Harmann (2003), aid flows are seven times less predictable than domestically generated revenue. For example, the US government's PEPFAR is a five-year HIV/AIDS financial intervention, which was started in 2003. In such a case, the self-sufficiency of recipient governments is critical, as the complete withdrawal of such funding would be especially disastrous where antiretroviral programmes depend upon such financial assistance.

Figure 1.7: Total HIV/AIDS resources allocated by foreign and domestic sources to countries under review, 2004/05

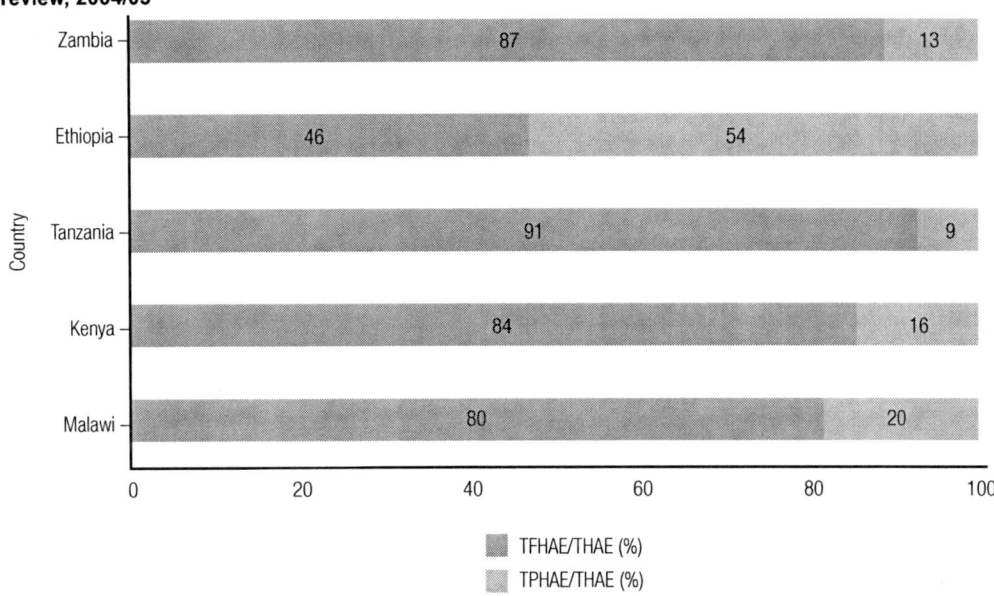

*TFHAE/THAE – the proportion of total HIV/AIDS resources allocated by foreign sources
*TPHAE/THAE – proportion of total HIV/AIDS resources allocated from domestic sources
Sources: Kenya, Malawi NHA report, 2006; Malawi NHA report, 2006; MoFED (Ethiopia), various years, 1997–2005; MoFNP, various years, 2002–2006; MoH, PER various years (Tanzania); RGoZ (Zanzibar), various years, 2004–2007. Calculations by author.

According to UNAIDS (2007a), $1.4 billion has been pledged by rich western countries to the fight against HIV/AIDS in Africa to date. Acknowledging the role that bilateral and multilateral institutions play in the HIV/AIDS response in Africa is also important. Figure 1.7 shows that Tanzania received the most foreign HIV/AIDS financing for the year 2004/2005 (91%), while Ethiopia had the least (46%). Based on the findings of the current study, African countries receive, on average, more than 80% of their HIV/AIDS resources from foreign donors.

Evidence has shown that currently much of the financing is donor-driven,[19] tending to negate the value of national policies and priorities, since donors prescribe what they want governments to do and tend to ignore national priorities, resulting in policy reversals.

Donors and African governments should, ideally, operate at the same level in terms of the determination of priorities, and complement one another when allocating resources to the various national priorities. Proper coordination and harmonisation of HIV/AIDS activities is required by all the stakeholders involved. In this regard, Hanlon (2005) also observes that donor financial assistance is often uncoordinated, adding up to a coherent whole, and not necessarily promoting government priorities. The main question relates to whether, if a government is donor-dependant, it can insist on its own priorities. While African countries and governments encourage donors to buy into their strategies, often unequal power relations result from a donor-driven agenda.

A second donor-related concern is one of duplication. Where lack of donor harmonisation prevails, duplication of effort is unavoidable. Improving aid effectiveness in Africa would entail sharing responsibilities among the different stakeholders. Aid donors need to improve the ownership of aid-funded programmes and projects by Africans and to ensure that aid is "demand-driven" rather than "donor-driven".[20] Increased aid must, therefore, be matched by homegrown policies and priorities.

According to a report by De Waal (2003), while aid works best when it forms part of an overall, coherent, nationally owned strategy, it works least well when it is assigned to a project that is specific to each individual donor, externally designed and poorly harmonised, and subject to complex and burdensome reporting and accounting requirements. The Paris Declaration (2005), which was signed by the different donor countries, alludes to the same principles and should be used as a basis for aid effectiveness. Cooperation between donor and recipient countries is key to improving the effectiveness of aid. Donors have, in the past, often imposed projects on African countries, causing recipient countries to have to contend with numerous missions from donor countries and agencies.[21] For instance, over the last decade, Tanzania, has had to cope with uncoordinated external aid, as have many other poor countries. From 2002 onwards, the government of Tanzania launched a framework for managing foreign aid resources, known as the Tanzania Assistance Strategy (TAS) (URT, 2005). TAS is an action plan for the harmonisation of procedures, including those channeling donor project funds through the exchequer system. An OECD–Development Assistance Committee (DAC) harmonisation group has also been formed to support the implementation of TAS, which is coordinated by the MoF in close collaboration with sector ministries, local governments, civil society and the DAC. Harmonisation efforts are focused on:

- Strengthening the link between the PRS and the budget;
- Reaching agreement on a common performance assessment framework for Poverty Reduction Support Credit (PRSC) and Poverty Reduction Budget Support (PRBS);
- Establishing sector working groups (SWGs) in all priority sectors, which respond to the need for harmonisation processes at sectoral level (ensuring that sectoral processes complement macro processes and are sequenced so as to merge smoothly); and
- Linking country/portfolio annual review processes to existing in-country review processes.

In Zambia, the government and donors contribute to the NAC basket fund initiated through the Joint Financing Agreement (JFA), which comprises the government, the Netherlands and Swedish embassies, Ireland, Norway and the Department for International Development (DFID). All other donors operating in Zambia comprise the JFA, showing that, though the Paris Declaration was adopted and signed, much still needs to be done at ground level in terms of its implementation. In Malawi, the government is in the process of finalising the domestication of the Paris Declaration. A Development Assistance Strategy has also been developed to promote national ownership by linking all development activities to the Millennium Development Goals.

The Effect of Inflation on HIV/AIDS Allocations (Nominal versus Real)

African countries also have to face the challenge of inflation. Inflation, which is measured as the percentage rate of change of a price, is the sustained, persistent, average increase in general price levels for certain sets of goods and services in a given economy over a prescribed period of time. Not all prices of goods and services necessarily increase at the same rate. Generally, when inflation increases, a household has to spend more money in order to maintain the same standard of living.

According to Piana (2001), *hyperinflation* is the most extreme inflation phenomenon, with yearly price increases of three-digit percentage points and an explosive acceleration. *Extremely high inflation* is when inflation ranges between 50% and 100%. *High inflation* is a situation of price increases of between 30% and 50% a year. *Moderate inflation* is when inflation ranges from 5% to 30%. *Low inflation* is characterised as ranging from 1% to 5%. A country is said to have achieved *price stability* when inflation is about zero. *Deflation* is when a country has below-zero inflation.

Inflation affects the ability and willingness of people to save.[22] The purchasing power of those who save money and those whose salaries are fixed is eroded when inflation is high. Over time, as the cost of goods and services increases, the value of a local currency falls, preventing people from purchasing as much with their dollar as they previously could. The general increase in the price of goods and services also hinders the implementation of HIV/AIDS initiatives, as the value of the local currency[23] is eroded.

In all the countries under review, HIV/AIDS allocations were severely affected by inflation rates (the general increase in the price of goods and services) for the FY 2004/05, with Ethiopia having the highest inflation rate of 18.4%, followed by Zambia, with 16.8%. Kenya had the lowest inflation rate of 10.3%. The real value of HIV/AIDS allocations lies in the value of the funds after adjusting for inflation, while the opposite is true for nominal allocations. The nominal allocations can only equate the real allocations rate when the inflation rate is equal to zero. With all the countries under review having an inflation rate greater than zero, their nominal allocations would be higher than real allocations.

When the Treasury formulates the budget, it makes assumptions/projections about macroeconomic variables, such as exchange rates, inflation, economic growth and unemployment. If the inflation projections are correct, it should be able to correctly adjust for inflation, resulting in little difference between the real and nominal allocations. A low real allocation means that the allocated resources have been eroded by inflation, allowing for the purchasing of relatively few goods and services in the current year in comparison with the previous year.

Figure 1.8: Nominal versus real HIV/AIDS allocations from domestic funds in countries under review, 2004/05

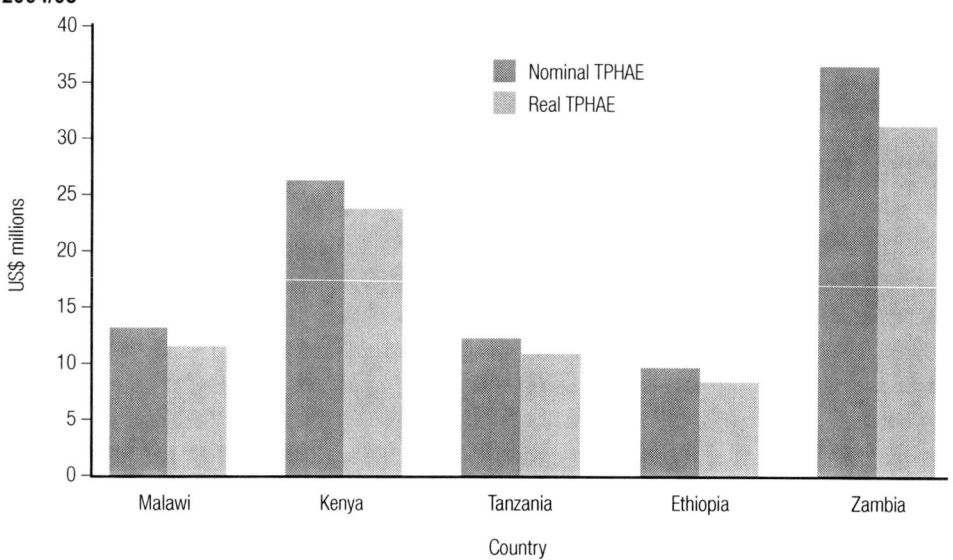

TPHAE – the total HIV/AIDS funds from domestic sources
Sources: Kenya, Malawi NHA report, 2006; Malawi NHA report, 2006; MoFED (Ethiopia,) various years, 1997–2005; MoFNP, various years, 2002–2006; MoH, PER various years (Tanzania); RGoZ (Zanzibar), various years, 2004–2007. Calculations by author.

ALLOCATIONS FOR HIV/AIDS INITIATIVES/FUNCTIONS

According to UNAIDS (2007c), the eight HIV/AIDS core functions on which service providers can spend HIV/AIDS resources consist of the following: prevention; treatment and care; OVC; research; programme management and administration strengthening; human resource incentives; social protection and the social services enabling environment; and community development. The assessment of how countries allocate their HIV/AIDS resources among the different functions is key, because it helps us to understand whether resources are allocated based on the policies and priorities of the country concerned. Such assessment helps with identifying cases of mismatch between policies and budgets.

Ideally, the allocations for the different functions should reflect the country's priorities, as reflected in the HIV/AIDS policy and the national HIV/AIDS strategic plans. Figure 1.9 illustrates the allocations for the different functions for Kenya, Tanzania and Ethiopia. In the case of Tanzania, the graph is based on the allocations to the 189 service providers that were sampled using the National AIDS Spending Assessments (NASA) framework.

Figure 1.9: Public and external HIV/AIDS allocations by function, 2004/05

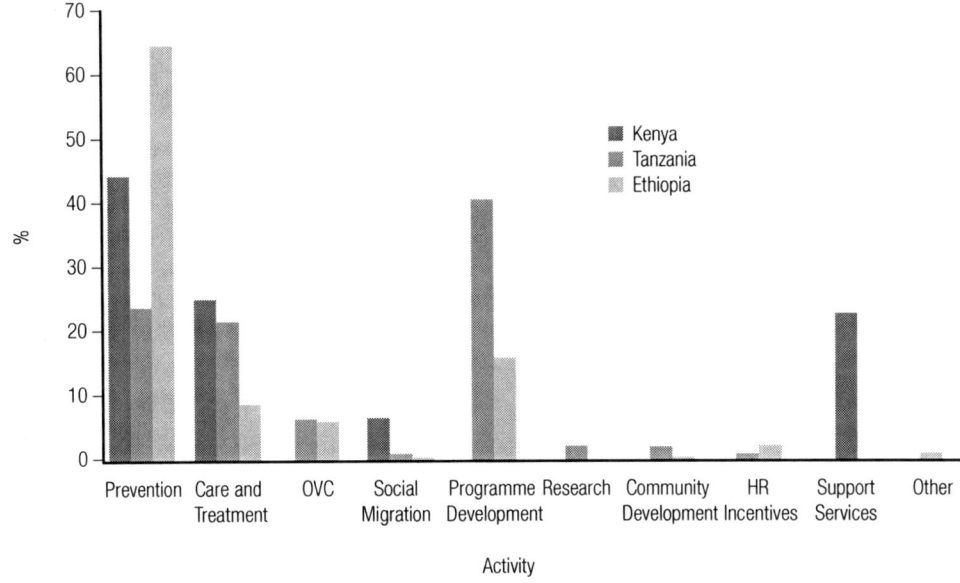

Sources: Ethiopia, Christian Social Services Commission, 2005; HIV/AIDS PER, 2005; Kenya, Getnet, 2006; MoH (2005; MoH–Global Fund accountability, 2005; NACC various income and expenditure statements; Tanzania. Calculations by author.

Zambia and Malawi could not provide information on the disaggregation of HIV/AIDS funds allocated for HIV/AIDS by function/activity. Most countries did not reveal the public HIV/AIDS resources disaggregated by function or beneficiary group as a result of inadequate government financial M&E systems. Figure 1.9 shows the disaggregated total domestic and external HIV/AIDS allocations for the different functions for Kenya, Tanzania and Ethiopia.

Though prevention is the leading priority in Tanzania, according to the HIV/AIDS policy, the resource allocations show a very different picture, with more resources being allocated for programme development. As discussed earlier, the allocation of resources should reflect, and be informed by, the priorities of a country, while budgets should be informed by policies.

There is a mismatch between Kenya's different HIV/AIDS priorities as outlined in the policy, and as implied from the costed KNASP (2005/06–2009/10). According to the policy, prevention is the top priority, followed by improvement of the quality of life. However, close analysis of the KNASP 2005/6–2009/10 shows that more funds are to be committed for the mitigation of socioeconomic impact, thus making it the leading priority.

Relatively more resources were allocated for prevention in the 2004/2005 budget, suggesting that Kenya is moving away from impact mitigation towards prevention as a priority. Kenya's allocations for 2004/2005 are consistent with its HIV/AIDS strategic plan (KNASP 2005/06–2009/10) priorities, which consist of prevention, improvement of the quality of life, and impact mitigation, in rank order. The motivation of such a prioritisation may be the consistent decline in HIV prevalence rates in Kenya over the past few years. The high allocation of resources to prevention activities may partly explain why Kenya has managed to record declining HIV/AIDS prevalence rates, suggesting that the Kenyan national budgets are indeed driven, or at least informed, by the policies concerned.

As Ethiopia has allocated the bulk of its resources to prevention activities, due to its very low HIV prevalence rates, resulting in relatively few people requiring treatment, it is critical for the country to ensure that infection does not occur.

TREATMENT

According to UNAIDS (2006a), the number of recipients of antiretroviral therapy in Africa more than doubled in 2005[24] alone, with roughly one in six PLWHAs receiving antiretrovirals by December 2005. Significant differences in progress between countries have occurred. While nearly 200 sites in Kenya were providing antiretrovirals by December 2005, in South Africa – the country with the largest population of PLWHAs – the number of people receiving antiretrovirals grew from fewer than 5 000 at the beginning of 2004 to roughly 190 000 by the end of the next year (UNAIDS, 2006a). Coverage levels of 50% or greater have been achieved in countries such as Botswana and Uganda, while, in others, the levels have remained at less than 10%. Worldwide, between 250 000 and 350 000 deaths were estimated as having been averted in 2005, as a result of increased treatment access (UNAIDS, 2005).

The "3 by 5" initiative launched by UNAIDS and WHO in 2003[25] served as a global target to provide three million PLWHAs in the low- and middle-income countries with life-prolonging antiretroviral therapy by the end of 2005. As such, it marked substantial progress towards the goal of universal access of HIV/AIDS prevention and treatment for those in need.

"All by 2010" describes the goal of universal access to antiretroviral treatment by the year 2010. According to the WHO "3 by 5" document, achieving such a target will entail administering treatment to a greater number than are currently in need. Such an increase is due to the fact that those who started treatment in previous years must continue to receive medication, with, each year, many hundreds of thousands of people progressing to the stage of disease at which treatment is required. Universal access to treatment can be regarded as having been achieved when 80% of all people in urgent need of treatment receive it.[26]

Figure 1.10 reflects the differences in the cost of recommended first-line regimens in the different countries under review. Malawi has the lowest cost per person per year, which is attributed to the availability of drugs from public hospitals that administer them free of charge. In Malawi, donors supported the extensive rollout of antiretrovirals, which were distributed for free by public hospitals. The cost of antiretrovirals is also relatively low in Kenya (US$150), which may be due to a local company being awarded a licence by GlaxoSmithKline for the local manufacture of generic antiretroviral drugs, which are cheaper than the branded drugs.

Figure 1.10: Cost differences of recommended first-line regimens in countries under review, 2005

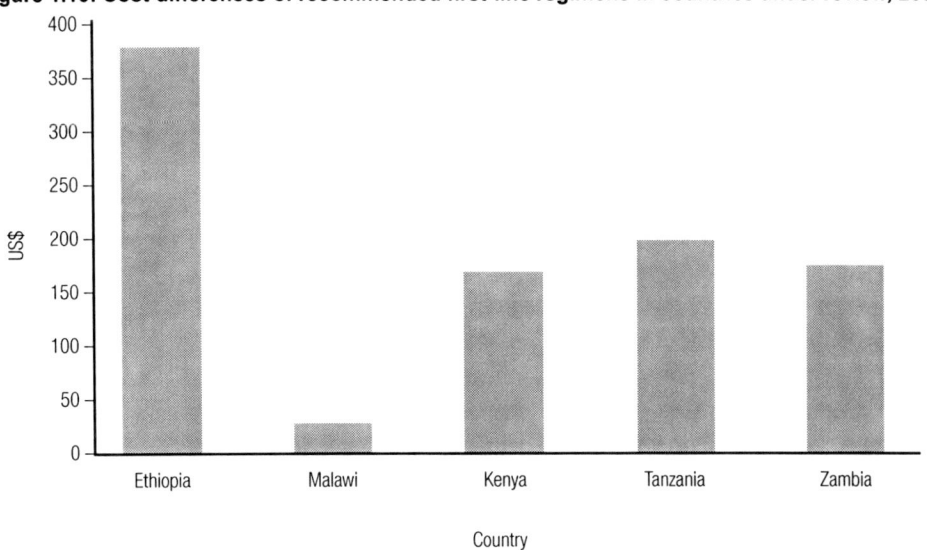

Source: WHO, 2005, Summary of country profile for HIV/AIDS treatment scale up – Kenya, Malawi, Zambia, Ethiopia, Tanzania. Calculations by author.

Figure 1.11 shows that, at the time of the survey, Kenya had the highest number of people in need of antiretrovirals, with which they were being provided (16.3%), while Tanzania had the least (3%). The extent of Tanzania's treatment programme is largely due to the increase in the GTAFM and the Clinton Foundation against HIV/AIDS' (CHAI) allocations to the treatment and care of PLWHAs. Private health-care providers also provide antiretroviral drugs, at a cost.

Figure 1.11: Relationship between provision of antiretrovirals and HIV prevalence

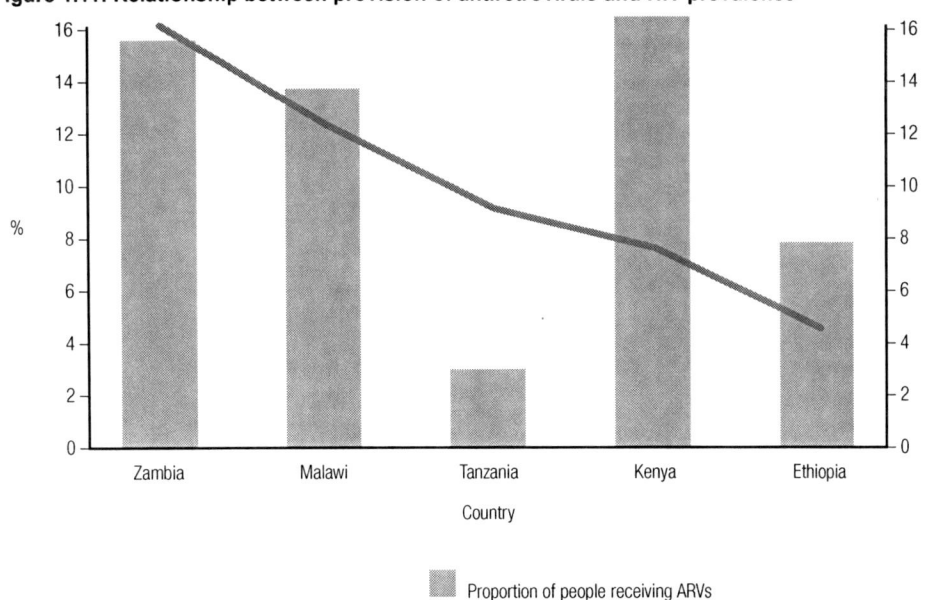

Source: WHO, 2005, Summary of country profile for HIV/AIDS treatment scale up – Kenya, Malawi, Zambia, Ethiopia, Tanzania. Calculations by author.

41

The availability of drugs is instrumental to the achievement of the "physical, emotional and psychological well being" of any PLWHA. Such achievement depends on appropriate political will. According to Peter Piot, the Executive Director of UN-AIDS: "Treatment is technically feasible in every part of the world. Even the lack of infrastructure is not an excuse...it is knowledge that's the barrier. It's political will" (XIV International AIDS Conference, Barcelona, 2002).

The current study shows the clear and strong positive relationship existing between HIV prevalence and antiretroviral provision. The higher the prevalence rate, the higher the number of people on antiretrovirals. However, despite Kenya's prevalence rate being lower than that of Tanzania, more Kenyans receive antiretrovirals than do Tanzanians, as antiretrovirals are cheaper in Kenya than they are in Tanzania, due to their being locally sourced in generic form. The high rate of antiretroviral provision in Kenya may also partly be explained by the fact that antiretrovirals are provided free of charge at public health and mission facilities, as well as at designated sites. Such provision has been enabled by consistent funding from PEPFAR, and by the government's importation of generic drugs.

Zambia has a relatively high percentage of people on antiretrovirals, which are 87% donor-funded. Zambia's treatment programme has only been made possible by an unprecedented amount of funding from the GFATM, PEPFAR and other financing sources. Zambia started providing free antiretrovirals to PLWHAs in 2005.

NUTRITION – AN IMPORTANT PART OF THE TREATMENT MATRIX

Antiretroviral therapy, which comprises a holistic process of HIV/AIDS treatment, is not limited to the provision of antiretrovirals According to UNAIDS,[27] a good diet containing a full range of essential micronutrients is key to bolstering the immune system, boosting energy levels and maintaining the body weight of PLWHAs. For those on ART, good nutrition and clean water make treatment more effective.[28]

Figure 1.12: The role played by nutrition in the treatment matrix

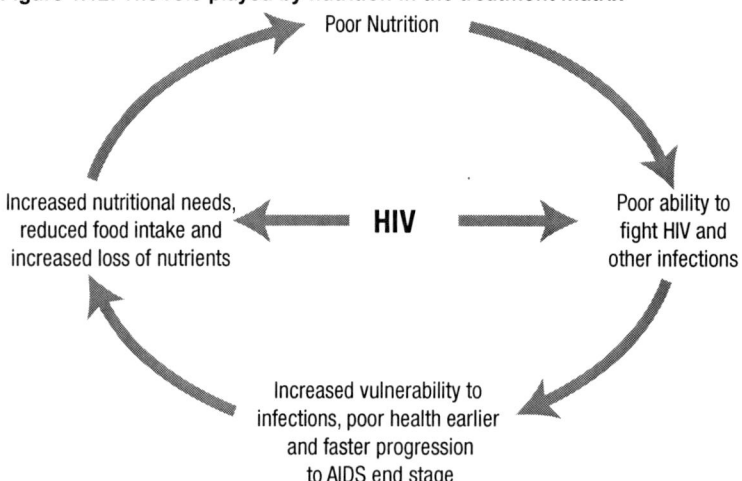

Source: Adapted from South African National Guidelines on Nutrition for People Living with TB, HIV/AIDS and other Chronic Debilitating Conditions (2001).

Of the countries under review, Kenya was the only country with a budget line item for nutritional supplements, with 3% of its treatment resources consisting of nutritional support. Though Ethiopia had 37% underweight children and 46.9% suffering from chronic malnutrition in 2004, none of its resources were earmarked for nutritional support.

The rollout of paediatric HIV/AIDS treatment and care has been slow in many countries, with, among the countries under review, only Malawi providing antiretrovirals to children infected by HIV at the time of the study. As explained earlier, the inability of this study to meet all NASA requirements means that information on the regional, age and gender disaggregation of the antiretroviral rollout was not available for each country.

Between 45% and 50% of people in Sub-Saharan Africa live below the international poverty line of US$1 per day (World Bank, 2005). Against such a background, African governments should seriously consider providing nutritional supplements to the poor who receive antiretrovirals, given the existence of such high poverty levels.

Figure 1.13: Breakdown of HIV/AIDS spending (%) on treatment in Kenya, 2004/05

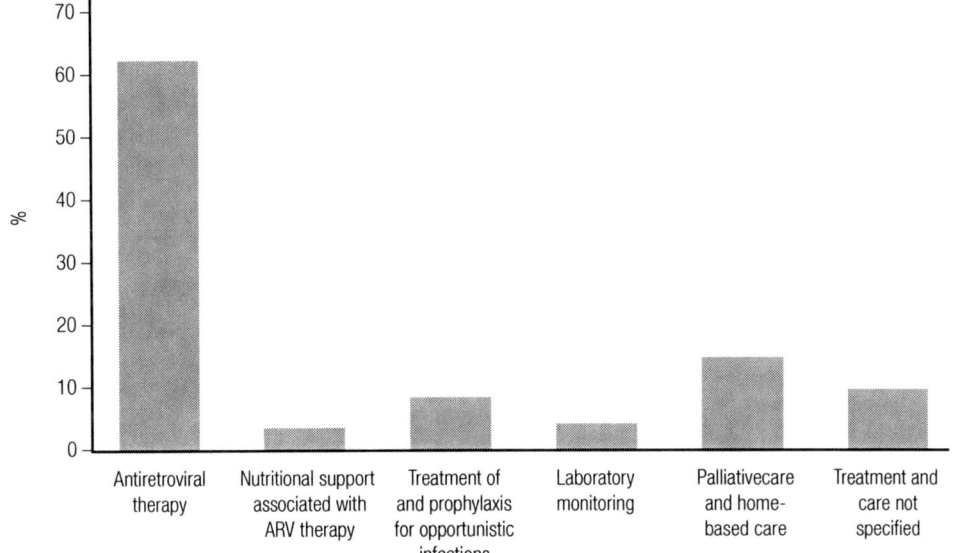

Sources: HIV/AIDS Public Expenditure Review; MOH, 2005; MOH – Global Fund Accountability Statement for the period 1 July 2005 to 31 December 2005; NACC, various statements of income and expenditure; UNAIDS, Kenya Office; UNDP, 2004.

The highest proportion of Kenya's treatment and care budget (62%) was earmarked for ART in 2004/2005, which is why there are more people on antiretrovirals in Kenya compared with the other countries under review. Though the proportion of funds allocated for nutritional support was low, the recognition that nutrition is a cornerstone to a successful treatment programme is a step in the right direction.

The Geographical Allocation of HIV/AIDS Funds

Though assessing how resources are allocated for the different HIV/AIDS spending categories (ASCs) is important, evaluating how resources are geographically allocated is also key. The spread of HIV infection is often associated with geographic factors, such as population mobility, the accessibility of, and proximity to, high transmission or urban areas, and the geographic distribution of those at a greater risk of infection (Montana et al, 2005). Evidence has shown that different regions have different prevalence rates and, as such, resources should be allocated on a needs basis. As mentioned earlier, the evidence from the countries under review shows that HIV prevalence is higher in the urban than in the rural areas, therefore we would expect more resources to be allocated to the former, where there is more need.

The allocation of resources to the different regions should reflect equity. Allocations can be based on the region's population size, the HIV prevalence, and the morbidity and mortality rates. However, such factors might not be used in practice due to the lack of harmonisation and coordination of HIV/AIDS initiatives. Those regions that tend to be more "attractive" to donors are likely to receive more resources than other regions. According to Thompson (2003), some areas may receive more aid than others due to media coverage. He argues that areas with the "CNN factor" tend to be granted more aid because of the extensive media coverage that they receive. According to Thompson (2003), some areas receive more aid due to national interest and donor country influence. Often several different CSOs provide HIV/AIDS services concentrated in a single district. In such cases, duplication of effort is inevitable. Decisions surrounding this are made either by the FS, FA or service providers.

Figure 1.14: Equity in HIV/AIDS resource allocation (%) in Kenya 2004/05

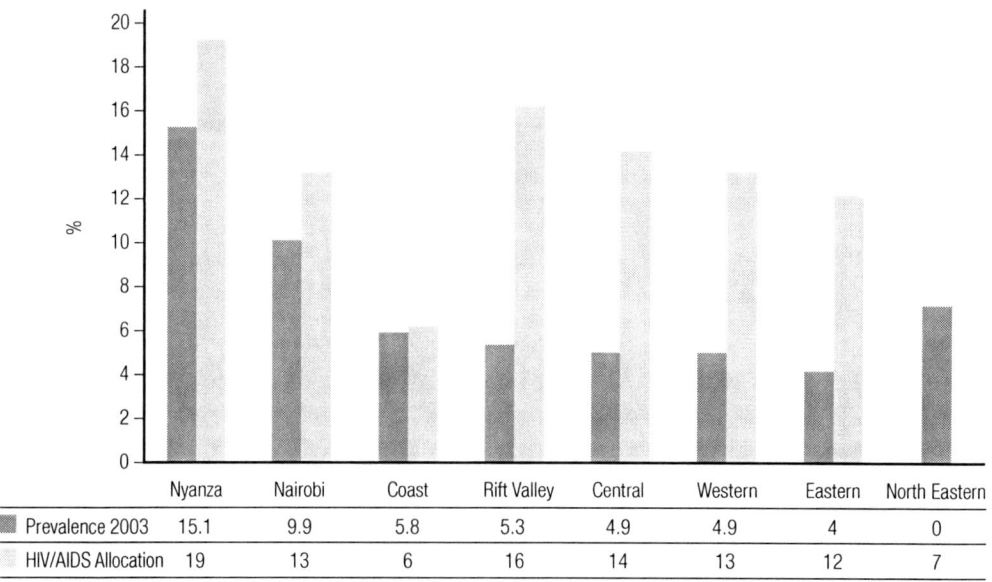

	Nyanza	Nairobi	Coast	Rift Valley	Central	Western	Eastern	North Eastern
Prevalence 2003	15.1	9.9	5.8	5.3	4.9	4.9	4	0
HIV/AIDS Allocation	19	13	6	16	14	13	12	7

Sources: NASCOP, 2003.

In Kenya, funds allocated by the WB are disbursed according to HIV prevalence, though this is not applicable to all the provinces. For instance, Nyanza, with the highest prevalence, received the largest share (19.4%) of the funding, while the Rift Valley, with a prevalence of 5.3%, received more funding (15.8%) than did Nairobi province (13.3%), with a prevalence of 9.9%. Paradoxically, the North Eastern province, with almost no prevalence, received more than the Coast province. Such a finding, though without clear justification, reflects inequalities in the distribution of donor funding, which is also outlined in the Kenya National Strategic Plan 2005/06 -2009/10, which calls for strengthening of equity in financing the fight against HIV/ AIDS.

SPENDING OF HIV/AIDS FUNDS

Absorptive capacity refers to the ability of HIV/AIDS service providers to spend all the resources that have been allocated to them within a specified time frame, as well as the capacity of a firm/organisation or institution to identify, assimilate and exploit knowledge from external sources (Cohen and Levinthal, 1990). The spending rate of any service provider, meaning the proportion of allocated funds/resources that is used for HIV/AIDS initiatives as intended, is affected by its absorptive capacity.

An assessment of HIV/AIDS resource use by the different government departments and CSOs confirms that not all that is allocated might be spent. Figure 1.15 shows that the spending rates are higher (86%) for donor allocations made directly to CSOs in Zanzibar, largely due to the strict donor reporting systems and to donor compliance being a prerequisite for eliciting more funds from the donors. According to Clemens and Radelet (2003), donor practices lie at the root of and exacerbate many absorptive problems by donors insisting on their own preferences, "short termism", the overdesign of projects, strict procedures and monitoring mechanisms, thus creating bottlenecks. Some of the challenges with respect to the use of donor funds include long delays in obtaining approval for projects and the disbursement of funds, and high transaction costs. According to Tayler (2005), much development aid is still "tied" to the FS in that fund recipients should procure assets or services from the donor country concerned.

Government funds allocated to the different ministries have the lowest spending rates due to the slow rate of disbursement and bureaucratic processes, as well as poor M&E and government financial information systems. No reprimanding mechanisms exist for nonperformers or for those who do not achieve their set objectives. Donor funds that are allocated to government departments have a slightly higher spending rate, though, which might be attributed to the strict reporting and accounting procedures required by the donors involved. The huge disparities in spending between government departments and CSOs may explain why most donors prefer channeling their funds through CSOs.

Figure 1.15: Spending rates of HIV/AIDS funds in Zanzibar, 2004/05

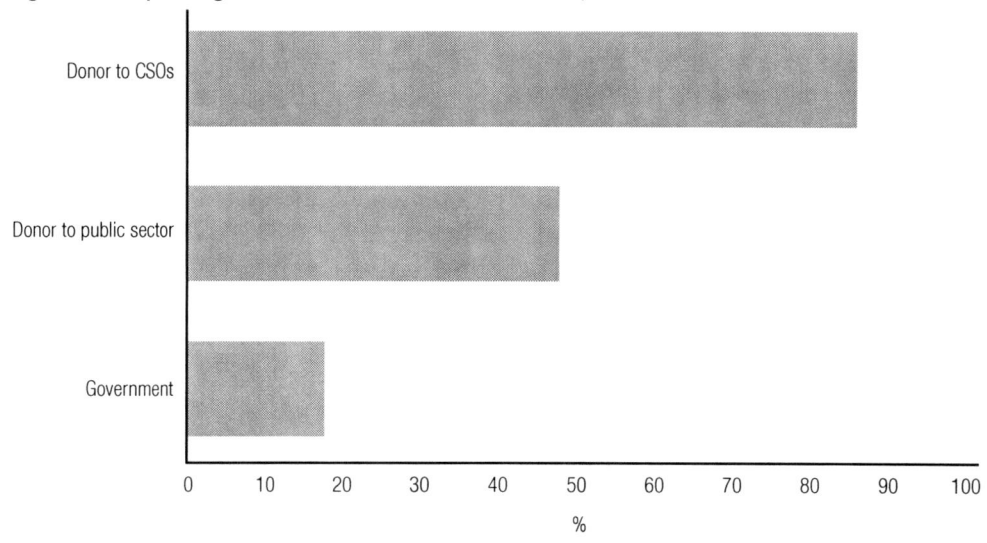

Source: RGoZ, 2007. Calculations by author.

The scenario presented in Figure 1.16 shows that, though the GTAFM has an agreement with the government of Zanzibar, CSOs are the major beneficiaries of the funds received.

Figure 1.16: Allocations versus actual expenditure of the Global Fund in Zanzibar, 2004/05

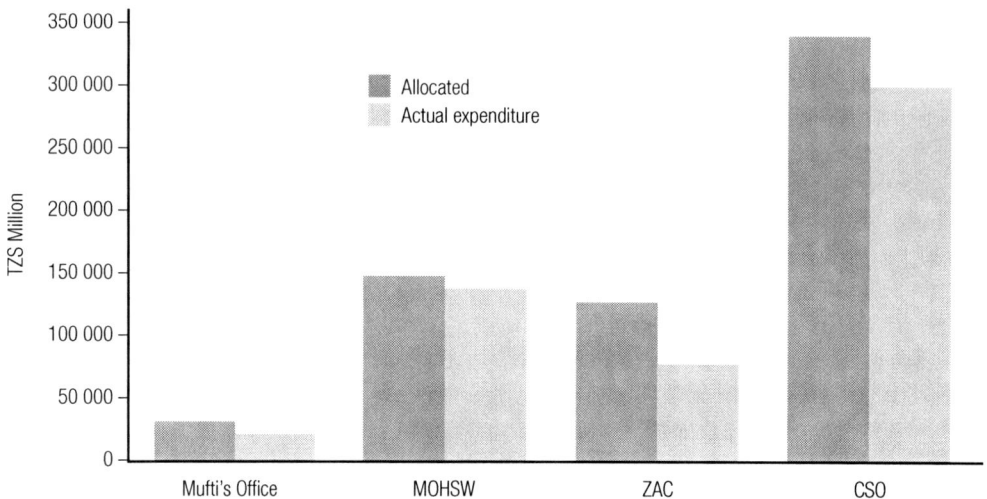

Source: RGoZ, 2007. Calculations by author.

The following reasons explain the low absorptive capacity:
- Lack of capacity of service providers, or the implementation of partners (staffing and systems for accountability) leading to lack of donor compliancy;

- Failure of implementing partners to deal with multiple donors with varied requirements;
- Slow disbursement of funds by the sources of finance and financing agents;
- Compromised implementation of the programmes by strict donor requirements and stringent reporting mechanisms; and
- Macroeconomic constraints (including high inflation rates; shortage of foreign currency; prohibitive tariffs on medical goods; high unemployment rates).

BENEFICIARIES OF HIV/AIDS FUNDING

Resources must be spent in a way that provides needed goods and services to targeted populations. According to Dmytraczenko et al (2006), it is not only the amount invested in the HIV/AIDS response that matters, but also how the funds are spent and whether those in need benefit from them. Policymakers need to be well equipped to make decisions regarding the optimal allocation of resources to meet the needs of vulnerable populations. Establishing how resources are distributed is important.

Figure 1.17: Beneficiaries of HIV/AIDS expenditure in Tanzania

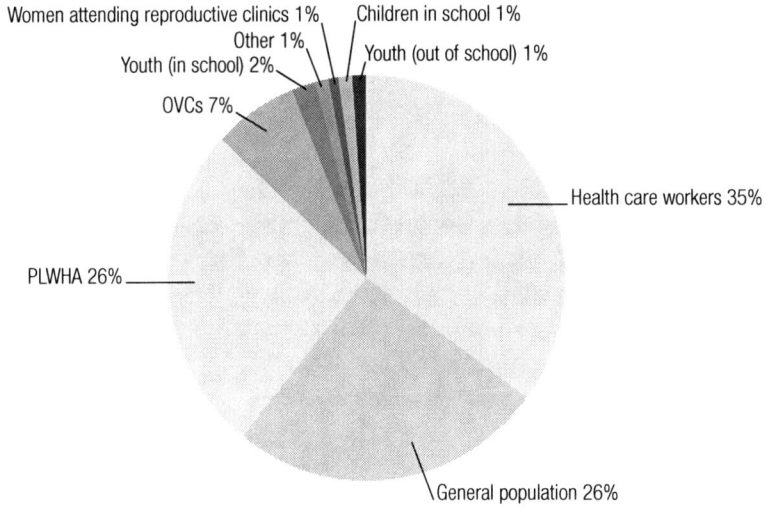

Figure 1.18: Prevention expenditure by target population in Kenya, 2004/05

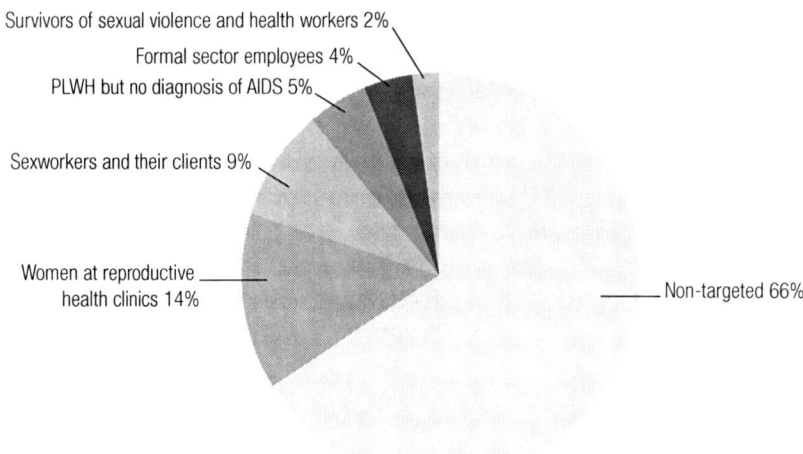

Survivors of sexual violence and health workers 2%

Formal sector employees 4%

PLWH but no diagnosis of AIDS 5%

Sexworkers and their clients 9%

Women at reproductive health clinics 14%

Non-targeted 66%

Though the countries under review endeavoured to disaggregate their allocation according to HIV/AIDS functions, disaggregation by beneficiary population is equally important. The Tanzanian information used is derived from the 189 service providers who were sampled in an attempt to use the NASA framework. While most of Kenya's prevention resources (65.6%) were not targeted, resulting in their benefiting the general population, only 26.5% of Tanzanian resources were not targeted.

MEN WHO HAVE SEX WITH OTHER MEN

Despite men who have sex with other men (MSMs) being widely considered to be a high risk group,[29] the Tanzanian and Kenyan findings showed that no resources were allocated for MSMs, prisoners and institutionalised persons. Such denial, stigma and lack of recognition by the authorities and societies prevails in many African countries. As a result, many MSMs feel ashamed of their sexuality, suffer from low self-esteem and attempt to keep their sexuality hidden from their families and the wider society, thereby increasing their risk of HIV infection.[30]

WOMEN AND CHILDREN

Violence against women is strongly linked to vulnerability to HIV (WHO, 2000). Women who survive domestic violence have a higher risk of being infected by HIV than their counterparts. Accordingly, Kenya allocated 1.97% of its prevention resources for victims of sexual violence, most of whom are women. In Tanzania, however, this study found that no resources were allocated for "women and children affected by trafficking and violence".

Though approximately 57% of those who are well documented as being PLWHAs in SSA are women, the evidence from the selected African countries still does not reflect the availability of HIV/AIDS programmes targeted specifically at women, apart from those directed at the prevention of mother-to-child transmission (PMTCT). Though some programmes that are in place target the "general population", women lack equal access to information on prevention and treatment, so they usually do not benefit from such programmes. Disaggregating expenditure in terms of the beneficiaries would enable policymakers to keep track of whether those most in need are benefiting from the funds and to assess the impact of the different HIV/AIDS programmes on those at whom they are directed.

CONCLUSION

The current study clearly shows that African countries need to ensure that the health sector is adequately funded with at least 15% of national resources, as it is only by doing so that commitments can be translated into action. PLWHAs already occupy more than 50% of public hospital beds.

SAPs are generally blamed for low government spending on the social sectors and for compromising Africa's ambition to reverse the effects of the pandemic within realistic targets, yet whether this is the only factor causing underspending is doubtful. Governments must be further interrogated to explain any shortfalls. The current research, while not indicating other causes, considers each case carefully, gauging prevalence against the resources committed. A relationship exists between the prevalence rates and the amounts allocated to fighting HIV/AIDS, as, for example, in Ethiopia, prevention receives more attention than do other aspects of the pandemic, which is possibly due to the relatively low infection rates.

The salient factor in the current study is the overreliance on donor funds by all the countries under review. While donor funds may be contributing to significant inputs into the national response, they appear to be disorganised, with allocations predetermined more by funders' preferences than local priorities. The absence of donor harmonisation in most countries clearly hampers aid effectiveness, resulting in the duplication of effort, as well as the marginalisation of areas alien to the donors' interests. With donors not yet working in unison, the beneficiary agencies, often consisting of civil societies, are likely to struggle with matters of absorption and delivery. While in Zambia, there is some level of donor cooperation, not all donors are likely to cooperate with one another despite being signatories of the Paris Declaration.

PEPFAR, the largest of the foreign pools of funds, continues to operate outside the global fund system, which, in itself, conflicts with the effective governance of the HIV/AIDS pandemic, despite its successes. In order to understand the effectiveness, efficiency and equity of HIV/AIDS funding, a common database is needed for all HIV/AIDS financing and spending throughout Africa. Only in this way can the impact of the different programmes be assessed.

Lastly, over-reliance on donor funds raises the question of sustainability. Beyond the current flow of aid, will African governments be able to sustain the huge treatment, care and support systems that have characterised responses in the recent past? Will governments be forced to make difficult choices, such as whether to prioritise prevention over treatment? What sort of political fallouts could such choices generate if certain sectors of society are neglected?

GENERAL RECOMMENDATIONS

ADEQUACY OF HIV/AIDS FUNDS AND DONOR DEPENDENCY

The current study found that, on average, more than 75% of funds meant for HIV/AIDS interventions are financed by bilateral and multilateral institutions. Nevertheless, HIV/AIDS resources are still inadequate to meet current needs. African governments should increase their health and HIV/AIDS allocations in order to achieve sustainability of such initiatives. In cases where governments receive the bulk of their resources from bilateral and multilateral organisations, donors should align their activities with national priorities.

DONOR COORDINATION AND HARMONISATION

Mechanisms aimed at improving donor coordination must be explored in order to minimise the current duplication, double funding, double counting and multiple reporting requirements. NACAs require a database on the sources of all HIV/AIDS funds, financing agents and service providers, the beneficiaries of such funds and the key priority areas being funded. NACAs lacking adequate financial and human resources must be recapitalised, strengthened and decentralised to the periphery, where most of the grassroots CBOs are located.

ABSORPTION CAPACITY AND EFFICIENCY

Despite increases in funding for HIV/AIDS in Africa, the ability of the countries under review to use the available HIV/AIDS resources productively has been hampered by several factors, ranging from the lack of procurement skills, human resources, reporting and efficient financial management, to strict donor requirements, and institutional and policy constraints. While donors should investigate the ability of service providers to absorb most – if not all – of the funds allocated to them, they should also revise their reporting requirements, as such requirements sometimes hamper the implementation of projects and related aid effectiveness. The service providers should also be encouraged to invest in human resource skills required for project and financial management. Proper reporting mechanisms should also be developed and implemented to track the impact of projects on the target population.

THE STRENGTHENING OF GOVERNMENT MONITORING AND EVALUATION AND FINANCIAL INFORMATION SYSTEMS

Participatory strategies should allow for continued assessment and feedback on the efficiency and effectiveness of HIV/AIDS strategies. Government departments and ministries should document the various activities undertaken during any specific FY. In addition, the monitoring and evaluation, and financial information systems require enforcing to ensure that ministries spend funds on the intended activities.

The absence of information relating to expenditure by ministries, and the lack of disaggregated data organised in terms of function and beneficiaries, makes it difficult for governments to track the impact of their spending on the lives of the intended beneficiaries. The monitoring role of CSOs should also be strengthened to enable assessment of the responsiveness of budgets to people's needs, as well as their sensitivity to poverty concerns. Such assessment will only be made possible when budget information is accessible and user-friendly for the public, and if CSOs, in their capacity as representatives of citizens, are allowed to participate in the budget process. Continued training of CSOs by regional institutions and international agencies with the requisite skills is emphasised in this regard.

STRENGTHENING THE HEALTH-CARE SYSTEM

The HIV/AIDS epidemic has further burdened the already ailing health-care systems, with over 40% of hospital bed occupancy being HIV-related. More resources than are currently available should be allocated for strengthening health-care systems. Health-care systems require adequate funding to ensure that the available resources are used effectively, equitably and efficiently, so as to reduce the effects of HIV/AIDS in Africa. Donors should ensure that they apportion a proportion of their resources for strengthening health-care systems. According to Oomman et al (2007), despite PEPFAR funding such strengthening, accounting systems make it difficult to determine the exact amounts spent on such activities.

TRANSLATING COMMITMENTS INTO ACTION

Though several governments have signed the different international and regional HIV/AIDS conventions and declarations, few have domesticated them, making it very difficult to hold the respective governments accountable. The declarations, policies and commitments, on their own, are not legally binding and, as such, the governments are not obliged to adhere to them. Though UN General Assembly Special Session on HIV/AIDS Declarations I and II require that reports be submitted biennially to the Special Session on HIV/AIDS, many countries submit incomplete reports very late.

Despite having signed the Abuja Declaration, African countries have yet to meet the targets set in the declaration. Despite the many donor resources, the governments concerned must also show their adherence to financial commitments by allocating at least 15% of their national budgets to the health sector. At a national level, the policies enacted have, in reality, been reduced to statements of intent due to the lack of costing and funding.

CSOs urgently need to hold governments accountable to their national, regional and international commitments and declarations, so that they can deliver on their promises through adequate and equitable resource allocation.

APPENDIX

Country information for 2004/05 used for the overview					
Country	Malawi	Kenya	Tanzania	Ethiopia	Zambia
Indicator					
Exchange rate	108.9	76.74	1076	8.66	4200
HIV prevalence rate	12	7.3	8.9	4.4	16
Inflation	15.5	10.3	13.6	18.4	16.8
GDP 2005 (US$ million)	2100	18700	12000	11200	3952
Population 2005 (million)	12.9	34.3	38.3	71.3	10.4
GDP per capita	162.7906977	545.1895044	313.3159269	157.0827489	380
TPE (local currency)	68769835000	3.88889E+11	3073266.939	24562000000	8.3473E+12
TPE (US$ million)	631.2448597	5067.616472	3315.8138	2836.258661	1987.452913
TPHE (local currency)	6417187218	28000000000	2.182E+11	1201400000	9.18203E+11
TPHE (US$ million)	58.90397214	364.8683868	202.7881041	138.7297921	218.6198205
Abuja target (%)	15	15	15	15	15
% of total budget allocated to health	9.3	7.2	6.1	4.9	9.3
TPHAE (local currency)	1505.46469	2129.535	14582	86773200	1.59041E+11
Nominal TPHAE (US$ million)	13.8	27.8	13.6	10.0	37.9
Real TPHAE US$ million	12.0	25.2	11.9	8.5	32.4
Nominal THAE (local currency)	7527323449	2225460000	1.80876E+11	160342617	1.25638E+12
Real THAE (local currency)	456201421.2	196943362.8	12388739726	8265083.351	70583002510
Nominal THAE (US $million)	69.1	181.0	168.1	18.5	299.1
Real THAE (US$ million)	59.8	164.1	148.0	15.6	256.1
Nominal TFHAE (US$ million)	55.3	152.0	153.5	8.5	261.3
Real TFHAE (US$)	47.9	137.8	135.2	7.2	223.7
TFHAE/THAE (%)	80	84	91	46	87
TPHAE/THAE (%)	20	16	9	54	13
TPHAE/TPHE (%)	23.5	7.6	6.7	7.2	17.3
Per capita THAE (US$ million)	5.4	5.3	4.4	0.3	28.8
Per capita TFHAE (US$)	4.3	4.4	4.0	0.1	25.1
Per capita TPHAE (US$)	1.1	0.8	0.4	0.3	3.6
Calculations by author.					

REFERENCES

Adetunji, J., 2000. *Trends in Under-five Mortality Rates and the HIV/AIDS Epidemic.*

African Union (AU), 2006. *Update on HIV/AIDS Control in Africa*, Abuja.

Arndt, C., 2000. "The Macro Implications of HIV/AIDS in South Africa: A Preliminary Assessment", *South Africa Journal of Economics.*

Baldeh, A , 2006. Response of Governments and International Institutions and Civil Society on Scaling up HIV/AIDS Financing.

Barnett, T., 2005. *HIV/AIDS Nutrition and Food Security: Looking to Future Challenges*, London School of Economics.

Barnett, T. and Whiteside, A., 1999a. *Guidelines for Preparing and Execution of Studies of the Social and Economic Impact of HIV/AIDS*, Geneva.

Barnett, T. and Whiteside, A., 1999b. *HIV/AIDS and Development: Case Studies and a Conceptual Framework*, Durban.

Booysen, F. le R. and Bachmann, M., 2002. HIV/AIDS Poverty and Growth: Evidence from Household Impact Study in the Free State Province, South Africa.

Bulir, A. and Harmann, J., 2003. Aid Volatility: An Empirical Assessment. IMF Staff Paper.

Buve, A., 1997. "AIDS and Hospital Bed Occupancy: An Overview", *Tropical Medicine and International Health*, 2 (2).

Byron, E., Gillespie, S. and Namgami, M., 2006. *Linking Nutritional Treatment of People Living with HIV: Lessons Being Learned in Kenya.*

Chossudovsky, M., 1995. "Structural Adjustment". In: *Notebooks for Study and Research*, 24/25.

Clemens, M. and Radelet, S., 2003. *Absorptive Capacity: How Much is Too Much, How Long is Long Enough? Challenging Foreign Aid*, Washington, DC: Centre for Global Development.

Cohen, D., 1998. Poverty and HIV/AIDS in Sub-Saharan Africa, HIV and Development Programme, (2).

Cohen, D., 2000. HIV and Development Programme: The Economic Impact of the HIV Epidemic, UNDP issue, Paper 2.

Cohen, W. and Levinthal, D., 1990. "Absorptive Capacity: A New Perspective on Learning and Innovation", *Administrative Science Quarterly*, (35).

Commonwealth Regional Health Community Secretariat for East, Central and Southern Africa.

Dickson, C., 2006. *Roles and Responsibilities of National AIDS Commissions: Debates and Issues.* Technical brief: HSLP Institute.

Dmytraczenko, T, De S., Chanfreau, C. and Kidane, L., 2006. The Value of Beneficiary Analysis: Who Benefits from Funds Targeted for HIV/AIDS?

Drimie, S., 2002. The Impact of HIV/AIDS on Rural Households and Land Issues in Southern and Eastern Africa.

EIP/FER/WHO, 2004. *Synergies between NAA and the National Health Accounts Framework*, Geneva.

Farmer, P., 1999. *Infections and Inequalities: The Modern Plagues*, Berkely, Cal.: University of California Press.

Foster, 2005. *Bottlenecks and Drip Feeds*, London:

Games, D. 2007. *Africa Beyond Aid*. Conference, 24-26 June 2007 Brussels, Belgium.

Goncalves, F., 1996. "Entangled in the Adjustment Web", *SAPEM*, 9 (12), September.

Guiness, L. and Alban, A., 2000. *The Economic Impact of AIDS in Africa: A Review of the Literature*, Geneva.

Guthrie, T., 2006. *An Introduction to Expenditure Analysis: An Overview of the NASA Methodology*, Istanbul.

Hallman, K., 2004. *Socioeconomic Disadvantage and Unsafe Sexual Behaviours among Young Women and Men in South Africa*, Population Council.

Human Rights Watch, 2005. *A Dose of Reality: Women's Rights in the Fight against HIV/AIDS*.

International Labor Organization (ILO), 2004. *HIV/AIDS and Work: Global Estimates, Impact and Response*.

Jayne, T.S., Villarreal, M., Pingali, P. and Hemrich, G., 2005. *HIV/AIDS and the Agricultural Sector in Eastern and Southern Africa: Anticipating the Consequences*, Michigan State University

Mann, J.M. and Tararitola, D.J.M., 1996. *AIDS in the World II Global Dimensions, Social Roots and Responses*, New York:

Mark, C., 2005, *Impact of AIDS: The Health Care Burden*,

Ministry of Planning and International Cooperation, 2006. *Aid Absorptive Capacity*.

Montana, L., Neumann, M., Mishra, V. and Hong, R., 2005. *Spatial Modelling of HIV Prevalence in Cameroon, Kenya and Tanzania*.

Moses, S., Plummer, F.A., Ronald, A.R., Ndinya, Achola J.D., 1989. *Geographical Patterns of Male Circumcision Practices in Africa: Association with HIV Seroprevalence*.

MRC, 2008. Sexual risk behaviour among men with multiple, concurrent female sexual partners in an informal settlement on the outskirts of Cape Town.

Ntuli, A., 2004, *HIV/AIDS and Health Sector Responses in South Africa: Treatment Access and Equity Balancing the Act*.

Oomman, N., Bernstein, M. and Rosenweig, S., 2007. *Following the Funding for HIV/ AIDS: A Comparative Analysis of the Funding Practices of PEPFAR, the Global Fund and World Bank MAP in Mozambique, Uganda and Zambia*.

2005. "Scaling up vs Absorptive Capacity: Challenges and Opportunities for Reaching the MDGs in Africa", *ODI Briefing Paper*.

Paris Declaration, 2005. *Paris Declaration on Aid Effectiveness*.

Pianna, V., 2001, Inflation, Economics, Web Institute.

Poku, N.K., Whiteside, A., Sandkjaer, B., 2007. *AIDS and Governance*. Aldershot, Ashgate.

Rajalakshmi, T.K., 2005. *The Importance of Nutrition as Part of a Holistic Treatment*.

Riddell, R.C., 1999. End of Foreign Aid to Africa? Concerns about Donor Policies.

Rugalema, 1999. HIV/AIDS and the Commercial Agricultural Sector of Kenya, Rome:

Salomon, J.A., Hogan, R., Stover, J., Stanecki, K., Walker, N., Ghys, P. and Schwarlander, B., 2005. *Integrating HIV Prevention and Treatment: From Slogans to Impact*.

Sichone, S.E.N., 2004. *HIV/AIDS and Economic Growth in Zambia.*

Southern African Regional Poverty Network (SARPN), 2006. *The Impact of Trade Policy on HIV/AIDS.*

Strand, P., 2007. *Comparing AIDS Governance: A Research Agenda on Responses to the AIDS Epidemic.*

Tayler, L., 2005. *Absorptive Capacity of Health Systems in Fragile States,* London:

Theodore, K., 2001. HIV/AIDS in the Caribbean: Economic Issues – Impact and Investment Response, *CMH Working Paper,* No. WG1:1.

Thompson, L. 2003. *Humanitarian Emergencies: Why Does Kosovo Get More Aid than Congo?* Geneva.

Treatment Action Campaign/AIDS Law Project, 2005. *Statement on World Health Organisation Consultation on Nutrition and AIDS in Africa.*

Toussaint, E. and Comanne, D., 1995. Globalization and Debt. In: Notebooks for Study and Research, 24/25.

UNAIDS, 2001. *Keeping the Promise: Summary of the Declaration of Commitment on HIV/AIDS,* Geneva: UNAIDS.

UNAIDS, 2005. *The "Three Ones" in Action: Where We Are and Where We Go from Here,* Geneva: UNAIDS.

UNAIDS, 2006a. *AIDS Epidemic Update,* Geneva: UNAIDS.

UNAIDS, 2006b. *Report on the Global AIDS Epidemic,* Geneva: UNAIDS.

UNAIDS, 2007a. *Financial Resources Required to Achieve Universal Access to HIV Prevention Treatment, Care and Support,* Geneva: UNAIDS.

UNAIDS, 2007b. *AIDS Epidemic Update,* Geneva: UNAIDS.

UNDP, 2004. *Building Dynamic Democratic Governance and HIV Resilient Societies.*

UNDP, 2005. *Human Development Report.*

UNDP, 2006. *Human Development Report.*

UNDP/SADC/SAPES, 2000. *SADC Regional Human Development Report: Challenges and Opportunities for Regional Integration.* SAPES Books: Harare.

UNFPA. 2005. *State of World Population.*

UN Habitat, 2002. *Management of the HIV/AIDS Pandemic at the Local Level.*

USAID, 2007. *Crosswalk from NHA to NASA: Achieving Harmonization.*

Waal, A., 2003. *The Links between HIV/AIDS and Democratic Governance in Africa.*

Weiss H.A., Quigley, M.A. and Hayes, R.J., 2000. "Male Circumcision and Risk of HIV Infection in SSA: A Systematic Review and Meta Analysis", *AIDS,* 14.

World Bank, 2005. *Millenium Goals: From Consensus to Momentum: Global Monitoring Report,* 2005.

World Food Programme, 2003. *The First Line Defense – Why Food and Nutrition Matter in the Fight against HIV/AIDS.* World Health Organisation (2000), Violence against Women and HIV/AIDS: Setting the Research Agenda - Meeting Report, Geneva, Zambia)

ETHIOPIA

ALEMU, G., BEDRI, A., HASSEN, Y. AND TEFERA, N.

EXECUTIVE SUMMARY

This research aims to establish how HIV/AIDS is prioritised by the Ethiopian government and its development partners in terms of budget allocation and spending. The findings from the study are hoped not only to stimulate great interest from the policymakers regarding HIV/AIDS financing, but also to assist with improving its effectiveness and efficiency.

The specific objectives of the study were:

- To track all donors and public HIV/AIDS resource allocations, funding flows and expenditures for financial year 2004/05 and to identify expenditure outputs (i.e. services provided and beneficiary groups);

- To work with donors, government and NGO research partners to develop a common framework for tracking HIV/AIDS resources and expenditure, possibly by institutionalising regular resource-tracking activities; and
- To make recommendations to policymakers on the effectiveness and efficiency of budgeting and funding mechanisms for government response to HIV/AIDS.

A budget tracking and expenditure monitoring approach was used as an analytical framework in an effort to analyse allocations and spending of HIV/AIDS resources. An attempt was made to use the UNAIDS NASA framework. The study undertook:

- Primary data collection based on the questionnaire developed by Idasa to map the flow of resources, budgetary allocations and expenditures for FY 2004/2005 (i.e. the total HIV/AIDS resource allocation (THAE) and actual expenditures and the breakdown by source, provider and functions); and
- Secondary data collection from the printed database of government documents for various years from the Ministry of Finance and Economic Development (MoFED), the MoH, the Federal HIV/AIDS Prevention and Control Office (FHAPCO), the Regional HIV/AIDS Prevention and Control Office (RHAPCO) and the Central Statistics Authority (CSA).

Though some donor funds that are channelled through central government are disbursed by FHAPCO, some donors also disburse funds directly to RHAPCOs; non-governmental service providers at federal, regional and local levels; and local governments. Though some funding from the central government budget goes directly to service providers, the actual expenditure is rarely reported.

Funds allocated by the government accounted for 48.8% of total funds allocated for HIV/AIDS in 2004/05, while external funds channelled outside FHAPCO accounted for 42.5%, with the balance being accounted for by local NGO donors, community contributions and unidentified sources. The external donors have the highest spending rates of 48%. The regional capacity to spend HIV/AIDS funds is generally poor, varying between regions. The average countrywide expenditure performance for HIV/AIDS was only 59% of the amounts allocated in 2004/05. The low spending rate is largely ascribed to the lack of human capacity, slow procurement, and the poor financial and project management of the federal, regional and further decentralised administrative units.

FHAPCO is responsible for disbursing funds to RHAPCOs, which, in turn, disburse funds to other stakeholders. Most public departments and NGOs delay submitting statements of expenditure (SOEs) and audit reports, which further hinders the disbursement of funds. Wide regional variations also exist in the allocation of funds not apportioned through RHAPCO. About 49.2% of the total external funds were allocated to Amhara regional state, while none was allocated to Gambela regional state in the same period under review. The capacity to spend external funds is, however, relatively sound, with a national level average of 79.8%, and a regional variation ranging from 61.8% at federal level to 100% in Dire Dawa and Tigray regional states, which might be due to stricter donor reporting requirements.

Nationally, prevention programmes accounted for 65.6% of the total expenditure on HIV in 2004/05. However, wide variations existed at regional level, ranging from

8.8% allocated to prevention interventions in Dire Dawa to 84.2% in Amhara regional state. Expenditure on treatment and care accounted for 8.5% nationally.

SOCIOECONOMIC SITUATION, POVERTY TRENDS AND DEVELOPMENT POLICIES IN ETHIOPIA

Ethiopia has a population of nearly 80 million people, with 80 distinct ethnic groups. It has the lowest gross national income (GNI) in the world, with per capita income of just US$100. While its GNI per capita is about 20% of the Sub-Saharan Africa average, its agricultural productivity is only 40% of the average. Access to education and health facilities is low. The economy is plagued by structural problems characterised by poor performance in the manufacturing sector, which contributed only 6.2% to the GDP in 2002 (WB, 2004).

The Ethiopian economy depends heavily on agriculture for its supply of food, raw materials, export earnings and other resources. Agriculture is a source of livelihood for about 85% of the total population, accounting for nearly 50% of GDP and about 85% of merchandise exports. The agrarian structure is dominated by subsistence smallholder farmers and plagued by land degradation, soil erosion, fragmented and small sized land holdings, and primitive farming methods.

The agricultural sector is rainfall-based, making both the population and the economy extremely vulnerable. As a result, recurrent droughts entail recurrent famines with increasing regularity. The overall growth of the economy is, therefore, largely dictated by what happens in the agricultural sector.

The economy has no internal engine that can move it to sustainable growth and development, therefore poverty is widespread. Though slight improvements have occurred in the poverty profile, particularly in respect to nutritional indicators and access to water and sanitation, the absolute levels of such indicators remains unacceptably low. A recent national household survey revealed that 44% of the population was living below the poverty line in 1999/00, compared with 45.5% in 1995/96 (see Table 2.1 below).

Table 2.1: Poverty data from household surveys			
	1995/96 (%)	1999/2000 (%)	2004/05 (%)
Rural	47.5	45.4	39.3
Urban	33.2	36.9	35.1
Total	45.5	44.2	38.7
Source: MoFED, 2006			

The country's Human Development Index is generally poor, being worse in the rural areas (see Table 2.2).

Table 2.2: Health and nutrition development indicators – Ethiopia versus the rest of the world							
	Prevalence of under nourishment (% of population)		Life expectancy at birth (years)		Access to improved sanitation facilities (% of rural population)		Adult literacy rate (% of population > = 15)
	1990/92	1999/2001	1980	2002	1990	2002	2001
Ethiopia	n/a	42	42	42	6	7	40
SSA	31	32	48	46	45	46	62
Low-income countries	26	24	53	59	20	31	63
World	21	17	63	67	27	38	Na
Source: World Bank, 2004; data for access to water and literacy rate from UNDP, 2003							

According to the UN, about 70% of the total population live in areas where they are at risk from malaria.[31,32] Childhood wasting and/or stunting are common, as is shown in Table 2.3.

Table 2.3: Prevalence of wasting, stunting and underweight by gender and survey year									
Survey year	Wasting			Stunting			Underweight		
	Boys (%)	Girls (%)	Average (%)	Boys (%)	Girls (%)	Average (%)	Boys (%)	Girls (%)	Average (%)
1996	7.8	6.9	7.3	68.1	65.1	65.7	47.8	42.9	45.4
1998	10.7	8.4	9.6	55.9	53.5	54.7	46.5	43.2	44.9
2000	10.2	8.9	9.6	58.1	55.3	56.7	45.9	44.1	45
2004	8.6	7.9	8.3	48.3	45.5	46.9	37.6	36.7	37.1
Source: MoFED, 2005									

Most (93%) Ethiopian children were delivered at home, according to the 2004 Welfare Monitoring Survey (WMS) survey, with births largely attended only by traditional birth attendants with no formal training. Countrywide, only 11% of total child births had been attended by a delivery nurse, a trained traditional birth attendant or other health personnel (7% in rural areas and 53% in urban) (MoFED, 2005). Access to clean water is also very low nationally, with about 64% of Ethiopian households using unclean drinking water in 2004. While 92.4% of the urban population has access to safe water, only 25.2% of the rural population has access to such a supply (MoFED, 2005).

THE HIV EPIDEMIC

The most common mode of transmission of HIV in Ethiopia is believed to be heterosexual, accounting for 75% of infections (Birhan, 2004). While mother–to–child transmission accounts for 20%, the rest are accounted for by blood transfusions and unsafe injections (Birhan, 2004).

PREVALENCE

The average adult HIV prevalence in Ethiopia was estimated at 4.4% in 2003. Large variances occur in terms of gender (male and female) and geography (urban and rural areas). The details are presented in Figures 2.1 and 2.2. As shown in Figure 2.1, indications are that the urban rate is on the decline, while that for the rural areas is on the increase.

Figure 2.1: HIV prevalence in urban and rural Ethiopia, 1983–2008

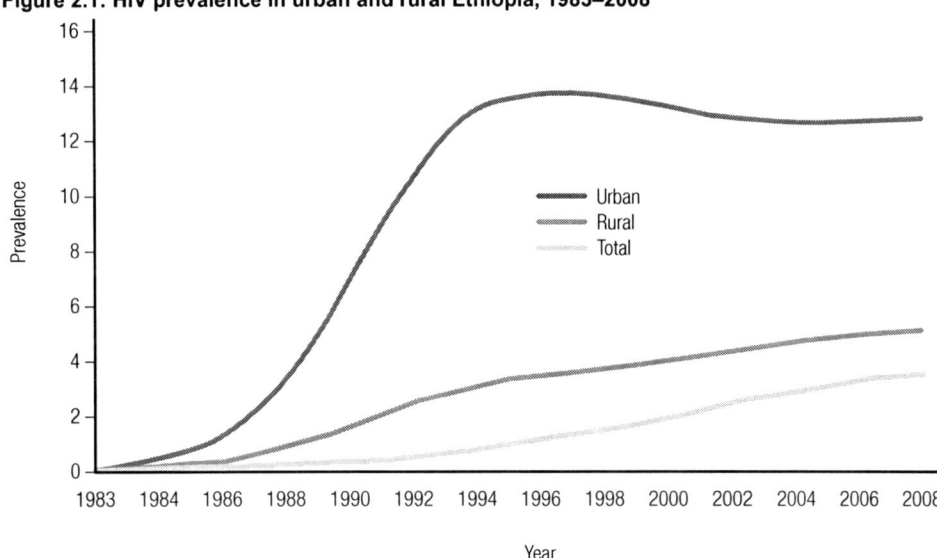

Source: MoH, 2004b

Figure 2.2: HIV prevalence in Ethiopia by gender, 1983–2008

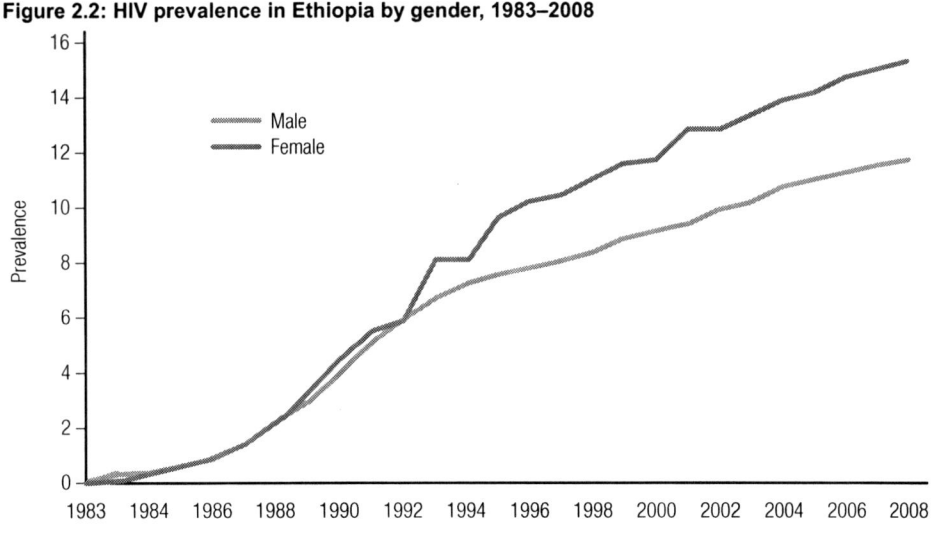

Source: MoH, 2004b

In 2003, 1.4 million Ethiopians were estimated to be HIV-positive, with the number expected to increase to 1.9 million by 2008. Nearly 100 000 people died of AIDS-related illnesses in 2004 (UNAIDS 2004 AIDS epidemic update). Since the late 1980s, HIV infection has been higher among females than males. About 100 000 children of up to 14 years of age were living with HIV in 2004 and AIDS-related deaths were estimated to be 25 000 for the same age group and year.

KNOWLEDGE, ATTITUDE AND PRACTICE

The first behavioural surveillance survey was conducted in Ethiopia in 2001/2002 (MoH, 2003), covering the following target groups: in-school youths, out-of-school youths (OSY) (15–24-year-olds), ground forces and the air force, transport workers, farmers, pastoralists, factory workers, and female sex workers.

The findings revealed that most people knew about HIV and its main modes of transmission. More than 66% of the youth knew at least one person living with HIV/AIDS, or someone who had died from AIDS. The survey also showed the high degree of HIV/AIDS-related stigma and discrimination.

RESPONSE TO HIV

SECTORAL RESPONSE

After the first AIDS case was identified in the country in 1984, Ethiopia established a National Task Force on HIV in the following year. The National AIDS Control Programme (NACP) was later set up at departmental level at the MoH in 1987. Two medium-term control and prevention plans were designed and implemented in 1989 and 1996 respectively. Information, education and communication (IEC) campaigns; condom promotion; surveillance; patient care; and the expansion of HIV screening laboratories in different health institutions were instituted. However, the impact was weak and the involvement of citizens minimal.

MULTISECTORAL RESPONSE

Government acknowledgement of the lack of sectoral coordination led to the establishment of the National HIV/AIDS Council (NAC) in April 2000. The Council, headed by the President of the Federal Democratic Republic of Ethiopia (FDRE), comprises members from the sector ministries, regional states, NGOs, religious bodies, civil society representatives and PLWHAs. The council oversees the implementation of federal and regional HIV/AIDS plans; examines and approves annual plans and budgets; and monitors the performance and impact of plans. The following are the major functions of the council:

- To promote HIV/AIDS policy development and updating;
- To develop a strategic framework and plans to enable an appropriate response to the onslaught of HIV/AIDS;
- To identify priority interventions and the actors involved;
- To coordinate HIV/AIDS responses;
- To build the partnership of stakeholders;
- To build the capacity for an effective response to HIV/AIDS;
- To establish national HIV/AIDS monitoring and evaluation;
- To promote the involvement of PLWHAs in activities; and
- To set research priorities.

The Board of Advisors appointed by the council meets monthly. The National Review Board (NRB), which was also established by the council, is composed of competent individuals representing the Ministry of Economic Development and Cooperation (MEDaC), the National AIDS Prevention and Control Secretariat, the MoH, MoFED, Women's Affairs Office, PLWHA Association, Catholic Relief and Development Agency (CRDA) (an NGO umbrella organisation), the Ethiopian Employers' Federation, the Ethiopian Social Rehabilitation and Development Fund, and the Ministry of Labour and Social Affairs. Similar structures were established at all tiers of government for the AIDS Council.

Woreda AIDS Councils, composed of members of the Woreda Administration who are responsible for social sector activities. At the lowest administrative tier, the Kebele AIDS Committees are composed of members of the Kebele Administration and residents. All line ministries and sector bureaus are represented on the National and Regional Advisory Boards (RABs).

The legal establishment of FHAPCO under the Prime Minister's Office office in June 2002 strengthened the coordinating efforts. Similar structures were set up in all regions, woredas and kebeles through the Ethiopian Multisectoral HIV/AIDS Programme (EMSAP). The multisectoral response has effectively mobilised resources and responses from various organisations, such as public bodies, multilateral and bilateral donors, national and international NGOs, CBOs, FBOs, the private sector, and PLWHA associations.

THE NATIONAL RESPONSE TO HIV

The National HIV/AIDS Policy (MoH, 1998c) focuses on prevention and care.
Specific objectives of the National HIV/AIDS Policy are:

- To establish effective HIV/AIDS prevention and control strategies to curb the spread of the epidemic;
- To promote a broad, multisectoral response to HIV/AIDS, including more effective coordination and resource mobilisation by the government, NGOs, the private sector and communities;
- To encourage government, NGOs, the private sector and communities to take

measures to alleviate the social and economic impact of HIV/AIDS;

- To support home- and community-based care and psychological support for PLWHAs, orphans and surviving dependents;
- To safeguard the human rights of PLWHAs and to avoid discrimination against them;
- To empower women, youth and other vulnerable groups to take action to protect themselves against HIV/AIDS; and
- To promote and encourage surveillance and research activities targeted at the preventative, curative and rehabilitative activities relating to HIV/AIDS.

Based on the national policy, the government launched a Strategic Framework (2001–2005) for the national response. The objective of the policy and strategic framework is to guide the implementation of successful HIV/AIDS programmes. In response, the government reviewed the five-year strategic plan and launched a new National Strategic Plan (NSP) (2004–2008) for intensifying the multisectoral HIV/AIDS response along with a free antiretroviral treatment programme. The focal areas of the new HIV/AIDS strategic plan are capacity-building; legal and human right issues; social mobilisation and community empowerment; the integration of HIV/AIDS activities with health programmes; the supply of safe blood; the mainstreaming of HIV/AIDS actions; coordination, networking and working with special target groups (commercial sex workers (CSWs), truckers, migrant labourers, those in uniform, teachers, students, and OSY). The objective of this programme is to reduce vulnerability to HIV infection among the identified targeted groups by encouraging the taking of all necessary preventive measures. The strategy also aims to improve the quality of life of PLWHAs and orphans and vulnerable children.

Figure 2.3 shows the intended budget for the NSP (2004–2008), broken down into targets for each programme/service area, with nearly two-thirds of the budget going to the strengthening of health facilities. Both health and nonhealth capacity-building claims about 31% of the budget.

Figure 2.3: Intended target budget for the strategic plan, 2004–08

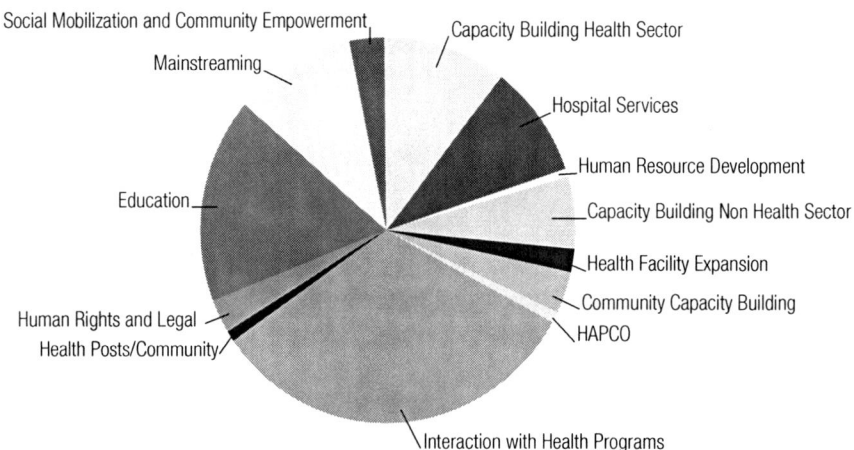

Source: MoH, 2004c

THE BUDGET PROCESS IN ETHIOPIA

STAGES OF THE BUDGET PROCESS/CYCLE

MoFED must first prepare a three-year rolling Macro Economic Fiscal Framework (MEFF),[33] providing a three-year forecast of economic growth, GDP, and government revenue and expenditure. The MEFF is reviewed and approved by the executive body, the Council of Ministers.

Ethiopia's budget process/cycle involves the following four stages at federal, regional, and woreda government levels of jurisdiction:
- Stage 1: budget preparation, consisting of the drafting/design process;
- Stage 2: budget approval and appropriation,[34] consisting of the legislative process;
- Stage 3: budget execution, consisting of the implementation process; and
- Stage 4: budget control, consisting of performance monitoring, entailing the audit and evaluation process.

STAGE 1: BUDGET PREPARATION

The first stage – budget preparation – comprises four phases:
1. During phase one, all public bodies[35] are required to perform all budget preparation activities, review the programme for the current year,[36] and prepare the unit costs and work plan for the coming year.
2. During phase two, MoFED/the Bureau of Finance and Economic Development (BoFED) issues a budget call letter to all public bodies. The letter reflects recurrent and capital budget ceilings, the priority or focal areas to be considered in preparing the budget, and the submission date for the budget request by public bodies to the respective finance and economic development institutions in all jurisdictions.
3. Stage three entails the conducting of a budget hearing. All public bodies, through their representatives, are required to defend their budgets before MoFED/BoFED.
4. During stage four, based on the budget hearing, government policies and priorities, the total expenditure ceiling, and the allocated ceilings for each public body, the requested budget is reviewed, adjusted and consolidated.

STAGE 2: BUDGET APPROVAL AND APPROPRIATION

Once the recommended budget is reviewed and adjusted by the respective executive body at all levels, it is presented to the respective legislative bodies, consisting of the Federal House of People's Representatives, the Regional House of People's Representatives and the Woreda House of People's Representatives, which review, amend and approve the budget.[37] Annual appropriation of the approved budget then follows.

STAGE 3: BUDGET EXECUTION

Budget execution involves the implementation of the budget by different public bodies carrying out their activities for the year. This stage involves the disbursement of the approved budget to the relevant agencies, the implementation of planned activities, and the recording of expenditure by the treasury.

STAGE 4: BUDGET CONTROL

Stage 4, budget control, involves monitoring activities in terms of the annual public bodies' reports and audit reports submitted to the House of People's Representatives at all levels. The Office of the General Auditor is in charge of auditing public bodies, for which it presents its findings to the House of People's Representatives.

STRENGTHS AND WEAKNESSES OF THE BUDGET PROCESS

PARTICIPATION

Participation is the level of involvement of all stakeholders/actors in the budget process, either directly or through legitimate intermediaries. The process of budget preparation, approval, implementation and control requires the participation of various stakeholders. Through the participation of people, their perspectives can be brought to the attention of the policymakers. Citizens can also hold their government accountable for identifying weaknesses in a budget, for building consensus,[38] and for mobilising the community effectively to meet a budget target (Shapiro, 2001).

In Ethiopia, participation in the budget process by citizens and civil society is limited. Citizens and civil society have no access to the monitoring of budget performance, in terms of which accounts for expenditures and audit reports are presented to the House of People's Representatives at federal, regional and woreda government level. The budget process is highly centralised at the different tiers of government.

TRANSPARENCY

Transparency involves the provision of user-friendly, comprehensive, accurate, timely and frequent information on a country's budget process. Budget decisions are made on the basis of clearly spelt out rules, procedures and forms. Such information should be made available and accessible to the general public, open to public scrutiny, clearly written and readily understandable by the public. Transparency on budget policies, expenditures and outcomes allows citizens and civil society to hold the government accountable, motivates the general public to participate in financial affairs, and helps to mobilise the community effectively to meet budget targets.[39] Though federal and regional budgetary laws and allocations appear in both the federal and regional *Negarit Gazetta*, the official law gazette of the government, neither of the gazettes is accessible to all citizens.

ACCOUNTABILITY

Accountability refers to the way in which decision-makers and implementers are held accountable for the formulation, approval, implementation and performance review of the budget by those whose interests it affects.

Accountability for budget approval involves:
- How closely the budget conforms with laws and the Constitution;
- The quality of budget documents;
- The criteria/process for allocating resources among regions: and
- Whether public input in budget preparation is respected.

Such accountability includes:
- Objects of expenditure (what the state spends the money on);
- State performance and results (the achievement of results or the meeting of objectives on which public funds are spent);
- The appropriateness and timeliness of audit reports; and
- The transparency of procurement (Shapiro, 2001).

Though there are public hearings at the House of People's Representatives at all tiers of government on budget performance, the participation of citizens and civil society is limited. In addition, budget reports usually focus on budget inputs and outputs, with very little on budget outcomes.

FINANCIAL AND REPORTING MECHANISMS IN ETHIOPIA

INTRODUCTION

Reports of financial performance are submitted both quarterly and annually to the agency that advanced the funds, which, in turn, reports to upper levels of government and donors until the final source of funds is reached. Internal auditing is expected to occur as spending is incurred and is followed by the external government's Auditor-General's audit of accounts, though delays of three years, on average, are likely with the latter.

GOVERNMENT FINANCING MECHANISMS

Federal, regional and, in some regions, zonal woreda and Kebele budget centres in Ethiopia. The federal budget centres consist mainly of ministries, commissions, the armed forces, the police, tertiary-level education establishments, referral hospitals and other institutions, under the control of the federal government. The next level of budgeting units comprises regions that are run by regional state councils, with some regions having zones with zonal councils. Below the regions are the woredas, which are the main service centres in the decentralised administrative structure.

The budget proposals from the executive bodies are compiled at the woreda level and presented to the woreda council, which amends them according to changing priorities. The regional or zonal council receives a copy of the proposed budget. The regional council, for its part, compiles plans based on proposals from bureaus and establishes the level of block grant to be allocated to each woreda or zone. Only after the federal government announces its budget do regions finalise their plans. In addition to the federal block grants, regional states and woredas also receive some budgetary resources from international NGOs, which, however, usually are neither recorded nor systematically kept.

The monthly mandatory reporting on government funding is largely adhered to, with the internal auditing of all financial transactions being done at least once a year. Auditing by the Auditor-General of federal funds is largely overdue, with external auditing being called for only when foreign funds are involved.

NAC receives donor funds directly, accounting for the funds to the sources. It distributes funds according to the decisions made by its board. Each receiving budget unit accounts for funds both to NAC and to the administrative tier to which it is answerable. The rules and regulations applicable to government budgetary resources also apply to funds received from NAC.

HIV/AIDS funds flow from the regional offices to home-based care centres at local levels, as shown in Figure 2.4.

Figure 2.4: HIV fund flow at local levels in Ethiopia

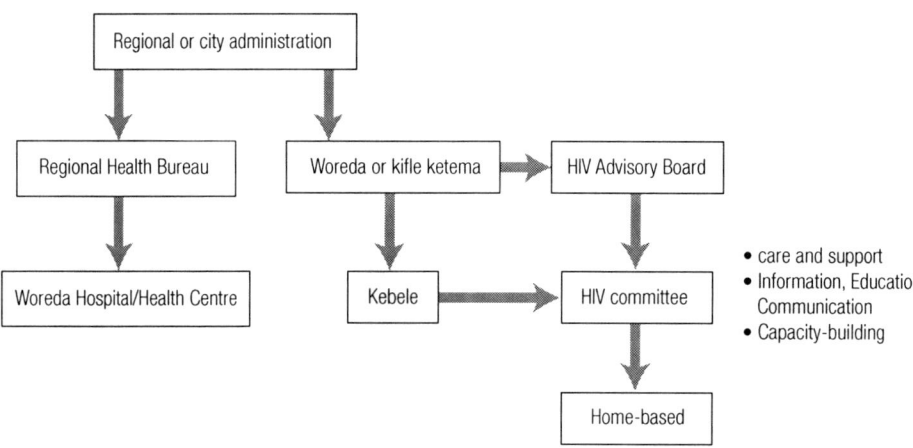

Donor funds disbursed by MoFED are largely treated as part of the government revenue, being governed by government financial regulations and reported "on budget" in the budget document. Accounting for the funds is dictated by the respective donors, though a major challenge exists with respect to the reporting period. While the Ethiopian Financial Year (FY) runs from June to May each year, most donor reporting periods run from January to December.

Intergovernmental Transfers

Constitutional provisions could enable a bidirectional flow from a lower tier of government to an upper tier and vice versa. However, the current flows tend to be unidirectional – from the regional down to the woreda (see Figure 2.4). Some regions have woredas run with surplus revenue that is sent to the regional finance bureau.

Donor Funds Flow

Donor funds are divided into grants and loans in the government budget document.[40] The federal subsidy includes central government domestic resources, grants and loans, as the classification also applies to federal ministries and agencies. Donor funds are associated with complicated procedures and guidelines that are time-consuming and involve extensive paperwork. The lack of expertise of implementing agencies has so far led to a slow and low utilisation rate of the disbursed funds. Donor funds from bilateral sources are largely disbursed through federal and regional administrations to civil society organisations (CSOs).

Public Spending on Health in Ethiopia

Public Allocations for, and Expenditure on, Health

Public spending on health in Ethiopia is very low, even by SSA standards. The share of expenditure on health from total public expenditure (TPE) has been less than 5% since 1997/8 (see Table 2.4).

Table 2.4: Time series data of countrywide public expenditure on health, 1997/98–2004/05								
Items	1997/98	1998/99	1999/00	2000/01	2001/02	2002/03*	2003/04*	2004/05*
Share from total public expenditure (%)								
Health	5.4	4.5	3.3	3.9	4.5	3.7	4.3	4.9
Share (excluding debt service)	5.7	4.8	3.8	4.4	4.9	4.0	4.7	5.2
Source: MoFED, various budget documents, 1997–2005 * audited data								

The relative share of health expenditure from total public capital expenditure suffered a disproportionate decline in 2000/01, which is largely due to the war waged with Eritrea. While Ethiopia is one of the countries with the highest proportion of public spending to Gross Domestic Product (GDP) in SSA, it has the lowest ratio of public health spending to both total public spending and the GDP. Ethiopia's public expenditure averaged about 25% of its GDP over the eight years preceding the current study, while its health spending tended to be less than 5% of TPE.

Nominal total public spending on health increased from Birr 618 million in 1997/98 to Birr 1 201.4 million in 2004/05 (a 94.4% increase), while overall public expenditure increased by 116% over the same period. Thus, nominal health expenditure has been growing more slowly than TPE. In real terms, health expenditure increased from Birr 657.7 million in 1997/98 to Birr 1 014.4 million in 2004/05, while overall public expenditure increased by 71.3%.[41]

The significant nominal and real increases, however, as the World Bank (2004:32) indicated, "have largely been eroded by population growth". Due to the high population growth, nominal per capita public spending on health has marginally increased from Birr 10.3 in 1997/98 to Birr 16.5 in 2004/05. In US$ terms, nominal per capita public health spending has increased from US$1.54 to $1.90 over the same period. The real increase in US$ terms, however, has declined from US$1.64 to $1.60.

UTILISATION OF HEALTH BUDGET – FISCAL ABSORPTIVE CAPACITY

The utilisation or spending rate can be calculated by expressing actual expenditure as a ratio of the allocated budget, with the spending rate being low to start with and declining further over the years.

Figure 2.5: Actual health expenditure as a ratio of the Ethiopian budget (%), 1997/98–2002/03

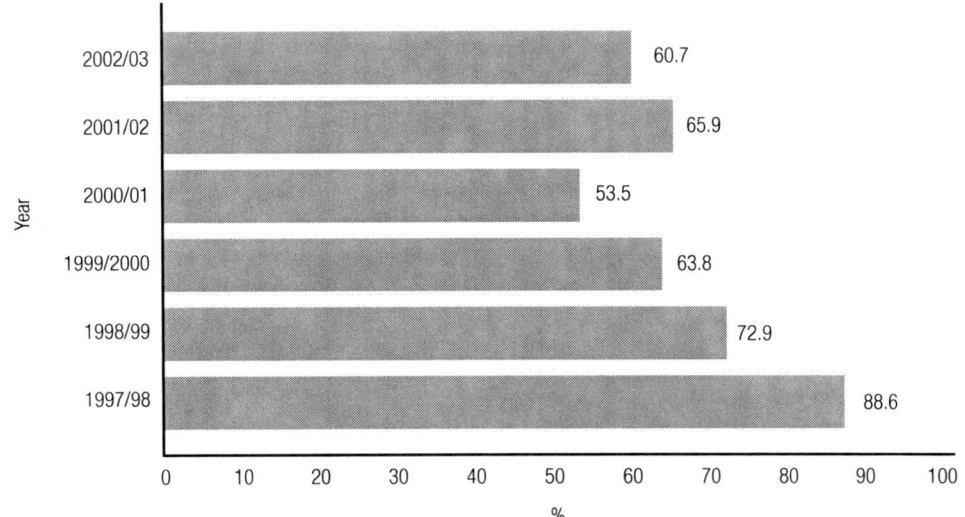

Source: Author's computation from MoFED, various budget books.

Actual expenditure of the total budget has been decreasing over the years (since 1997/98) although there was a slight improvement in 2001/02. The low utilisation rates are a reflection of low absorptive capacity within the government departments thus making it difficult to achieve socio-economic objectives. Utilisation rates for the budget have been marred by procurement bottlenecks, lack of information, contracting lags, insufficient contracting capacity and lack of adequate human capacity.

GOVERNMENT BUDGET ALLOCATIONS AND EXPENDITURE FOR HIV/AIDS IN ETHIOPIA

The government budget refers to funds from the federal government treasury, the regional government and the woreda government treasury, as well as donor funds that are channeled through government basket funding. As such, government controls the allocation and utilisation of such funds. The FHAPCO is the financial agent for these donor funds, which are largely sourced from the Global Fund and Ethiopian Multi-Sectoral HIV/AIDS Programme (EMSAP) through the WB. The government allocated Birr 86.7732 million (US$10.02 million) for HIV/AIDS initiatives in 2004/05, while it contributed 54% to the HIV/AIDS response in 2004/05.

71

Figure 2.6: Government budget allocations for HIV/AIDS, 2004/05

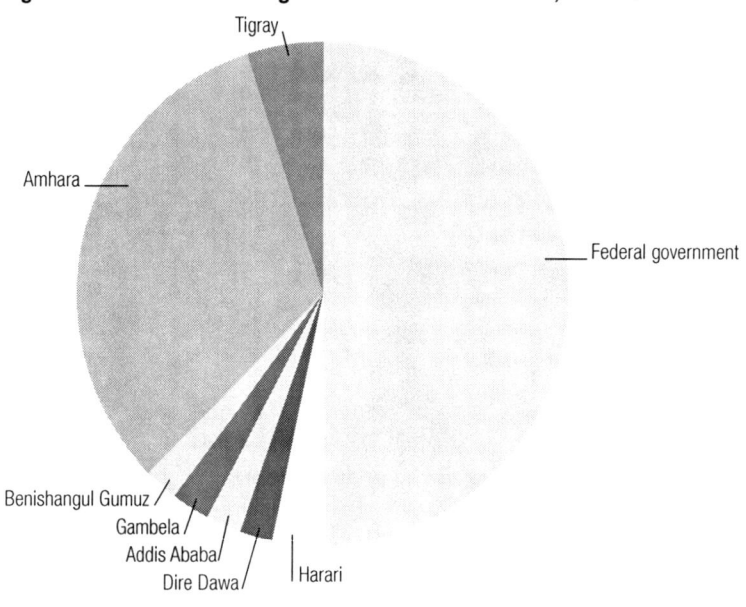

Source: Computation by authors.

EXTERNAL HIV/AIDS FINANCING SOURCES IN ETHIOPIA

INTERNATIONAL BUDGET ALLOCATIONS

International budget allocations refer to the flow of funds from external sources that are not channelled through FHAPCO. The total external funds allocated in 2004/05 amounted to Birr 73.61 million (about US$8.5 million), accounting for about 46% of the total resources mobilised for HIV/AIDS in Ethiopia in the same financial year.

Table 2.5: Funds received (Birr '000) from various donors in support of HIV/AIDS efforts, 2004/05			
	Amount received	Share of the total (%)	Amount received in real values (1999/2000 prices)
Federal government	25 092	36.9	21 186.6
Regional states			
Harari	196	0.3	165.5
Dire Dawa	1 082	1.6	913.6
Tigray	5 270	7.7	4 449.7
Gambela	0	0.0	0.0
Benishangul Gumuz	756	1.1	638.3
Amhara	33 521	49.2	28 303.6
Addis Ababa	2 153	3.2	1 817.9
Total	68 070	100.0	56 881.2[42]

SPENDING RATES OF HIV/AIDS FUNDS

Of the total amount allocated for HIV/AIDS response, only Birr 113.26 million (US$13.08 million) was utilised in 2004/05, with the national average spending rate for HIV/AIDS funds standing at 74.6%.

The national average spending rate of donor funds was 79.8%, compared with 74.6% for the government budget, which may be explained by the strict reporting requirements of the donors. The regional spending rate for donor funds varied from 61.8% at federal level to 100% for Tigray regional state and Dire Dawa administration council. The variation in the spending rate might be explained by the relative differences in institutional capacity.

Figure 2.7: Spending rate from donor allocations (Birr '000), 2004/05

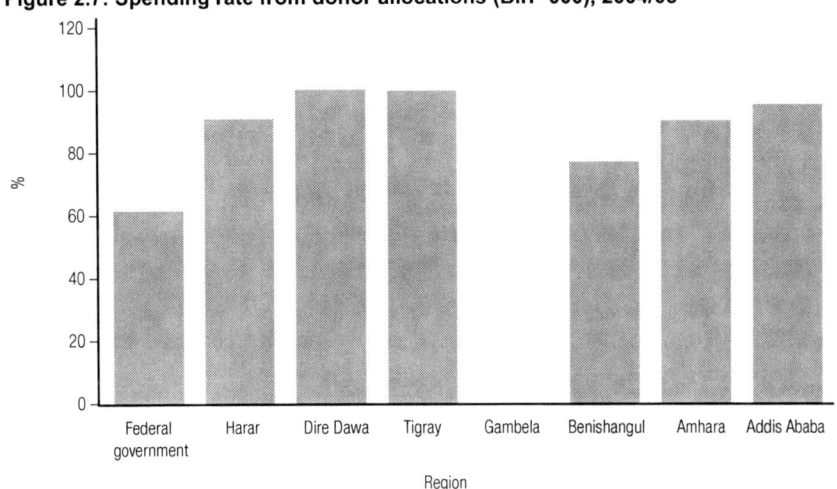

Table 2.6 depicts various regional spending rates from government allocations in 2004/5. Spending rates from the government allocations varied greatly across regions. For instance Tigray and Addis Ababa have high spending rates of 100% and 98% respectively compared to Amhara and Gambela with low spending rates of 20% and 55% respectively. Low spending rates hamper efforts to fight HIV/AIDS.

Table 2.6: Spending rate from the government allocations, 2004/05			
	Amount received (Birr '000)	Amount spent (Birr '000)	Spending rate (%)
Federal government	38 875	29 924	77
Regional states			
Harari	2 752	1 753	64
Dire Dawa	1 651	1 523	92
Tigray	1 689	1 689	100
Gambela	1 849	1 022	55
Benishangul Gumuz	1 397	1 271	91
Amhara	26 064	5 248	20
Addis Ababa	3 964	3 884	98
Source: Calculations by authors			

According to the WB (2003:35), performance of the Ethiopian multisectoral HIV/AIDS project (EMSAP) managed by FHAPCO is unsatisfactory due to lack of absorptive capacity in procurement, financial management and project management at the regional and woreda administrative units. The following were identified by the WB (2003; 2005) as explanations for the slow disbursements:

- Decentralisation of the management of the project at woreda level, at which level capacity is extremely limited;
- Delays in submitting Statements of Expenditure;
- The limited capacity of FHAPCO and RHAPCOs;
- Capacity problems in procurement, financial management and project management at the regional and woreda administrative units; and
- The absence of pre-existing administrative structures and insufficiently qualified staff at all tiers of government.

COMPOSITION OF HIV/AIDS EXPENDITURE IN ETHIOPIA

An aggregate amount of Birr 113 million (US$13.05 million), including public and external sources, was spent on HIV/AIDS by the different regions on various programmes in 2004/05. Approximately two-thirds of HIV/AIDS resources was spent on prevention, in conformity with Ethiopia's HIV/AIDS policy. Though programme development is not a major priority in the policy, many resources were earmarked for that activity.

Table 2.7: Aggregate expenditure on HIV/AIDS (public and external) by function (Birr million), 2004/05										
Region	Expenditure by function									Total
	Prevention programmes	Treatment and care	Orphans and vulnerable children	AIDS programme development	Human resources	Social mitigation	Reduced vulnerability	HIV-related research	Other	
Harari	0.24	0.53	0.25	0.85	0.00	0.13	0.05	0.01	0.00	2.06
Dire Dawa	0.32	0.90	0.51	0.44	1.21	0.01	0.06	0.00	0.14	3.59
Tigray	3.63	0.08	1.46	3.40	0.01	0.01	0.08	0.00	0.00	8.67
Gambella	0.46	0.00	0.35	0.21	0.00	0.00	0.00	0.00	0.00	1.02
Benishangul Gumuz	0.20	0.03	0.26	0.33	0.07	0.00	0.00	0.00	0.97	1.86
Amhara	29.87	1.69	0.73	2.92	0.00	0.09	0.00	0.00	0.15	35.45
Addis Ababa	2.71	1.22	1.16	0.89	0.00	0.02	0.12	0.00	0.00	6.12
Federal	35.94	5.40	2.16	9.23	1.14	0.27	0.19	0.18	0.00	54.51
%	64.77	8.69	6.07	16.13	2.15	0.47	0.43	0.17	1.12	100.00

A regional analysis of the functional spending rates shows that Amhara and Tigray spent more than 75% of their budget on prevention, while the emerging regions (Gambella and Benishangul Gumuz) spent only 25%. The federal government spent two-thirds of its funds on prevention during the period under review. The analysis in the above tables clearly shows the mismatch between the regional budget allocations and the HIV/AIDS strategic plan. Though different expenditure categories provided by National AIDS Spending Assessments (NASA) and National Strategic Plans (NSP) make comparison difficult, commitments need to be translated into action in accordance with the HIV/AIDS policy.

CONCLUSION

Despite concerted efforts by the various stakeholders (the government, donors and the private sector), several challenges still require attention in terms of HIV/AIDS financing and spending in Ethiopia. Channels and mechanisms for the efficient flow of funds need to be tailormade to suit the principles of the Paris Declaration. Resource allocation among regions must take place based on the need to achieve equity. HIV/AIDS policy priorities must be aligned with resource allocation in order to achieve consistency. The government must put M&E in place to aid the assessment of the impact of existing HIV/AIDS programmes. The absence of effective monitoring systems, especially within government departments, makes it difficult to track progress and to assess whether the target population for any HIV/AIDS intervention is securing maximum benefit from the funds.

REFERENCES

Bollinger, L., Stover, J. and Eleni, S., 1999. The Economic Impact of AIDS in Ethiopia, September 1999, The Futures Group International, in collaboration with: the Research Triangle Institute (RTI) and the Centre for Development and Population Activities (CEDPA).

Central Statistics Authority (CSA), 1998. *The 1994 Population and Housing Census of Ethiopia: Results at Country Level*, Vol. 1, Statistical Report.

FDRE, 1995. *Proclamation* No. 1/1995.

Garbus, L., 2003 "HIV/AIDS in Ethiopia", *Country AIDS Policy Analysis Project*, San Francisco: AIDS Policy Research Center, University of California.

Getnet, A., 2002. *Aid-driven Import Substitution and the Agriculture–industry Nexus: Conceptualising the Aid-growth Relationship in Ethiopia*, Maastricht: Shaker Publishing.

Getnet, A., 2006. *Problem of Low/Slow Disbursement in the World Bank Funded Projects in Ethiopia*, Paper commissioned by AERC.

Kello, A.B., 1998. "Impact of AIDS on the Economy and Health Care Services in Ethiopia", *Ethiopian Journal of Health Development*, 12 (3).

Ministry of Finance and Economic Development (MoFED), 2006. *Ethiopia: Building on Progress: A Plan for Accelerated and Sustained Development to End Poverty (PASDEP) (2005/06–2009/10)*, Volume I: Main Text, Addis Ababa.

Ministry of Finance and Economic Development (MoFED), 1997–2005. Various budget documents.

Ministry of Health (MoH), 1995a. *Health Strategy*, Addis Ababa: MoH.

Ministry of Health (MoH), 1995b. *Health Policy*, Addis Ababa: MoH.

Ministry of Health (MoH), 1998a. *Health and Health-related Indicators*, Addis Ababa: MoH.

Ministry of Health (MoH), 1998b. *Program Action Plan for the Health Sector Development Program*, Addis Ababa: MoH.

Ministry of Health (MoH), 1998c. *HIV/AIDS Policy*, Addis Ababa: MoH.

Ministry of Health (MoH), 2000. *AIDS in Ethiopia: Background Projectors, Impacts, Intervention and Policy*, 3rd edn., Addis Ababa: MoH.

Ministry of Health (MoH), 2001. *National AIDS Council: Strategic Framework for the National Response to HIV/AIDS in Ethiopia*, Addis Ababa: MoH.

Ministry of Health (MoH), 2003. *HIV/AIDS Behavioural Surveillance Survey (BSS)*, 2003, Round One, Addis Ababa: MoH.

Ministry of Health (MoH), 2004a. *Health and Health-related Indicators*, Addis Ababa: MoH.

Ministry of Health (MoH), 2004b. *AIDS in Ethiopia*. 5th edn. Addis Ababa: MoH.

Ministry of Health (MoH), 2004c. *Ethiopian Strategic Plan for Intensifying Multisectoral HIV/AIDS Response, 2004–2008*, Addis Ababa: MoH.

Ministry of Health (MoH), 2004d. *Technical Document for the Fifth Report AIDS in Ethiopia*, Addis Ababa: Disease Control and Prevention Department, MoH.

Rahel, T. G., [No Date]. National Response to HIV/AID in Ethiopia. (unpublished).

Shapiro, I., 2001. *A Guide to Budget Work for NGOs*, Washington, DC: International Budget Project.

Streak, J., 2003. *Monitoring Government Budgets to Advance Child Rights: A Guide for NGOs*, Cape Town: Idasa.

UNDP, 2003. *Human Development Report*, Oxford University Press.

World Bank, 1998. *Participatory Poverty Assessment for Ethiopia*, World Bank Discussion Paper, Africa Region.

World Bank (WB), 2001. *Ethiopia: Focusing Public Expenditures on Poverty Reduction*, Vol. II, Report No. 23351-ET.

World Bank (WB), 2003. *Country Assistance Strategy*, Report No. 25591-ET.

World Bank (WB), 2004. *World Development Indicator*.

World Bank (WB), 2005a. *Implementation Completion Report (IDA-30770) on a Loan/Credit/Grant to the FDRE for an Education Sector Development Project*, Report No. 30706.

World Bank (WB), 2005b. *Implementation Completion Report (TF-25158 IDA-30320) on a Credit to the FDRE for a Road Sector Development Program Support Project*, Report No. 34485.

World Bank (WB), 2005c Ethiopia: Country Portfolio Performance Review for Fiscal Year 2004.

Kenya

Odundo, P., Njeru, E., Kioko, U. and Korir, J.

Executive Summary

To launch an effective and targeted campaign against HIV/AIDS, policy-makers, planners and stakeholders require a clear understanding of the total resources available for HIV/AIDS response in the country. Clear knowledge of the total HIV/AIDS resources and expenditure allows for greater transparency and accountability in resource utilisation for domestic effective oversight in assessing whether expenditure is appropriately targeted at both social groups and regions. The current period of political commitment allows for the formulation of innovative policies based on reliable data, particularly with regard to current HIV/ AIDS financing and expenditure. The overall aim of the study is to contribute to the improvement of national policy in order to address the HIV/AIDS epidemic. Such improvement is made possible through the collecting of information on HIV/AIDS allocations, expenditure and programming, as well as through making that information available to policy-makers, government officials and donor agencies; and improving the capacity of civil society NGOs and government officials to track, monitor and improve resource allocation and expenditure on HIV/AIDS.

To achieve the above broad aim, the study tracks the flow of funds for HIV/AIDS interventions in the country and the complex financial flows from source through the providers to the beneficiaries. In addition, public and donor health-care expenditure is quantified, based on routinely published data sources.

The findings of the current study indicate that health-care expenditure and total government expenditure have increased in nominal value in terms of both the allocations and actual budget out-turns. The proportion of actual Ministry of Health (MoH) recurrent expenditure relative to total government expenditure increased from 2001/02 to 2003/2004, but declined in FY 2004/2005. While the utilisation of recurrent allocations exceeds 90% in the MOH, development allocation use was low (5% in 2003/04 and 13.3% in 2004/05).

The proportion of public-health allocations in the government budget, as a share of total government expenditure with debt service (both domestic and foreign) in 2004/05, accounted for 4.5%. The actual public-health sector allocation, excluding debt servicing, ranged from 7% in FY 2001/02 to 5.8% in FY 2004/05. The total health expenditure (THE), including debt servicing, decreased from 7% in 2001/02 to 5.7% in 2003/04. The total health allocation, as a share of GDP, was 1.5% in FY 2001/02, but decreased slightly to 1.4% in FY 2004/05, perhaps due to poor macro-economic conditions and a decline in donor funding.

In real terms (after adjusting for inflation) total public-health expenditure (TPHE) in 2001/02 increased marginally from KES 14,032 million in 2001/02 to KES 14,930 million in 2002/03, but declined in the following FY (expressed in 2001/02 terms), representing an increase of 1% in 2004/05. In nominal per capita terms, MoH expenditure increased steadily from KES 450 in 2001/02 to KES 533 in 2004/05. In real terms, however, per capita expenditure declined by 3% between 2001/02 and 2004/05.

The analysis further shows that HIV/AIDS expenditure in the national budget increased significantly from US$37.46 million in 2002/03 to US$54.95 million in FY 2003/04, representing an increase of 46.6%, partly due to increased financial support from the development partners concerned. In the 2002/03 national budget, the MoH received the bulk of the budget allocations (69.3%), followed by the Office of the President (OP) (29.4%), the Ministry of Education (MoE) (1.1%) and Home Affairs (0.2%). The allocations to the MoH increased by 2.5% between 2002/3 and 2003/4. However, allocations to the MoE decreased by 0.7%, while those to Home Affairs decreased by 0.1%.

In 2004/5, donors spent approximately KES 12.33 billion (US$151.66 million) on HIV/AIDS interventions. The US government contributed the largest share of HIV/AIDS funds, accounting for about 59.48% (US$90.2 million) of the total donor funding, with other significant contributions coming from the World Bank (11.14%), the Global Fund (9.47%), Japan International Cooperation Agency (JICA) (8.78%) and Department for International Development (DFID) (5.90%). Overall, a total of US$181 670 342 was spent on HIV/AIDS-related interventions in 2004/05. Analysis by provider and by function reveals that prevention programmes received most of the total HIV/AIDS funding (37%), followed by the treatment and care component (36.8%). Support services and the mitigation of socioeconomic impact accounted for 5.1% and 21.1% respectively.

In 2004, donors spent US$40.37 million (KES 3.1 billion) on treatment and care, US$71.5 million (KES 5.5 billion) on prevention, US$10.7 million (KES 0.8 billion) on mitigation of social and economic impact, and US$36.8 million (KES 2.8 billion) on support services. Prevention of mother-to-child transmission (PMTCT) accounted for the largest proportion of funding at 13.9% (US$9.17 million), followed by voluntary testing and counselling (12.4%).

Given the findings of this exercise, inadequate absorptive capacity, and lack of systems and accountability frustrate programme implementation. The volume of resources flowing to the population targeted in each priority area remains minimal if the challenges are not addressed by all partners and systems instituted to document and disseminate the lessons learnt by, and the experiences of, all partners in the utilisation of whatever resources are available in Kenya.

SOCIOECONOMIC ENVIRONMENT

According to the 1999 census, the total population of Kenya was estimated at 28.7 million. Of the total population, 80% live in rural areas. The urban population has increased from 3.8 million in 1989 to 9.9 million in 1999, and was projected to grow to 16 million in 2005 (MoPND, 2003). Results of the 2003 Kenya Demographic Survey indicate that infant mortality increased from 74/1 000 live births in 1998 to 78/1 000 live births in 2004, while the under-five mortality rose slightly from 112/1 000 births to 114/1 000 births in the same period. Trends in the nutritional status of children under three years show that the percentage of stunted children increased to 31% in 2003 from the 29% reported in 1993.

EDUCATION TRENDS

The provision of quality education is a major priority for the Government of Kenya (GoK), as stated in its Economic Recovery Strategy Paper of 2003. This priority is in line with the Millennium Development Goals (MDGs) that call for Universal Primary Education (UPE), and the elimination of gender disparity in primary and secondary education preferably by 2005, and in all levels of education by no later than 2015. Since 2003, the number of students enrolled at various levels of education has substantially increased. However, the primary school enrolment rates vary widely across regions and gender, being particularly low among girls in the arid and semi-arid regions. Enrolment in secondary education has also substantially improved, with enrolment increasing from 30 000 students in 1963 to over 862 907 students in 2003.

Despite the increased budget allocations to primary education by the government, enrolment at various levels is characterised by regional and gender disparities and declining GERs (Central Bureau of Statistics, 2006). Nevertheless, various achievements have been recorded, especially in increasing primary school enrolment, decreasing primary school repetition, improving quality of information and increasing availability of learning materials. However, the transition rates are still low, coupled with gender and regional disparities. The completion rate for girls is very low, as they tend to drop out of school to care for their parents and relatives infected by HIV. In order to achieve the education-related MDGs, the government needs to address overstretched facilities, overcrowding, the high pupil-teacher ratio (PTR), and regional and gender disparities.

ECONOMIC SITUATION

Between 1997 and 2001, the economy grew by an annual average rate of only 1.5%, below the population growth estimated at 2.5% per annum, thus leading to a decline in per capita incomes. Real GDP growth was 2.8% in 2003, increasing to 4.3%, 5.0% and 6.7% in 2004, 2005 and 2006 respectively. The main contributors to the impressive growth were manufacturing, government services, agriculture and tourism. However, economic growth is far below the recommended growth rate of about 7% required to support the implementation of MDG-related activities until 2015 (MoPND, 2003).

Bad governance, the inefficient use of public resources, corruption and structural adjustment programmes have significantly worsened the poor economic performance, as can be seen in Table 3.1.

Table 3.1: Selected key economic indicators for Kenya, 2001–05					
Indicator	2001	2002	2003	2004	2005
GDP growth rates	4.5	0.6	3	4.9	5.8
GDP at market prices (Ksh billion)	1 020	1 022.20	1 136.30	1 282.50	1 415.20
Wage employment ('000)	1 677.10	1 699.70	1 727.30	1 763.70	1 807.70
GDP per capita (current) KES	33 767	32 434	35 327	39 091	42 313
GDP per capita (constant) KES, 2001=100)	33 767	32 549	32 845	33 764	35 045
GDP per capita (constant) US$, 2001=100)	450	433	437	450	467
Gross National Product (KES billion)	1 010.50	1 010.90	1 129.60	1 272.50	1 406.90
Inflation rate (% change in CPI)	5.80	2.00	9.80	11.30	10.30
Source: Central Bureau of Statistics (CBS) Kenya, Ministry of Planning and National Development (2005), Economic Survey 2005, Nairobi, Kenya. Note: 2001 = 100, 2001 is the base year.					

POVERTY

The decline in economic growth, coupled with increased inequality in the distribution of income, has led to a rise in poverty levels. Poverty increased sharply during the early 1990s, declined during the mid-1990s, and rose steadily after 1997. By 2003, over 56% of the population was living below the poverty line[43] (CBS, 2003). Regionally, pockets of very high poverty exist that exceed the national average. For instance, the rural absolute poverty situation was 59.6% by 2003, with urban absolute poverty standing at 51.5% in the same year. Falling per capita income, as well as its uneven distribution, has led to an increase in poverty levels (PRSP, 2001–2004).

Figure 3.1: Poverty trends in Kenya – percentage of population living in poverty

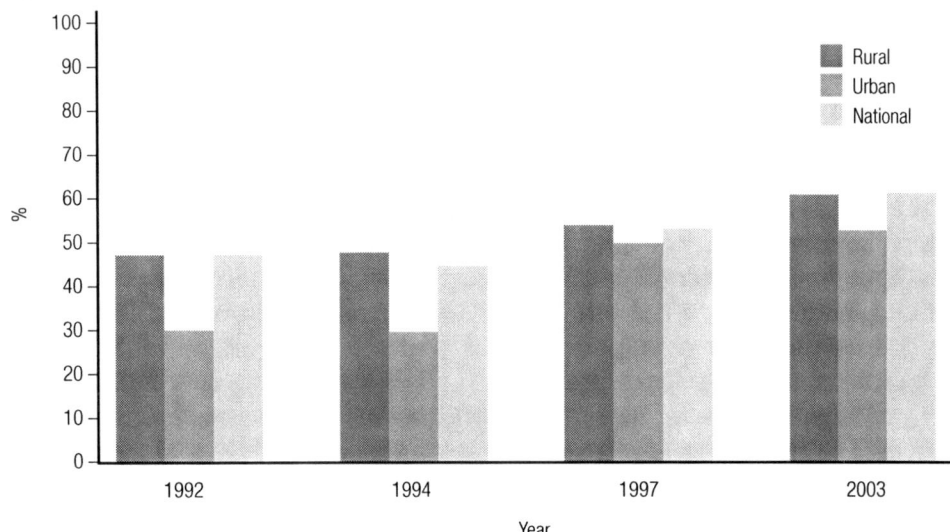

Sources: CBS, 1994; CBS, 1997; CBS, 2004; CBS, 2006; Kenya Macroeconomic Evolution Since Independence; MoPND, 2004; PRSP, 2001–2004; WB, 2003

Women tend to be more vulnerable to poverty than men. About 70% of the active female labour force work as subsistence farmers, compared with 43% of men. Subsistence farmers are well documented as being among the very poor, thus empowerment of women in terms of resource allocation is pivotal to breaking the vicious cycle of poverty. Such empowerment would enable them to enjoy the benefits of economic development and would also reduce their vulnerability to HIV/AIDS.

GENERAL HEALTH CARE SYSTEM

Kenya's health care system is pluralistic, with a wide range of players, including the MoH and parastatal organisations, and the private sector, consisting of private for-profit, NGO and FBO facilities. The MoH, operating a nationwide system of health facilities, is the largest provider and financier of health-care services in the country. The bulk of financial support for the public health-care system is received from the exchequer, which is supplemented by user fees and donor funding (off-budget support). The health services are provided through a network of over 4 700 health facilities countrywide, with the public sector system accounting for about 52% of the health facilities in the country. The private sector, mission organisations and the Ministry of Local Government run the remaining 48% of such facilities. The NGO sector predominantly provides health clinics, and maternity and nursing homes, with medical centres accounting for 85% of such facilities.

The health system is implemented through a network of facilities organised in a pyramidal pattern, from the dispensaries and health centres at the base of the pyramid, through subdistrict hospitals, district hospitals and provincial general hospitals, and, at the apex, referral hospitals. The *health centres* generally provide preventive and curative services, mostly adapted to local needs, while the *dispensaries* act as the health system's first line of contact with patients, providing a wider range of preventive health measures, which is a primary goal of Kenya's health policy. The *district hospitals* oversee the implementation of health policy at the district level, maintain quality standards, and coordinate and control all district health activities. The *national referral hospitals* provide sophisticated diagnostic, therapeutic and rehabilitative services. The two national referral hospitals are Kenyatta National Hospital in Nairobi and Moi Referral and Teaching Hospital in Eldoret. The provincial hospitals act as referral centres to support the district hospitals, providing highly specialised care.

The government health service is supplemented by privately owned and operated hospitals and clinics, and FBO hospitals and clinics. The mission health facilities are mainly located in the rural areas, as well as in the underserved parts of the urban centres. While they rely on donations and user fees, private hospitals and clinics operate for-profit health services, often providing specialised curative and preventive care. The private health-care delivery systems include pharmaceutical outlets and community pharmacies distributed countrywide.

The country is plagued by high mortality rates, low and declining life expectancy, high infant mortality and death rates, and declining population growth rates, which could be attributed to the HIV/AIDS epidemic. Infant mortality in 2003 was 77/1 000 live births, while under-five mortality[44] was 115/1 000 live births, and maternal mortality was estimated at 414/100 000 live births. According to the Kenya Demographic Health Survey (KDHS, 2003), only 40% of births occur in a health facility. Traditional birth attendants play a vital role in delivery, assisting close to 28% of births. The distribution of nurses and personnel is totally inadequate, with the reported nurse–patient and doctor ratio standing at 49/100 000 and 4/100 000 respectively.

HIV/AIDS Epidemic

NACC (2005) estimates that 2.2 million Kenyans have been infected with HIV, and more than 1.5 million have so far died from the disease, leaving over 2.3 million children orphaned. In addition, several million children live with parents who are ill, often being forced into the role of primary care-givers for their parents, young siblings and other dependants. Over 60% of those infected live in the rural areas, where the socioeconomic conditions are steadily worsening due to poverty and unemployment. Many more PLWHAs are estimated to be housebound, unable to access health care and impoverishing their households still further.

Evidence from Kenya shows the epidemic peaked in the late 1990s, with an overall HIV prevalence of 10% in adults, which declined to 7% in 2003 (KDHS, 2003), to 5.9% in 2006, and to 5.1% in 2007. This is only the second time in more than two decades that a sustained decline in national HIV infection levels has been reported in a Sub-Saharan African country. Such a decline has partly resulted from changes in sexual behaviour, increased use of preventive methods among women, fewer sexual partners, and increasing abstinence from sex by young women and men. However, despite the significant declines, HIV prevalence still remains high among young people.

Figure 3.2: Prevalence of HIV/AIDS epidemic in Kenya, 1990–2006

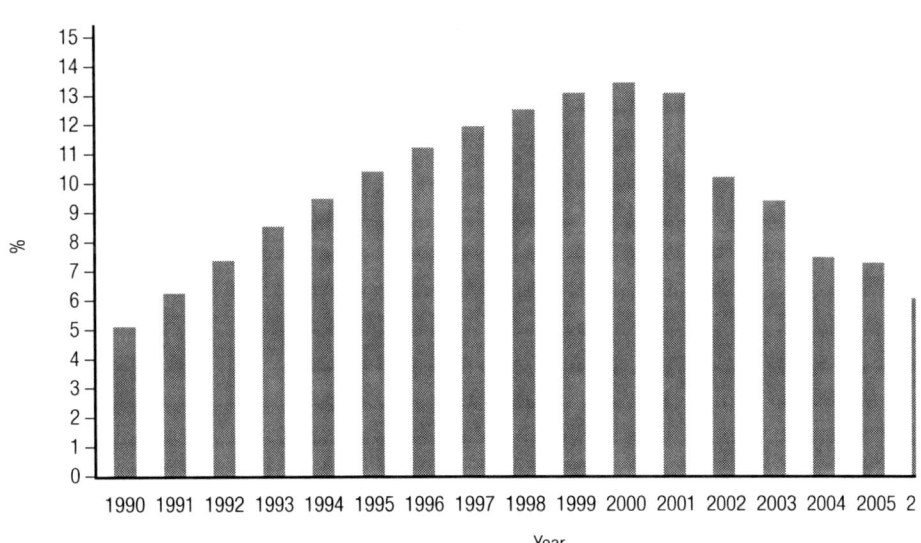

Source: NACC, 2004; Sentinel Surveillance, Kenya, 1990–2005

GENDER AND GEOGRAPHIC BREAKDOWN

The KDHS (2003) report indicates that the prevalence among women aged 19 to 49 is nearly 9%, while for men aged 15 to 54 the prevalence level is under 5% (the equivalent of 0.9 million men in the same category). The female–to–male ratio of 1.9 to 1 is higher than that in most African population-based studies, reflecting the vulnerability of young women to HIV infection. Such vulnerability is largely due to their inability to negotiate for safer sex, their economic dependency, and their limited access to information on prevention and treatment. The circumcision of most Kenyan males reduces their chance of infection.

Of women aged 15 to 19, 3% are HIV infected, compared with 0.4% of men aged 15 to 19, while HIV prevalence among women aged 20 to 24 is over three times that of men in the same age group (9% and 2.4%, respectively). The prevalence among women peaks at age 25 to 29 (12.9%), while among men the prevalence rises gradually with age, reaching its peak at age 40 to 44 (8.8%). Only in the age group 45 to 49 is the HIV prevalence higher among men (5.2%) than women (4%).

The prevalence of HIV infection varies widely across Kenyan provinces. Nyanza and Nairobi provinces, with a prevalence of 10.8% and 10% respectively, have the highest prevalence rates, while the Eastern province (3.4%) and North Eastern province (2%) have the lowest prevalence rates.

Table 3.2: HIV prevalence by province, adults aged 15–49 years, 2005 (%)			
Province	Male	Female	Total
Nairobi	7.9	12.0	10
Central	2.1	7.9	5
Coast	5.1	7.0	6.1
Eastern	1.3	5.4	3.4
North Eastern	1.4	2.6	2
Nyanza	8.4	13.2	10.8
Rift Valley	2.8	5.4	4.1
Western	3.7	5.6	4.7
Total	4.0	7.7	6.1%
Sources: Kenya HIV/AIDS Draft Data Booklet; NACC, 2006			

IMPACT OF THE HIV/AIDS EPIDEMIC

The HIV/AIDS epidemic is devastating, in that it primarily affects the economically active members of the population (those aged 15–49 years), threatening national and personal well-being by negatively impacting on individual health, life expectancy and productive capacity.

HIV also undermines development across all sectors of the economy and society. Major challenges include the following:

1. Productivity of the agricultural sector, upon which the majority of Kenyans rely for their livelihood, is being undermined by negative impacts on the supply of labour, crop production, agricultural extension services, and the loss of knowledge and skills. For example, a recent study by Kimalu et al (2003) found that HIV/AIDS impacts negatively on agricultural production by reducing the area of land under cultivation. At the household and community levels, the epidemic threatens food security, and the nutritional and health status of smallholders and their families. Further evidence indicates that the commercial agricultural subsector, a major source of employment and foreign exchange earner, is severely depleted by increasing health costs, increased morbidity and the mortality rates of key workers.

2. HIV/AIDS hinders intellectual development through enforcing absenteeism from school, and decreasing long-term learning capacity and the accumulation of human capital. According to NACC (2006), prolonged absenteeism from school not only reduces the future earnings of an individual, but also future variations in productivity and scope of specialisation. The debilitating effects of HIV/AIDS on the labour force have serious consequences for productivity. In addition, HIV/AIDS causes considerable loss in household production and reduction in the GDP due to the enforced increase in health-care expenditure.

3. The negative impacts on education in the country are felt in the numbers of teachers dying of AIDS and children dropping out of school due to the death of their parents and loss of household income. A baseline Government/UNICEF report (UNICEF, 2006) on the impact of HIV/AIDS on education in Kenya asserted that teacher performance was affected adversely by their absence due to HIV-related illnesses. The same report further found that teachers who are dying of AIDS are either not being replaced or are taking time to be replaced. Girls from infected and affected households also often have to drop out of school to take care of their relatives.

4. The HIV epidemic has also added to the burden on the health infrastructure in Kenya, with increasing cases of TB and HIV-related illness. According to the MoH, over 50% of government hospital beds are occupied by people with HIV/AIDS-related illnesses (HMIS report, 2004), crowding out patients suffering from other diseases. The impact on the health sector is felt both through direct costs (the expense of medical treatment, supplies and personnel) and indirect costs (the death of trained medical personnel). HIV/AIDS is also usurping health sector resources needed to treat other health problems. The increased need for the care of PLWHAs is especially problematic, given the inability of Kenya to meet the World Health Organisation (WHO) requirement of US$35 to US$40 per capita per year to finance the minimum general health services packages, which include antiretroviral therapy (ART) for PLWHAs, is undermining health workers' morale as the health worker–patient ratio increases.

5. At household level, the disease impacts on individuals and their families in terms of loss of income and high medical expenses. A study by the Kenya

National AIDS Control Council (2006) showed that those infected by HIV spend over 60% of their income on medical bills. Many families were found to be using up their savings, while others were forced to resort to borrowing money or to selling their assets in order to be able to pay for treatment (Kenya National AIDS Control Council, 2006). The KDHS (2003) showed that the economic burden of HIV/AIDS tends to fall most heavily on poor households, which have to spend a significant proportion of their total income on treatment and care. The epidemic is also responsible for the increase in child- and female-headed households, as well as the feminisation of poverty.[45]

6. Many private companies are experiencing increased levels of absenteeism and high medical and funeral insurance, absenteeism, recruitment and training costs due to HIV/AIDS.

The Role of Research and Costing Analysis in Drawing Up the Budget

Until recently, information on the total resource requirements for an effective response to HIV/AIDS was not based on the sound estimation of unit costs. However, since 2005, numerous costing studies have been undertaken to determine the total resources required to implement the key priority areas of the Kenya National HIV/AIDS Strategic Plan (KNASP). The costing of HIV interventions is aimed at providing a more accurate assessment of the amount of resources required to mount an effective response to the epidemic. To determine the resource requirements to meet the 2005–2010 Strategic Plan, a costing analysis was undertaken. The estimation of resource requirements was accomplished using the Resource Needs Model,[46] which estimates required resources for a given set of targets in line with the four broad categories of interventions contained in the KNASP, namely prevention of new infections, improvement of the quality of life, the mitigation of socioeconomic impact. In addition, ART costing was undertaken to determine the resources required for the various ART components.

Table 3.3 summarises the resources required for each intervention, with the total accumulated cost for the three priority areas being estimated at KES 177,453 million. Of the total, 24.3% is allocated for the prevention of new infections, while 29.4% is earmarked for improvement of the quality of life. Of the total resource requirements earmarked for the latter purpose, about 66% is spent on ART, while 14% is used for the treatment of opportunistic infections. Scaling up the provision of ART to PLWHAs will help to prolong life and reduce mortality. The protection of human rights has also been recognised as a critical component, consuming 7.8% of the total amount of resources available to improve the quality of life. Mitigation of socioeconomic impact accounts for 30.4% of the total resources, while 15.9% is taken up by the support services.

The bulk of estimated resource requirements for the mitigation of socioeconomic impact will be spent on mitigating programmes (59%), while livelihood and social security and mitigation policy will account for 12% and 9.5% respectively. For 2007/08, approximately KES 36 billion was required to achieve the results and targets specified in the KNASP for that FY.

KES, million	2005/06	2006/07	2007/08	2008/09	2009/10	Total
Total prevention	5,740	7,765	8,661	9,788	11,173	43,127
Improving quality of life	7,229	8,832	10,898	12,041	13,155	52,155
Mitigation of socio-economic impact	7,252	9,221	10,865	12,126	14,441	53,905
Support services	5110	4303	6202	6024	6627	28266
Overall Total (KES million)	25,331	30,121	36,626	39,979	45,396	177453

Table 3.3: Estimated financing requirements for KNASP (KES million), 2005/06–2009/10

Sources: Kenya National HIV/AIDS Strategic Plan, 2005/6–2009/10; NACC, 2005

OUTLINE OF GOVERNMENT RESPONSE TO HIV/AIDS

HISTORY OF GOVERNMENT RESPONSE

The first case of HIV in Kenya was identified in 1985 and the national response saw the establishment of departments within the MoH to prevent and control the spread of the epidemic. For over 15 years the national response to HIV/AIDS was led by the health sector, since HIV/AIDS was viewed as a health problem. During that time, minimal resources were allocated by the government for managing the epidemic. However, the national response did not make much progress and the country saw the epidemic spread in every sector and at every level. Some of the perceived reasons for this rising trend are:
- The failure to involve all sectors in the national response;
- The failure of the HIV/AIDS programme to take adequate account of the socio-cultural factors affecting the spread of the epidemic;
- Use of the health sector as both an implementer and coordinator of HIV/AIDS programmes;
- Insufficient commitment and leadership to fighting the epidemic both internally and externally; and
- Inadequate human and financial resources.

In 1999, the GoK, declaring HIV/AIDS a national disaster, established NACC and earmarked financial resources for the cause. The establishment of NACC facilitated the development of the KNASP 2000–2005, which devised a multisectoral response to the epidemic, jointly agreed on by stakeholders within government, civil society, the private sector and development partners (KNASP, 2005/06–2009/10).

The national response to HIV/AIDS in Kenya has consisted of three distinct phases, the first lasting from 1984 to 1991, the second from 1992 to 1997, and the third from 1998 to 2005.

87

The Initial Phase (1984–1991)

During this initial period, the epidemic was identified and the National AIDS Council (NAC), was established under the MoH. The focus during this phase was on policy development under the guidance of the MoH.

The Second Phase (1992–1997)

During the second phase, the National HIV/AIDS and STD Control Programme (NASCOP) was established and Sessional Paper No. 4 of 1997 on AIDS in Kenya developed. The Paper provided a policy framework within which AIDS prevention and control efforts could be coordinated for the next 15 years (GoK, 2003). The Paper recognised the fact that responding to the HIV/AIDS crisis required strong political commitment at the highest level; the implementation of a multisectoral prevention and control strategy prioritising the needs of the youth; the mobilisation of resources financing HIV prevention, care and support; and the establishment of a NACC to provide leadership at the highest level possible. The Paper clearly showed the political will of the government to support effective programmes to control the spread of HIV, to protect the human rights of those with HIV, and to provide care for those infected with and affected by HIV.

The Third Phase (1999 to 2005)

The government declaration of HIV/AIDS as a national disaster paved the way for a substantial flow of funds from both the government and its development partners. The establishment of NACC in 2000 added impetus to the fight against HIV, prompting the development of KNASP 2000–2005, which set out a multisectoral approach to fighting the epidemic. Both NACC and NASCOP provided the national institutional framework within which liaison and the coordination of HIV/AIDS-related activities could take place in Kenya. To mainstream HIV/AIDS activities in all government sectors, NACC initiated the setting up of AIDS Coordinating Units (ACUs) in various line ministries, recognising AIDS as a multisectoral, rather than a health, problem, embracing a wide range of strategies, and recognising the role of other sectors, such as private and civil society, in combating AIDS.

The GoK launched a Joint AIDS Programme Review (JAPR) to assess and develop mechanisms enabling multisectoral collaboration, and the capacity of NACC to support and manage ACUs and stakeholders focused on implementing the strategic plan. The establishment of the second KNASP 2005–2010 (A Call to Action) in 2005 set the targets to be achieved by stakeholders, reflecting still further GoK's commitment to the "Three Ones"[47] principles of the International Conference on AIDS and STDs in Africa (ICASA) Conference (2003). The government has clearly shifted from a sectoral response to a comprehensive multisectoral national strategy involving all relevant stakeholders (KNASP, 2005/06–2009/10) embracing institutional and programmatic reforms. To strengthen policy formulation and oversight, the government established a cabinet subcommittee on HIV/AIDS to coordinate and oversee the implementation of HIV programmes in Kenya.

At the programme level, the government implemented a new policy focused on decentralising response to the community level of the individual constituencies. To provide for an explicit legal framework for the national response to the HIV epidemic, the government promulgated a Bill on HIV/AIDS. Once enacted, it will provide the legal framework needed to enable a comprehensive response to the epidemic. Increased stakeholder participation in the planning and operationalisation of new policies, the establishment of a joint agreed strategic plan, jointly supported institutional arrangements, and a joint national M&E framework and HIV/AIDS programme review mechanism, all serve to reflect government commitment to maintaining an openly productive dialogue with all the stakeholders concerned.

GOVERNMENT HIV/AIDS POLICY

Key components of the policy response include the prioritisation of certain areas for the prevention of HIV/AIDS, as well as mechanisms for the mitigation of socio-economic impact at individual, family, community, sectoral and national levels. The adoption of such an approach has facilitated the investment of significant amounts of resources at the provincial, district, community and household levels, where both the main determinants and the main impacts of the disease lie. The three priority areas highlighted in the plan include prevention and advocacy; treatment along a continuum of care and support; the mitigation of socioeconomic impacts. All these priority areas fall within, and are consistent with, the interventions developed for meeting the MDGs. Given the above situation, the interventions that have been proposed for scaling up towards meeting the set targets are now discussed.

HIV/AIDS PRIORITY AREAS

The different priority areas consist of:
- Priority area 1: Prevention of new infections;
- Priority area 2: Improvement of the quality of life; and
- Priority area 3: Mitigation of socioeconomic impact.

PRIORITY AREA 1: PREVENTION OF NEW INFECTIONS

Prevention strategies to be implemented include:
- Increasing the availability of, and access to, counselling and testing;
- Condom promotion;

- Strengthening STI and HIV programme linkages;
- Expanding the PMTCT of HIV;
- More effective targeting of behaviour change communication (BCC);
- Improving the availability of safe blood supply;
- Ensuring safety and expanded access regarding post-exposure prophylaxis (PEP);
- Universal precautions; and
- Ensuring that prevention and treatment efforts are mutually supportive.

PRIORITY AREA 2: IMPROVEMENT OF THE QUALITY OF LIFE

This priority area focuses on:
- Improving the availability of, and access to, treatment and care; and
- The more effective protection of human rights.

PRIORITY AREA 3: MITIGATION OF SOCIOECONOMIC IMPACT

The objective of this priority area is to adapt existing programmes and develop innovative responses to reduce the impact of the epidemic on communities, social services, and economic productivity. The components of this priority area comprise:
- Undertaking impact studies;
- Advocacy;
- The development of mitigation policies;
- The implementation of mitigation programmes;
- Community empowerment; and
- Human resource planning.

SUPPORT SERVICES

In addition to the above priority areas, several support services have been identified to ensure effective delivery of the KNASP strategies, including:
- M&E;
- Research;
- The Financing and Procurement Framework;
- Institutional capacity-building; and
- Communication, coordination and networking.

STRUCTURES AND INSTITUTIONS FOR IMPLEMENTING GOVERNMENT HIV/AIDS PROGRAMMES

The success of the national response to the epidemic depends on the maintenance of a strong, effective strategic partnership between the national and international stakeholders, government, civil society and the private sector. In Kenya, the HIV/AIDS epidemic is addressed primarily through NACC, an entity established in terms of Legal Notice No. 170 of 1999, which operates through multisectoral implementers under a structured consultative leadership. NACC is mandated to coordinate and supervise all HIV/AIDS activities in Kenya, as well as to mobilise resources, and to formulate and promote policies. In addition, NACC is responsible for the production and circulation of annual reports to stakeholders, development partners, civil society, and the private sector, as well as being responsible for organising a Joint AIDS Programme Review (JAPR), a forum in which all stakeholders involved with HIV/AIDS convene and discuss their achievements, lessons learnt and existing HIV/AIDS-related challenges. NACC also spearheads the mainstreaming of HIV/AIDS through the MTEF process in order to improve resource allocation and to ensure the sustainability of HIV/AIDS programmes.

To promote a multisectoral approach, each government ministry has an ACU, which is responsible for mainstreaming HIV-related efforts in all core functions of the planning process. The ACUs act as advocates for NACC policies in order to ensure that the HIV/AIDS strategic interventions are fully integrated into the mainstream ministry functions. In the new structure, CACCs are the foci for spearheading the fight against the epidemic at grassroots level. In addition to mainstreaming AIDS in core activities, the ACUs are supposed to mainstream HIV/AIDS into constituency development activities. Specifically, the CACCs were designed to emphasise community-based activities through both CBOs and individuals. The active participation of Members of Parliament (MPs) in launching such committees catalysed open discussion about HIV at the community level. MPs also have to encourage the communities to generate proposals and to approve proposals submitted by CBOs for NACC funding and the coordination of HIV/AIDS-related activities in their respective constituencies. In addition, MPs are responsible for setting up networks and supervising stakeholders involved in implementing HIV/AIDS-related activities in their constituencies.

The Ministry of Planning and National Development's (MoPND's) mandate entails coordinating planning in general, as well as working jointly with NACC in mainstreaming HIV/AIDS-related efforts at all levels through establishing and maintaining linkages with national policy development, planning and budgeting. The MoPND, by way of the central planning and coordination department and the central planning units (CPUs) in all ministries, is expected to influence the mainstreaming of HIV/AIDS into core sector priorities through interministerial and multisectoral HIV/AIDS policy formulation, review, implementation, budgeting and resource allocation (NACC, 2006).

The Budget Process

Overview

The budget process in Kenya comprises three main stages:
- budget planning and formulation;
- budget approval and execution; and
- budget monitoring.

The formulation of long-term development strategies and policies precedes the start of the process. The Ministry of Finance and Economic Affairs and the budgetary supply departments (BSDs), together with the MoPND, are responsible for the technical reviewing of various economic aggregates, including the growth rate of the GDP, inflation trends, money supply and balance of payments (BoP). The process culminates in a budget outlook paper providing the macroeconomic projections and policy directions for the FY ahead, indicating the expected revenue and expenditure that form the basis for the establishment of sector ceilings. The growth projections determine the overall revenue that the economy can realise. The External Resources Department (ERD) of the Ministry of Finance and Planning captures data relating to external resources, consisting of grants and loans from development partners.

The budgeting process in Kenya has undergone various reforms aimed at addressing fiscal discipline and efficiency in relation to the use of government resources. Key among such reforms was the introduction of an MTEF, consisting of a rolling three-year budget, in 1999/2000. The reforms are aimed at:
- Linking policy-making to planning and budgeting;
- Maintaining aggregate fiscal discipline;
- Improving inter- and intrasectoral resource allocation, based on the cost of priority programmes and projects aimed at increasing the effectiveness of public expenditure; and
- Increasing efficiency by achieving desired outcomes cost-effectively.

The key components of the MTEF include:
- The definition of a global resource envelope;
- The determination of intersectoral allocations based on core functions; and
- Proposals of intrasectoral allocations based on outcomes, activities, outputs and operational efficiency.

The transparency of such an approach to budgeting allows the participation of the public and private sector in public hearings during budget preparation. During the MTEF process, the ministries/departments concerned have to focus on the expected outcomes of expenditures and programmes. The annual budget and three-year rolling MTEF provide a mechanism for evaluating realisation of the outputs and outcomes, and their contribution to the overall economic growth of the economy.

Stages of the Budget Process

Stage 1: National and District Development Planning

The Ministry of Finance and Planning sets the long-term macro and micro targets at the desired growth levels, followed by the various ministries developing strategic plans indicating their overall objectives, programmes and activities. The preparation of such plans involves a wide range of stakeholders, including private sector representatives and the relevant NGOs, development partners and civil societies. The plans form the reference points guiding national development and provide the budgetary direction to be followed throughout the planned period.

Stage 2: Preparation of Budget Outlook Paper (BOPA)

Stage 2 involves projecting anticipated revenue and expenditure levels. The Economic Affairs Department of the Ministry of Finance (MoF) and the Budgetary Supplies Department (BSD), jointly with the MoPND, prepares a budget outlook paper which gives the macroeconomic projections and policy direction for the FY. Such projections indicate the expected revenue and expenditure that form the basis for sector ceilings, determining the overall revenue that the economy can realise. The external resources, consisting of grants and loans from development partners, are captured by the External Resource Development (ERD) of the Ministry of Finance and Planning. The process of determining the resource envelope is coordinated by the Ministry of Finance and Planning, and allows for the participation of the Central Bank, development partners and other stakeholders. However, the representation of marginalised groups is minimal at this stage, as the civil societies presumed to represent them are rarely involved at this point in the process.

Stage 3: Resource Allocation to Sectors and Bidding

During December, the treasury issues a circular regarding the preparation of the budget, which sets the stage for the preparation of the ministerial public expenditure reviews[48] (MPERs). For budget purposes, the government is divided into eight different sectors, with core ministries[49] bidding for resources. The chairman of each sector and the secretariat meet at the Budget Steering Committee (BSC) level, which is chaired by the Permanent Secretary. The MoF has to decide on the amount to be allocated to each sector. Other key stakeholders outside government are drawn mainly from the donor community, the private sector and other stakeholders. Sector resource bidding usually takes place in January.

Stage 4: Working Out Ministerial Ceilings

After each sector receives its allocation of resources, how much each ministry will get from the different sectors consisting of the key ministries, development partners, civil society, the private sector and other stakeholders is determined. The Sector Working Groups (SWGs) prioritise programmes/projects and activities within each sector and allocate resources to high priority areas in line with the government's overall strategic objectives. The MTEF sector paper highlights each ministry's policy priorities, for which they have to compete in terms of resources. The ministry whose policies are thought to have the greatest impact on poverty reduction, and are most essential to the survival of the people, receives the highest allocation, justifying the prioritisation of the social sector in terms of resource allocation.

Stage 5: Ministerial Itemised Budget Proposals

After each ministry has received an allocation from various envelopes, the sum total of which form the ceilings for the respective ministry, a Ministerial Budget Committee is convened, consisting of departmental heads and chaired by the PS. Each department prepares its preliminary budget estimates under the coordination of a ministerial MTEF forum. The ministerial budget committee reviews the proposals and makes the necessary adjustments to ensure that they fall within the budget ceilings stipulated in the treasury circular.

Stage 6: Submission of Ministerial Proposals

After the allocation of resources to various programmes and projects, including those which are HIV/AIDS-related, the sectoral reports are finalised and submitted to the MoF for further review and consideration. The Sectoral Group then ascertains whether the ministerial proposals meet the expenditure ceilings for the ministries concerned and sees that items have been charged against the correct sector resource envelope. The MoF then reviews the ministerial estimates and prepares the detailed budget and MTEF documents to be tabled in parliament during the annual budget speech made by the Minister for Finance in June.

Stage 7: Finalisation of the Budget Proposals

The proposals are finalised and submitted to the MoF together with the budget speech, which is a summary of the consolidated budget proposals, for presentation to parliament. The final preparation of the draft budget must be completed by the end of May.

STAGE 8: BUDGET PRESENTATION AND APPROVAL BY PARLIAMENT

Once the minister is satisfied with the budget proposals submitted by the BSC, they are presented to parliament before 21 June, as is required by the Constitution. The parliament usually approves the budget between August and October, with each ministry presenting its budget, with accompanying justification, for approval. However, before such approval is granted, each ministry is allowed to spend, at most, a quarter of the allocation in the budget, mainly on personnel emoluments, transport costs and other essentials.

THE LINK BETWEEN THE NATIONAL RESOURCE ENVELOPE FOR HIV/AIDS AND THE MEDIUM-TERM EXPENDITURE FRAMEWORK

In terms of the MTEF process, government funding for HIV programmes is included in the core poverty programmes under the Office of the President. Once the NACC National Resource Envelope (NRE) has been finalised, the funding for HIV/AIDS activities is linked to the MTEF, which facilitates policy dialogue and eventually leads to HIV/AIDS mainstreaming within each government ministry and/or department.

SYNCHRONISATION OF DONOR AND NATIONALLY-SOURCED FUNDS

The on-budget HIV/AIDS support from donors (mainly in the form of grants) is channeled through the MoF to a special account controlled by the Treasury. The ministries receive the donor commitment document from the MoF. The External Resources Department (ERD) in the MoF keeps records of the amounts committed for specific projects within the budget year. The commitment documents also show the nature of disbursements commonly referred to as Appropriation in Aid (AIA) or revenue, and the government commitment, if any. The information is captured in the budget according to the donor commitment register.

ROLE OF PARLIAMENT IN THE BUDGET PROCESS

While parliament has the responsibility of approving budgetary allocations, its role in the budget process is relatively limited. It plays an indirect role in the budget process by deciding on government priorities through debating and passing policy documents and legislation relating to various ministries or sectors. However, the presentation of the budget to Parliament during the annual minister's budget speech is the only time that Parliament actually participates in the budget process.

In addition to the limited opportunities for its involvement in the budget process, Parliament rarely examines the budget proposals for HIV/AIDS activities, as such items are included in the health budget as a whole, and insufficient time and resources are available in which to break it down into specific line items. The MPs are, therefore, responsible for ensuring that the government allocates a certain percentage of the budget for HIV/AIDS-related activities, and that every department can show what percentage of its budget is directed towards HIV/AIDS initiatives.

ACCESSIBILITY OF BUDGET INFORMATION BY THE PUBLIC

The main entry point for the public to budget information is the Sector Hearing of the MTEF process, during which members of the public are invited to contribute to Sectoral Policy Papers. In addition, the Treasury has a website via which MTEF sectoral documents are made available to the public, though such documents tend to be too detailed and technical to be user friendly. Both the print and the electronic media also publish the information, though most people, who live in the rural areas, lack access to such sources. With the information only being published long after the budget presentation, it is inadequate for evaluating and/or monitoring budget implementation. While the rigorous monitoring that occurs at the macro-aggregate level helps to ensure adherence to set macro targets, little is done to monitor the budget in terms of its effectiveness, efficiency and equity. With the budget information usually being published in English, those citizens who are illiterate are effectively excluded from the process.

HEALTH-CARE FINANCING AND REPORTING MECHANISMS

THE GOVERNMENT OF KENYA BUDGET

The GoK's contribution to the health sector is channeled through the budget as an instrument for allocating public finances for health. As noted earlier, equity and efficiency principles are the main drivers of the government's policy on public spending within the health sector. The key spending and resource allocation objectives include the increased allocation of resources to rural health services; increased spending on drugs and nonpharmaceuticals; and reduced spending on curative services and tertiary care facilities. As noted above, GoK contributes an estimated 30% of the total health-care financing of the country. Table 3.4 shows that the government's contribution to the health sector has continued to increase in absolute terms, from Ksh 12 billion in FY 2000/01 to Ksh 33 billion in FY 2006/07. However, in real terms, the contribution from government has been decreasing. Public health expenditure as a percentage of the GDP varied only minimally over the same period.

The analysis of public health expenditure reveals that recurrent expenditures are consistently and substantially higher than that spent on development, both in absolute terms and as a percentage of the GDP. For instance, recurrent expenditure increased from KES 15.4 billion in FY 2003/04 to KES 15.9 billion in FY 2004/05, representing an increase of 3.3%. In per capita terms, the health expenditure per capita increased from KES 481.97 in FY 2002/03 to KES 712.67 in FY 2004/05, to KES 681.78 in FY 2005/06, being projected at KES 970.4 for the FY 2006/07. The per capita expenditure is, however, below the WHO's recommended level of US$34 per capita,[50] falling short of the GoK commitment to spend 15% of the total budget on health, as agreed on in terms of the Abuja Declaration. Such a trend reflects the inability of the government to ensure adequate service provision to the population.

Table 3.4: Ministry of Health expenditure, 2000/01–2006/07 (KES million)							
	2000/2001	2001/2002	2002/2003	2003/2004	2004/2005	2005/2006	2006/2007
Recurrent	11 041	12 715	14 405	15 438	15 952	19 765	21 611
Development	1 032	2 519	945	1 003	7 659	3 242	11 716
Total	12 073	15 234	15 350	16 441	23 611	23 007	33 327
Per capita KES	395.49	488.44	481.97	506.05	712.67	681.78	970.4
Per capita US$	5.05	6.28	6.29	6.52	9.10	9.47	13.6
Ministry of Health expenditure (gross) as % of total government expenditure							
Recurrent	7.67	8.23	8.69	7.76	7.22	6.29	7.63
Development	4.49	17.18	5.12	2.77	8.83	3.73	8.5
Ministry of Health expenditure (gross) as % of the GDP							
Recurrent	1.32	1.38	1.40	1.41	1.29	1.29	1.28
Development	0.12	0.27	0.09	0.09	0.62	0.21	0.70
Total	1.44	1.65	1.49	1.50	1.91	1.5	1.98
Source: MoH PER, Republic of Kenya, various years							

FINANCIAL FLOWS FOR HIV/AIDS IN THE PUBLIC SECTOR

The funds earmarked for HIV/AIDS activities are transferred directly by the Treasury to the ACUs in each ministry. In the case of on-budget donor funding, the MOH prepares and submits to the Treasury/ERD special exchequer requisitions (SERs), which are based on work plans, after which the treasury confirms the availability of the funds and requests the Central Bank of Kenya to transfer such funds to an Exchequer account. The funds are then transferred to the ministry's development account by way of an Exchequer Issue Notification. The funds intended for district-based projects, including those relating to HIV/AIDS (on-budget), are transferred to the district reimbursement suspense account operated by the Treasury, and immediately transmitted to the district project bank accounts according to the list provided by the ministries implementing HIV/AIDS activities.

Government funding follows the government budget and financial procedures, with the funds for HIV/AIDS being channeled through the MoH and NACC in the

OP. HIV/AIDS funding to MoH forms part of its budgetary allocations for the delivery of health services. The budget allocations to NACC are aimed at providing support for NACC efforts to coordinate and mobilise resources for a multisectoral response to HIV/AIDS, including administering intergovernmental transfers under the CACCs, and transfers to line ministries for specific HIV/AIDS-related expenditure items and programmes.

The funding flows occur as follows:

1. MoF transfers HIV/AIDS funds to the MoH, NACC and the line ministries. The MoH is responsible for implementing a range of HIV/AIDS-related activities through the public health facilities and NASCOP. In addition, the ministry acts as a conduit for Global Fund and MAP funds earmarked for HIV/AIDS activities. The beneficiaries for these funds are The general population benefits from such funds.

2. Donor funds in Kenya are channeled through both on-budget and off-budget support. On-budget support is channeled through a special account held by NACC under the OP and is disbursed though the MoF. NACC disburses funds from the special account to ACUs, NGOs, FBOs, the private sector and CBOs through the community initiative fund. In addition to the above funds disbursed through NACC, many NGOs, FBOs and CBOs receive funds directly from donors both inside and outside the country, the amounts of which are difficult to quantify.

3. The MoE is a conduit for funding HIV/AIDS interventions within the education sector. In addition to budget allocations to the ministry, it receives funds from Kenya's development partners to support the implementation of HIV/AIDS interventions. The ACUs in the ministry are responsible for overall ministry HIV/AIDS policy and service coordination; awareness creation; the prevention and control of infections; and health education and promotion.

4. The OP NACC is responsible for overall HIV/AIDS policy formulation; resource mobilisation; service coordination; the identification of strategic partners at all levels; and the identification of lead agencies for specific interventions and provision. NACC is a conduit for funding CBOs, local NGOs, CACCs and ACUs in line ministries. The budgetary allocations are also meant to facilitate intergovernmental transfers under the CACCs, as well as transfers to line ministries for specific HIV/AIDS-related expenditure items and programmes.

5. Until the end of June 2005, the ACUs were mainly funded from the Kenya HIV/AIDS Disaster Response Project (KHADREP), funded by the WB to the tune of US$50 million credit. The funding of ACUs in the line ministries was aimed at supporting the mainstreaming of HIV/AIDS within the ministries.

6. Most local and international corporate organisations have an HIV/AIDS financing scheme for their infected and affected employees. The funds involved are specifically earmarked for HIV/AIDS prevention, and the treatment of OIs, as well as for antiretrovirals.

7. Direct household expenditure includes all forms of 'out-of-pocket' payments for the treatment of OIs and drugs, such as consultation and laboratory fees paid to hospitals/health-care providers, the purchase of antiretrovirals (especially from

providers), and the copayments required by medical specialists.

8. Other sources of financing come from NGOs and the private sector, including private foundations, which are increasingly becoming a major source of funding for HIV/AIDS in Kenya. Most of the NGOs receive their funding from charitable organisations. Charitable donations are usually channeled to specific institutions, such as mission hospitals or to local NGOs providing health care to HIV/AIDS-infected and affected clients.

OVERVIEW OF ALLOCATIONS FOR HIV/AIDS IN THE 2004/5 NATIONAL BUDGET

The total HIV/AIDS allocations (comprising both the MoF budget allocations and on-budget support) for Kenya can be analysed in terms of the allocations granted to line ministries.Table 3.5 provides details of the Total HIV/AIDS Expenditure by the government.[51]

THE MINISTRY OF HEALTH

The MoH budget estimates indicate that the total government expenditure on HIV/AIDS increased from US$25.05 million in 2003/04 to US$27.75 million in 2004/05. Overall, the MoE was allocated a total of KES 20 million between 2003/04 and 2004/05, with the GoK accounting for approximately 0.4% of the total public HIV/AIDS financing in the two FYs. The allocations are made to the MoE for the promotion of school-based prevention services, including life skills and HIV/AIDS education, and teacher education (pre-service and in-service) aimed at building up positive attitudes and skills for HIV/AIDS prevention and control. Such services are provided in primary, secondary and tertiary institutions. In addition, the ministry has an ACU with a line item for HIV/AIDS intended for the support of workplace-based prevention activities.

The OP (especially NACC) is responsible, in broad terms, for policy formulation and the coordination and supervision of the implementation of HIV/AIDS-related programmes, the M&E of national response, the mobilisation of stakeholders, and for overseeing the utilisation of HIV/AIDS funds. The total HIV/AIDS allocation in FYs 2003/04 and 2004/05 was KES 161 million and KES 174 million, respectively. On average, such an allocation accounted for 7.5% of the total HIV/AIDS allocations by the Treasury.

The Office of the Vice-President (OVP) is largely concerned with the implementation of programmes targeting OVC, women and youth. Part of its budget is used for prevention interventions at headquarters (HQ), while the rest is transferred to various government departments in the provinces and districts, earmarked for community- and home-based care and support programmes run by the provincial administration, prisons, the police and the armed forces. For FYs 2003/04–2004/05, the government allocated a total of KES 10 million for HIV/AIDS interventions.

Figure 3.3: Percentage share of HIV/AIDS allocations by ministry for 2003/04–2004/05 national budgets

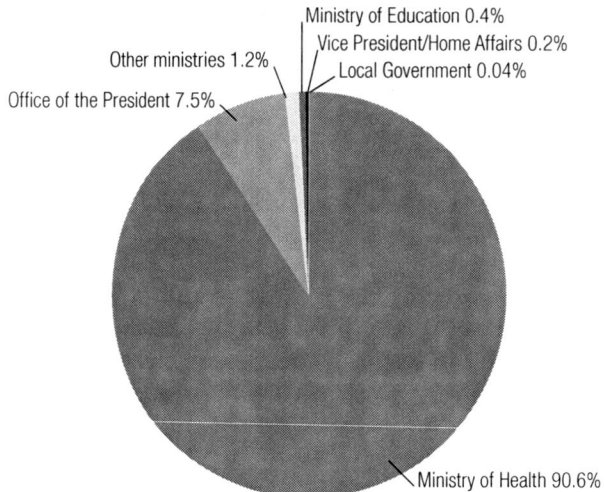

Source: GoK, Estimates of Recurrent Expenditure of the Government of Kenya, 2004/05, 2005/06; Kenya NHA, 2001–2002
Note: a) The MoH expenditure on HIV/AIDS was estimated based on information in the Kenya NHA 2001–2003, which indicated that the MoH spent KES 1 637 million (US$20.9 million) of funds from the central government revenue (Treasury) in FY 2001/02. The figures for FYs 2003/04 and 2004/05 are derived from this amount, taking into consideration only the changes in price level (inflation) experienced since FY 2001/02.
b) The exchange rates used were: US$1 = KES 76.6 for 2003/04 and US$1 = KES 76.74 for 2004/05.

SOURCE OF HIV/AIDS FUNDS FOR ON-BUDGET SUPPORT

Out of the total HIV/AIDS funding for FY 2002/03, the contribution by the GoK accounted for 65.5% of the total budget, followed by the WB, which accounted for about 31% of the total amount. The government contribution includes the expenditure on human resources, and infrastructure and systems development. UNDP and UNICEF each accounted for 0.1% and 1.1% of the total budget support, respectively. The same pattern applies to FY 2003/04 and 2004/05.

The HIV/AIDS allocations increased from US$54.95 million to US$75.139 million in FY 2004/05, representing an increase of 36.7%. Over the three years, the largest share (US$107.498 million) went to the MoH. However, the budget allocation to the MoE decreased from US$396 988 in FY 2002/3 to US$214 084 in FY 2004/05.

The analysis shows that the GoK is by far the largest source of funding for the 2002/03 to 2004/05 period, accounting for 49% of the total. The WB accounted for 25%, while UNDP, UNICEF, the Global Fund and JICA accounted for 1%, 1%, 16% and 8% respectively. Table 3.5 indicates the total HIV/AIDS allocations in the national budget according to government source and blocks of development partners in support of the national response over the three-year period from 2002/03–2004/05.

Table 3.5: Total funds (US$) specifically allocated for HIV/AIDS in national budgets, 2004/05							
Agent	Source of funds						
	GoK	World Bank	UNDP	UNICEF	Global Fund	JICA	Total
OP	34 890						34 890
MoH	26 404 645	1 535 137		210 168	12 930 853	984 777	42 065 580
NACC	2 149 345	15 944 141	287 813		1 690 291		20 071 590
MoE	130 423			83 545			213 968
Home Affairs	65 212						65 212
Others	359 786						359 786
KEMRI						12 328 624	12 328 624
Total	29 144 301	17 479 278	287 813	293 713	14 621 144	13 313 401	75 139 650
Sources: GoK, Estimates of Recurrent Expenditure of the Government of Kenya, 2004/05, 2005/06; NACC, Kenya National Health Accounts, 2001/02. Real calculations based on GDP inflation figures; 2001/02 base year							

Figure 3.4: Total HIV/AIDS allocations in the national budget, 2002/03–2004/05

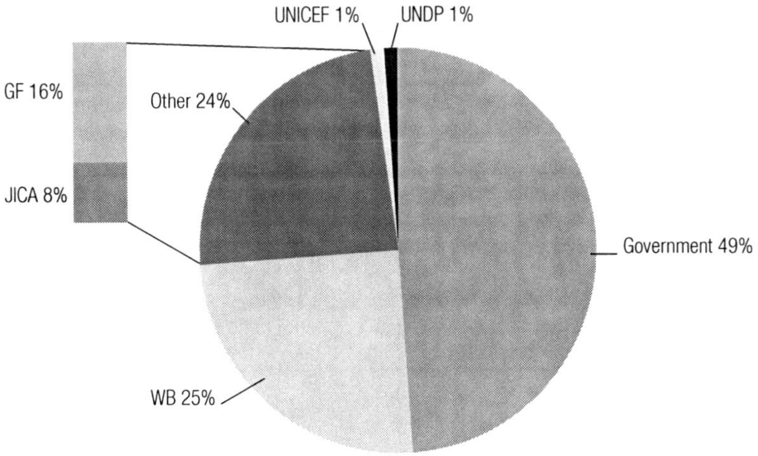

HIV/AIDS Expenditure by Donors

As noted earlier, donor funding comes from either bilateral or multilateral agencies. According to the Public Expenditure Review (2005), funds from the Global Fund are channelled through the MoH and NACC. In the 2004/2005 budget, a total of KES 12.33 billion (US$151.66 million) was specifically allocated for HIV/AIDS by donors. The US government contributed[52] the largest share of HIV/AIDS funds, accounting for about 59.4% (US$90.2 million) of total donor funding, with other significant contributions coming from the WB (11.1%), the Global Fund (9.4%), JICA (8.7%) and DFID (5.9%).

Table 3.6: HIV/ AIDS expenditure (KES million) by donors, 2004/05	
Donor	% of total
United Nations Development Programme (UNDP)	0.6
United Nations Population Fund (UNFPA)	1.3
United Nations High Commission for Refugees (UNHCR)	0.22
United Nations Children's Fund (UNICEF)	0.7
United Nations Fund for Women (UNIFEM)	0.04
United Nations Office on Drugs and Crime (UNODC)	0.04
World Food Programme (WFP)	0.9
World Health Organisation (WHO)	0.4
World Bank	11.1
Food and Agricultural Organisation (FAO)	0.03
Department for International Development (DFID)	5.9
United States Agency for International Development (USAID)	59.5
Finnish NGOs	0.11
Swedish International Development Agency (SIDA)	0.7
Japan International Cooperation Agency (JICA)	8.7
European Union (EU)	0.2
Global Fund for AIDS, TB and Malaria	9.5
Total	99.94

Sources: MoH, HIV/AIDS Public Expenditure Review, 2005; MOH-Global Fund Accountability Statement for the period 1st July 2005 to 31st December 2005; NACC, various statement of income and expenditure; UNAIDS, Kenya Office; UNDP, 2004

Note: (a) The expenditure by USAID was computed as annual (in terms of calendar year), based on the data from HIV/AIDS PER, MoH, 2005. The calculated amount is close to the US$91 million given in the PEPFAR annual report for 2004. As the annual report did not break down the expenditure by function, the sole figure on which to rely was the PER.
(b) The total expenditure on HIV/AIDS in the table should be regarded with caution, due to double counting, especially with respect to the PEPFAR funds channeled mainly through such UN agencies as UNICEF. However, the problem is not large, due to the small proportion of funds attributed to the agencies..

FLOW OF FUNDS FROM SOURCE TO AGENTS

Table 3.7 presents the flow of funds from source to agents in FY 2004/05. Almost US$182 million was designated for HIV/AIDS interventions by the government, and bilateral and multilateral agencies. As noted earlier, the 2004/05 national budget shows some serious commitment to making financial resources available for the HIV/ AIDS response. The contribution by the government through budgetary allocations supports interventions implemented by the ACUs in line ministries and government departments. The ACUs act as agents for the transfer of funds to the respective departments within the ministry's departments at national, provincial, district and divisional levels. In addition, transfers occur between ministries and NACC. While the resources for the public HIV/AIDS response financed from government revenue are channeled through government ministries, some of the ministries also receive direct funding from donors in support of specific HIV/AIDS programmes. Table 3.7 highlights the flow of funds from the Government of Kenya, bilateral and multilateral sources to various agents.

Table 3.7: Flow of funds from source to agents, 2004/05		
Source	Agent	Amount (US$)
Ministry of Finance	NACC	26 574 957
Ministry of Finance	Office of the President	65 212
Ministry of Finance	Other ministries	359 785
World Bank	NACC	15 944 141
World Bank	Ministry of Health	1 535 137
UNDP	NACC	287 813
UNICEF	Ministry of Education	210 168
UNICEF	Ministry of Education	83 545
Global Fund	NACC	1 690 291
Global Fund	Ministry of Finance	12 930 853
MoF	NACC	2 149 345
UNDP	UNDP	697 384
United Nations Population Fund	UNFPA	1 930 544
UNICEF	UNICEF	805 148
United Nations Office on Drugs	UNODC	63 700
WHO	WHO	627 000
WFP	Other multilateral from UN	1 297 000
Office of the United Nations High Commission	OUNHC	338 878
UNIFEM	Other multilateral from UN	98 600
UK government	DFID	8 941 442
US government	USAID	90 204 438
Government of Japan	MoH	984 777
Government of Japan	Parastatal organisations	12 328 624
Commission of the European Commission	Country office for bilateral agencies	304 081
Government of Finland	Finnish NGOs	173 000
Swedish government	SIDA	1 044 479
Total		181 670 342
Sources: Expenditure data obtained from various sources, including UN agencies, GoK printed estimates, local NGOs and the private sector. Other sources include the PEPFAR database and PER, 2005.		

FINANCIAL FLOWS FROM FINANCING AGENTS TO SERVICE PROVIDERS

Within the public sector, NACC and the MoH are the principal financial agents for transferring funds to providers, with NACC coordinating and financing community/ household-based HIV/AIDS initiatives as part of the national response to HIV/AIDS. The disbursement of funds takes place through both the CBOs and such a mechanism to empower community involvement in the HIV/AIDS response. Since 2002, NACC has disbursed funds to over 1 500 CBOs, NGOs, FBOs and private sector organisations. Some of the organisations act both as financing agents and service providers, with the funds being transferred from the agents through several service providers (NGOs, CBOs, FBOs, and public and private health-care providers).

Table 3.8 shows that a total of US$165 990 623 was transferred by the agents to such providers. The amount is lower than the total amount allocated for HIV/AIDS initiatives (US$181 670 342) due to:

- The inability to track all funds transferred from agents to service providers;
- The poor record-keeping of providers and agents;
- The administrative costs of the FAs;
- The failure of providers to supply information on their source of funding;
- Donor unwillingness to release information on the various CBOs, NGOs and private organisations that benefited from their funding; and
- A lack of transparency among the different CBOs, NGOs and donors.

Table 3.8: Financial flow from agent to provider		
Agent	Provider	Amount (US$)
NACC	CACCs and ACU training	1 808 938
Office of the President	Office of the President	34 890
Ministry of Finance	Ministry of Home Affairs	130 423
Ministry of Finance	Ministry of Home Affairs	65 212
Ministry of Finance	ACUs	359 785
Ministry of Health	Hospitals, nursing and residential service providers	41 080 803
NACC	NGO involved in advocacy	11 602 383
NACC	NACC	6 660 289
Ministry of Education	Primary and secondary schools	213 968
JICA	KEMRI	12 328 624
UNDP	Health promotion and prevention service providers	92 334
United Nations Office on Drugs and Control	Health promotion and prevention service providers	63 700
Ministry of Health	Hospitals, nursing and residential service providers	984 777
Country Office for Bilateral Agencies	Other providers	304 060
USAID	Other providers	90 204 437
UNIFEM	Advocacy and awareness NGOs	56 000
Total		165 990 623
Sources: Expenditure data obtained from various sources, including GoK printed estimates, local NGOs, the private sector and UN agencies. Other sources include the PEPFAR database and PER, 2005.		

The study also identified many challenges in tracking resources disbursed at various levels, which may partly be explained by the absence of a system to monitor the flow of funds from source through agents to beneficiaries. The lack of disaggregated data shows the functions, beneficiaries (by region, age and gender) and objects of expenditure.

COMPOSITION OF HIV/AIDS ALLOCATIONS

Figure 3.6 shows the contribution of funding from donors. In FY 2004/05, donors spent US$37.9 million on treatment and care, US$68.2 million on prevention, US$10.6 million on the mitigation of socioeconomic impact, and US$34.9 million on support services. USAID was the single largest source of funds in all the prevention-related categories, accounting for 62.4% of the total, followed by the WB (23.7%), the Global Fund (4.9%), UN agencies (3.9%), and DFID (3.5%), among others. In terms of treatment and care interventions, USAID was again the largest source, contributing 62.5% of the funding for treatment and care, with the other major contributors of funds for treatment and care interventions being the Global Fund (22.1%), DFID (8.2%) and the World Food Programme (WFP) (3.2%). The donor contribution made to the mitigation of socioeconomic impact was as follows: USAID (60.5%), WB (26.5%), SIDA (4.9%), UNICEF (3.6%) and the Global Fund (1.9%). Overall, 45% of donor funding was spent on prevention programmes, 25% on treatment and care, and 23% on support services. The mitigation of socioeconomic impact received the smallest allocation (7%) of donor funding.

The current study shows that most donors prioritise prevention and treatment. However, funding levels can be seen to be widely disparate when the total donor funding by priority area/function and the KNASP funding guidelines are compared. The 2005–2010 KNASP estimates that the prevention of new infections should take 24% of the national HIV/AIDS resource envelope (NRE), and treatment and care 29%. Donor expenditure on prevention, treatment and care for 2004/05 stood at 45% and 25% respectively, clearly showing that most donors differed in their priorities from the national priorities, according to the KNASP costing resource requirement guidelines. Overspending might, therefore, occur in some priority areas, whereas other areas might be underfunded. Figure 3.6 compares the KNASP financing guidelines in terms of priority area and HIV/AIDS donor expenditure. The graph shows that prevention and support services were overfunded by 21% and 6% respectively. Improving quality of life and the mitigation of socioeconomic impact were underfunded by 4% and 23% respectively.

Figure 3.5: Comparison of donor expenditure on HIV/AIDS and KNASP financing estimates, 2004/05 (%)

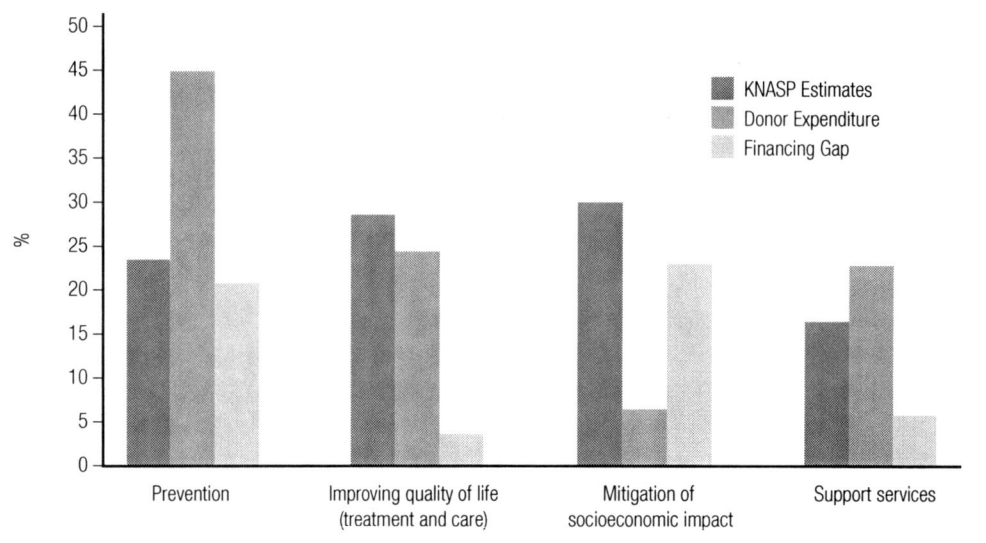

Sources: MoH,2005, HIV/AIDS Public Expenditure Review; MoH-Global Fund Accountability Statement for the period 1 July 2005 to 31 December 2005; NACC, various statements of income and expenditure; UNAIDS, Kenya Office; UNDP, 2004

Donor HIV/AIDS Expenditure on Prevention by Function (2004/05)

Table 3.9 presents the allocation of HIV/AIDS expenditure by function. Of the total foreign HIV/AIDS resources for prevention purposes, "other prevention" accounted for the largest proportion of funding, 37.8% (US$25.8 million), followed by abstinence and being faithful (14.1%), PMTCT (10.9%), VCT (10%) and behavioural change programmes (6.6%). The largest contribution came from bilateral organisations. The share of government contribution for prevention interventions amounted to US$9.3 million, with the largest share being spent on behaviour change and abstinence interventions.

Donor HIV/AIDS Expenditure on Prevention by Target Population (2004/05)

Of the donor THAE, 65.8% was spent on activities targeting the general population, mainly (13.9%) for awareness campaigns for women attending reproductive health (RH) clinics, with 8.9% being spent on creating awareness and condom distribution among commercial sex workers and their clients. PLWHA and formal activities targeting formal-sector employees received 5.4% and 3.9% respectively. Table 3.10

shows that the amount of US$65.9 million is lower than the amount given in Table 3.9. As noted earlier, it was not possible to track all the flows from sources to beneficiaries. The data in Table 3.10 shows only those funds that could be tracked up to the beneficiary level.

Table 3.9: HIV/AIDS expenditure on prevention by function and source, 2004/05 (US$ millions)	
Function	%
Mass media	0.4
Community mobilisation	6.0
Voluntary counselling and testing	10.0
Programmes focused on sex workers and their clients	5.4
Harm reduction programmes for injecting drug users	0.1
Workplace activities	1.2
Prevention programmes for people living with HIV/AIDS	3.2
Condom social marketing	1.7
Prevention of mother–to–child transmission	10.9
Blood safety	0.7
Post-exposure prophylaxis	1.6
Safe medical injections	0.4
Behaviour change	6.6
Abstinence and Be Faithful	14.1
Other prevention	37.8
Total	100
Sources: MoH, 2005, HIV/AIDS Public Expenditure Review; MoH-Global Fund Accountability Statement for the period 1 July 2005 to 31 December 2005; NACC, various statements of income and expenditure; UNAIDS, Kenya Office; UNDP, 2004	

Table 3.10: Prevention expenditure by target population, 2004/05		
Beneficiary	Amount in US$ (million)	Percentage of total
General population	43.3	65.61
Sex workers and their clients	5.9	8.94
Injecting drug users	0.1	0.15
Formal sector employees	2.6	3.94
People living with HIV, but not diagnosed with AIDS	3.6	5.45
Women at reproductive health clinics	9.2	13.94
Victims of sexual violence and health care workers	1.3	1.97
Total	65.9	100
Sources: MoH, 2005, HIV/AIDS Public Expenditure Review; MoH-Global Fund Accountability Statement for the period 1st July 2005 to 31st December 2005; NACC, various statements of income and expenditure; UNAIDS, Kenya Office; UNDP, 2004		

HIV/AIDS EXPENDITURE ON TREATMENT BY TARGET POPULATION (2004/05)

Of the total amount of donor funding for HIV/AIDS treatment and care, 62% was spent on ART, while treatment of opportunistic infections, laboratory monitoring and palliative and home-based care each respectively accounted for 8.2%, 3.6% and 14.2%. Expenditure on treatment and care and nutritional support each respectively accounted for 9.3% and 3%. As noted earlier, a significant proportion of donor funding for HIV/AIDS is channeled directly to specific programmes implemented mainly by NGOs, civil societies, government ministries and/or intermediary organisations. That part of donor funding earmarked for home-based care is allocated directly to the NGOs/CBOs providing home-based care. Also, the GoK, through the Ministry of Home Affairs, disburses funds to families caring for orphans.

Figure 3.7 shows the total donor funds allocated for treatment and care by source. As noted above, five categories of expenditure on treatment and care exist. The largest share of funds for antiretrovirals and palliative care comes from USAID, while the nutrition associated with ART is supported by the WFP. The figure further shows that the Global Fund supports HIV/AIDS-related laboratory monitoring. Though the government contributes to treatment and care, how much is unknown.

Figure 3.6: Breakdown of HIV/AIDS spending on treatment and care, 2004/05

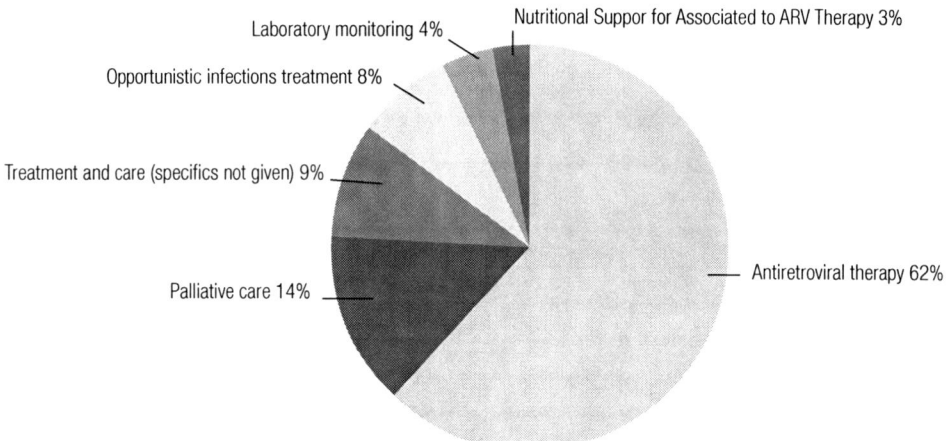

Sources: MoH, 2005, HIV/AIDS Public Expenditure Review; MoH-Global Fund Accountability Statement for the period 1 July 2005 to 31 December 2005; NACC, various statements of income and expenditure; UNAIDS, Kenya Office; UNDP, 2004

HIV/AIDS EXPENDITURE ON THE MITIGATION OF SOCIOECONOMIC BY FUNCTION (2004/05)

Funds for the mitigation of socioeconomic impact fall into three categories:
- the funds transferred to NGOs/CBOs and FBOs by donors and those disbursed by NACC;

- the funds transferred to households through the Ministry of Home Affairs to families taking care of orphans; and
- the funds transferred to the provincial health departments for OVC support.

In 2004/05, approximately US$10.7 million was spent on the mitigation of socio-economic impact of HIV/AIDS, with approximately 64% (US$6.8 million) coming from USAID. The largest share of this amount (73%) was spent on OVC support education, while 19% was used to support families caring for orphans. While the expenditure on income-generating activities accounted for 5%, community support for OVC activities and human rights received 2% and 1% respectively.

Figure 3.7: Distribution of mitigation expenditure by function, 2004/05

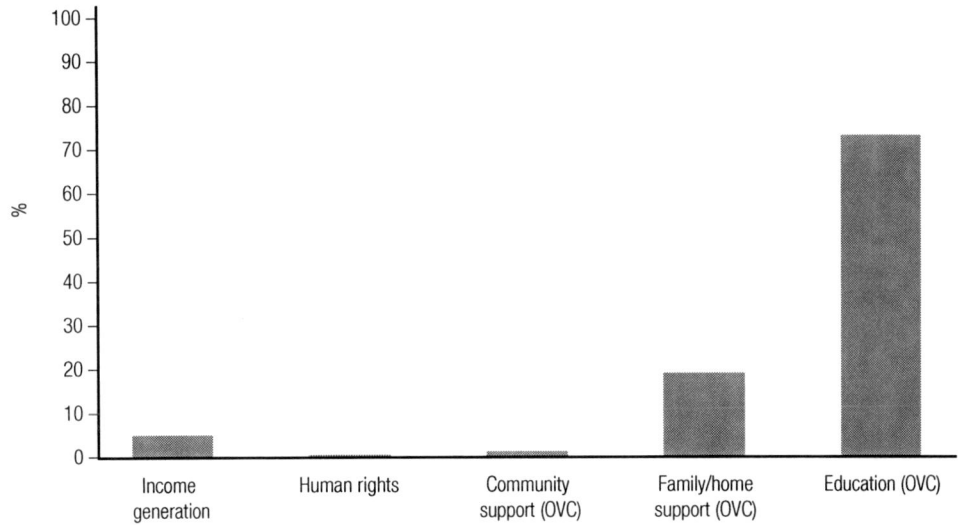

Sources: *MoH, 2005, HIV/AIDS Public Expenditure Review; MoH-Global Fund Accountability Statement for the period 1 July 2005 to 31 December 2005; NACC, various statements of income and expenditure; UNAIDS, Kenya Office; UNDP, 2004*

THE FLOW OF HIV/AIDS EXPENDITURE THROUGH THE NATIONAL AIDS CONTROL COUNCIL

In line with the mandating of NACC with the coordination of the national strategic response, as outlined in the strategic plan 2005–2010, the council has coordinated the disbursement of on-budget and off-budget funds to various implementing organisations. Between FYs 2001/02 and 2004/05, NACC received a total of US$57.07 million, of which donors contributed a major portion (85%). The WB contributed 74.5% of the total funding channeled through NACC, followed by the UNDP (4%) and the Global Fund (6%). Though donor funding is important for the national response, public funding should form the primary source of finance. The need for public funding arises due to many preventive services comprising public goods (e.g.

IEC). Government commitment to the fight against the epidemic should be reflected in the amount of resources allocated to HIV/AIDS. Figure 3.9 presents a summary of the donor flow of funds to NACC.

Figure 3.8: NACC HIV/AIDS expenditure by source of funding

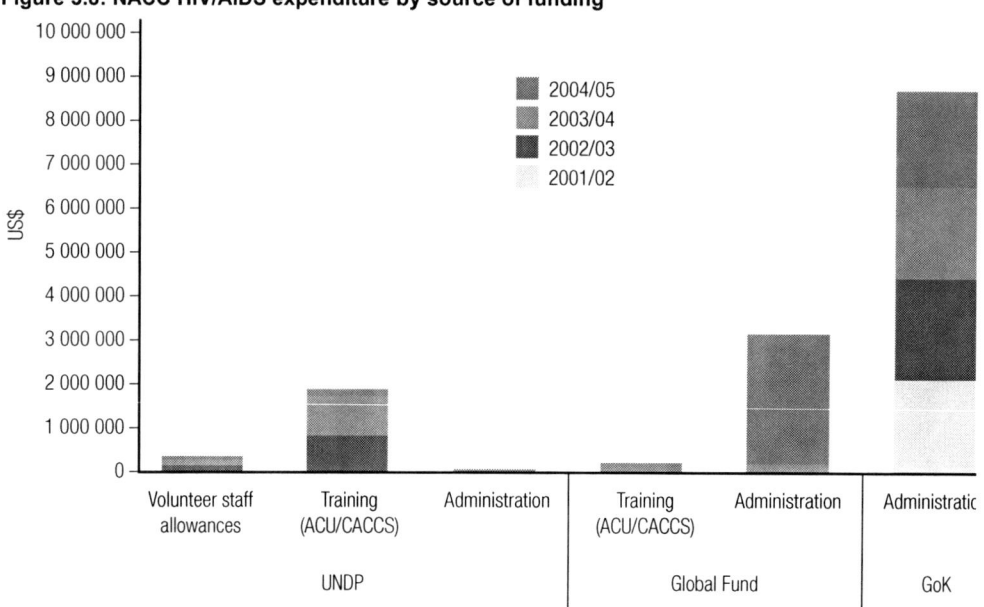

THE ABILITY/CAPACITY TO SPEND HIV/AIDS RESOURCES (EFFICIENCY)

As noted earlier, NACC coordinates and finances community/household-based HIV/AIDS initiatives as part of the national response. In FYs 2001/02–2004/05, such funds were disbursed through CBOs. Of the KES 2 363.4 million committed for disbursement by NACC to the CBOs, approximately KES 1 857.2 million had been spent by the end of FY 2004/05, with KES 506.2 million unspent by the end of that FY. Of the funds earmarked for the CBOs operating at the national level, only 8% were spent by the end of FY 2004/05. Nyanza province was the least efficient in terms of spending, with 4.2% of the HIV/AIDS funds unspent by the end of FY 2004/05, followed by the Coastal province (4%), the Rift Valley province (3.2%) and the Western province (3%). North Eastern province, which has the lowest rate of HIV/AIDS prevalence in the country, spent almost all of its funds committed for that year.

Such variations in HIV/AIDS-related expenditure might either be linked to NACC's delay in disbursing funds or to the lack of capacity of civil societies to meet the requirements set by NACC. Though NGOs and FBOs have contributed to the national response, numerous challenges hinder the efficient disbursement and spending of resources earmarked for HIV/AIDS at the lower levels. Most of such institutions lack systems and functional structures to support the disbursement of funds to CBOs and the efficient spending of HIV/AIDS funds.

EFFICIENCY IN HIV/AIDS SPENDING BY COMMUNITY-BASED ORGANISATIONS AND NON-GOVERNMENTAL ORGANISATIONS

Figure 3.9: Percentage of HIV/AIDS funds unspent by CBOs and NGOs

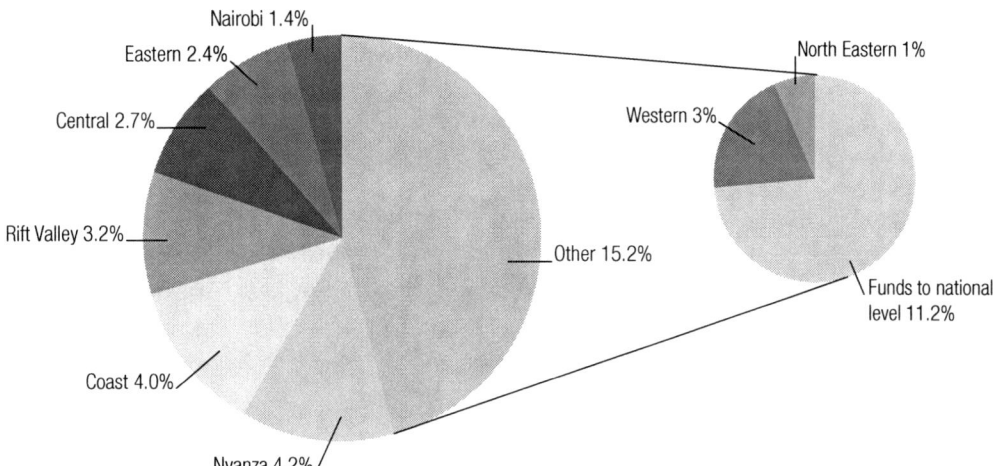

PROCESSES, STRUCTURES AND OBSTACLES IN SPENDING

As noted earlier, the existing institutional framework of the multisectoral response is expected to facilitate the flow of financial resources and to minimise duplication, to facilitate synergy across programmes and to allow for cross-pollination of ideas. However, the disbursement of funds, either through on-budget or off-budget support, is likely to create challenges that may result in inefficient spending. The study findings revealed that the following factors might be contributing to such inefficiency.

LOW ABSORPTIVE CAPACITY AMONG IMPLEMENTERS, ESPECIALLY AT LOWER LEVELS

Some development partners have expressed concern at the low absorptive capacity of implementing agencies receiving funding for the HIV/AIDS response. A key concern is the lack of human capacity, infrastructure development and expertise in development programmes intended to meet the targets set in the KNASP and its subsequent Joint Programme Review reports, especially at the lower levels at which CBOs and some NGOs receive financial support.

Furthermore, some international NGOs have only disbursed and spent money with great care, fearing the irrational use of resources where capacity is lacking or in cases in which compliancy, accountability and the transparency of the recipient CSOs appear inadequate.

In addition, where the financing mechanism or arrangement for the flow of resources is based on reimbursable expenditure, the problem of lack of cash flow to be spent in advance was also found to be a bottleneck in the utilisation of resources by some NGOs. Such a bottleneck contributed to the slow disbursement of resources by some key partners, especially where contractual arrangements were made on the basis of the reimbursement of expenses incurred in agreed programmes of work (PoWs) and expenditure by results-oriented activity.

Logistical Challenges to the Flow of Funds

As indicated earlier, the NRE shows how much has been disbursed to priority areas of the National AIDS Strategic Plan. However, issues of delineation of financial resource flows at lower levels remain a major challenge. Once funds are disbursed to NGOs and CBOs, their use must be monitored to ensure that the resources are used in accordance with the agreed priority areas. Unfortunately, the mechanism for ensuring that this happens is either ineffective or has not yet been instituted, though NACC has finalised an M&E framework that will not only capture data relating to technical outputs, but also on the resource flow. Notwithstanding, the capacity-building process envisaged is long overdue.

Most development partners provide data that is not disaggregated into specific functions or target populations, making it difficult to track the flow of resources using NASA. Moreover, some development partners found it difficult to provide information on delineated allocated funds according to the priority areas or in broad areas contained in NASA, given that some of their support for Kenya comes through their contribution to the GFATM. Similarly, some international development partners fund the CBOs and NGOs directly, so that it is difficult to track the resources. A significant number of CBOs and NGOs surveyed were reluctant to disclose their HIV/AIDS expenditure data.

Duplication of Reporting of Resource Flow

The issue of the duplication of reporting on financial flow has been cited as a major impediment, especially for a central-level organisation with multiple levels of implementation or multiple implementing partners. Such a hindrance has been recognised in the NRE as a major issue. Efforts should be taken to minimise the duplication of reporting through joint reviews at national level and by the decentralisation of M&E systems. Developing and standardising financial reporting tools by means of participatory processes involving all stakeholders is key.

Under-reporting is also a major issue emanating from the sensitivity of budgets and funds received by CBOs and other implementing agencies. While some CBOs were able to disclose both their budgets and the amount that they received from donors and NACC, others withheld crucial information from the study team. Under-reporting also resulted in only a few CBOs being included in the sample.

TRANSPARENCY AND ACCOUNTABILITY

The current research was complicated by numerous instances of incomplete, and sometimes conflicting, data. The increased level of funding for HIV/AIDS from multiple sources presents a major challenge with regard to transparency and accountability in the flow and utilisation of resources. The government and development partners have tried to ensure that any concerns about institutional transparency and accountability are adequately addressed.

NATIONAL PRIORITIES VERSUS "POPULAR" ISSUES

The issue of prioritisation has been cited by a number of development partners as a critical one, due to the tendency to shift resources from one priority area to another in response to whatever is popular. The advent of ART received substantial attention, and therefore financial resources, resulting in fears that the issue of prevention might be neglected. Even within the ART programme, most resources are spent on the provision of drugs, with little attention being paid to strengthening the systems and laboratory support, including monitoring drug sensitivity in order to avoid the emergence of drug resistance.

Notwithstanding issues associated with the lack of effective coordination, commitment by all the partners and government officials, such as the ACU heads, is critical to effective implementation. Improvements are needed, particularly in regard to financial management and staffing, so that absorption capacity and efficiency can be enhanced. In the absence of an impact analysis, reviewing the outcomes of expenditure is impossible.

CHALLENGES IN RELATION TO COMMUNITY FINANCING

NACC coordinates and disburses community/household-based HIV/AIDS initiatives as part of the national response to HIV/AIDS. The disbursement of funds, channeled through CBOs has enabled NACC to empower communities and increase grassroots involvement in the continued war against HIV/AIDS. Since 2002, NACC has funded over 1 000 projects in various ministries, CBOs, NGOs, FBOs and private-sector organisations.

The survey findings revealed major challenges in measuring and documenting the resources disbursed to such organisations, as well as in measuring the output of the activities implemented by the CBOs, in terms of what difference they make to the prevention, care and support services in contributing to the national targets. No system yet exists to generate priority and impact-disaggregated data from the lower levels of implementation in the community.

OVER-RELIANCE ON EXTERNAL DONOR FUNDING

The fight against the HIV/AIDS epidemic relies heavily on external donor funds for most of its programmes. Few organisations visited were resourced by domestic sources. However, the Kenya AIDS NGOs Consortium, the Kenya Network of Women with AIDS, and Women fighting AIDS in Kenya have undertaken fund-raising. The ACUs rely heavily on funding from the KHADRE Project under NACC, with domestic funding mainly covering personnel and infrastructure costs. Such organisations prioritise prevention advocacy, the care and support of PLWHAs and activity-related commodity supply.

EQUITY OF BUDGET ALLOCATIONS FOR HIV/AIDS INTERVENTIONS

The current analysis of equity in the financing of HIV/AIDS-related budget allocation is based only on WB KHADREP allocations, because donor funding is, in most cases, not disaggregated by province, age or gender. Notwithstanding such a limitation, assessing such equity using WB funding channelled through NACC as a case study is possible. The study found that Nyanza province accounts for the largest share of total funding, amounting to 19.4% of the HIV/AIDS resources, followed by the Rift Valley with 15.8%, Central province with 13.7%, and Nairobi province with 13.3%. Coastal province received the least share of total funding, amounting to 5.6%.

Figure 3.10: KHADREP/MAP HIV/AIDS allocation by province, 2000–2005 (KES million)

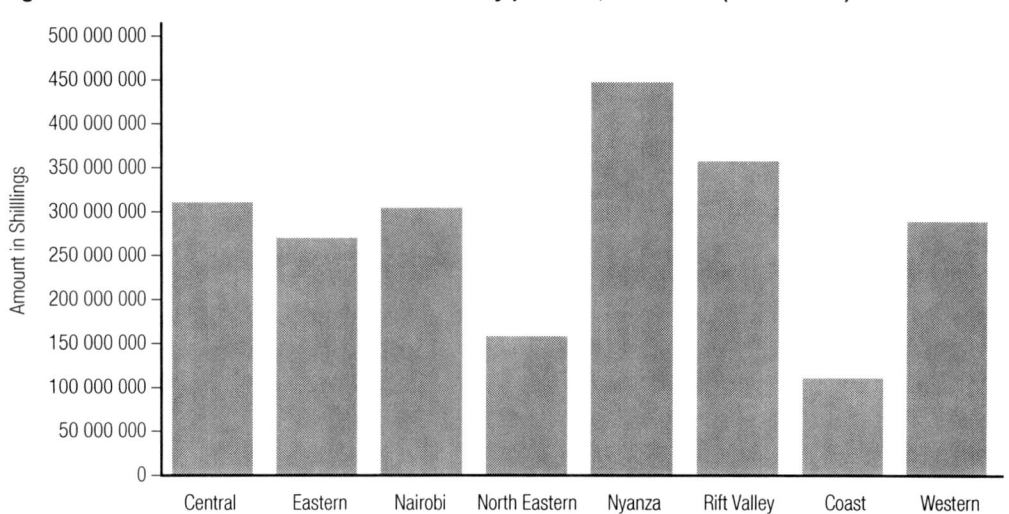

Source: KHADREP, 2000–2005. www.worldbank.org/operation/disclosure

The WB allocation is consistent with the HIV prevalence only in some provinces. For instance, Nyanza, with the highest prevalence, received the largest share (19.4%) of the funding. The Rift Valley, with a prevalence of 5.3%, received more (15.8%) than Nairobi province (13.3%), with a prevalence of 9.9%. Paradoxically, North Eastern province, with almost nil prevalence, received more than Coastal province. The situation reflects the inequalities in the distribution of donor financing. The emerging picture indicates that the allocation of funds does not necessarily address the epidemiological needs experienced. The problem is also underlined in the KNASP 2005/06-2009/10, which calls for strengthening of equity in financing the fight against HIV/AIDS.

Figure 3.11: Equity in HIV/AIDS resource allocation (%)

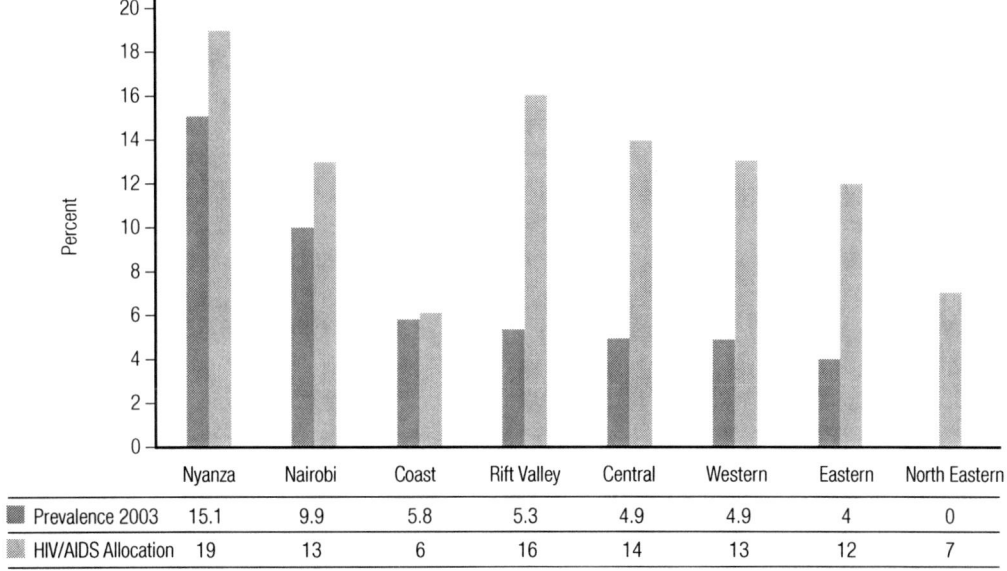

	Nyanza	Nairobi	Coast	Rift Valley	Central	Western	Eastern	North Eastern
Prevalence 2003	15.1	9.9	5.8	5.3	4.9	4.9	4	0
HIV/AIDS Allocation	19	13	6	16	14	13	12	7

Sources: KHADREP, 2000–2005; NASCOP, 2003

Though the HIV/AIDS expenditure analysis by level of disease burden gives some insight into sufficiency and equity considerations in resource allocation across provinces, it should be treated with caution. This is because it neither takes into account HIV/AIDS spending from other sources, nor includes the off-budget support to CBOs and NGOs, which receive funds directly from international development partners.

CONCLUSION

Since the declaration of AIDS as a national disaster by the GoK in 1999, substantial amounts of financial and human resources have been committed and disbursed by government, development partners, local organisations, communities and the private sector. However, information on the flow of such resources from the sources of finance to HIV/AIDS service providers is not centralised, helping to induce a environment that fosters duplication of effort by different actors. Some of the challenges detracting from the efficient and effective use of HIV/AIDS funds further include low absorptive capacity, and the lack of effective financial and M&E systems. While the Kenyan possession of a costed strategic plan is commendable, consistency between priorities and the budgets is necessary.

REFERENCES

Ayieko, M.A., 1997. *From Single Parents to Child-headed Household: The Case of Children Orphaned by AIDS in Kisumu and Siaya Districts*, Study Paper No. 7, New York: UNDP.

Central Bureau of Statistics (CBS), Kenya, 2005. Ministry of Planning and National Development. Economic Survey 2005, Nairobi, Kenya.

Cohen, D., 1992. *The Economic Impact of the HIV Epidemic*, Issue Paper No. 2, New York: UNDP.

Cohen, D., 1999. *The HIV Epidemic and the Education Sector in Sub-Saharan Africa*, Issue Paper No. 32, New York: UNDP.

Cohen, D., 1999a. *Responding to the Socio-Economic Impact of the HIV Epidemic in Sub-Saharan Africa: Why a Systems Approach is Needed*, New York: UNDP.

Enos, H.N., Njeru, and Kioko, U., 2004. *The Impact of HIV/AIDS on Primary Education in Kenya.*

Enos, H.N., Njeru, P.M. and Nguli, M.N., 2004. *Gender Aspects in HIV/AIDS Infection and Control in Kenya.*

Government of Kenya (GoK), 2003a. *Development Estimates, 2003/2004*, Nairobi: Government Printer.

Government of Kenya (GoK), 2003b. *Economic Recovery Strategy for Wealth and Employment Creation, 2003–2007*, Nairobi: Government Printer.

Government of Kenya (GoK), 2003c. *Kenya Demographic and Health Survey, 2003.* Nairobi: Government Printer.

Government of Kenya (GoK), 2003d. *Kenya Demographic Survey, Ministry of Planning and National Development: Preliminary Report*, Nairobi: Government Printer.

Government of Kenya (GoK), 2004. *Estimates of Recurrent Expenditure of the Government of Kenya, 2004/05.* Vol. II (Votes R15–R46), Nairobi: Government Printer.

Government of Kenya (GoK), 2005a. *CBS Geographical Dimension of Well-Being in Kenya. Who and Where are the Poor? A Constituency Level Profile*, Vol. II, Nairobi: Government Printer.

Government of Kenya (GoK), 2005b. *Estimates of Development Expenditure of the Government of Kenya, 2005/06*, Nairobi: Government Printer.

Government of Kenya (GoK) and UNICEF, 2002. *Impact of HIV/AIDS on Education in Kenya and Potential for Using Education in the Widest Sense for Prevention and Control of HIV/AIDS.*

Human Development Report, 2003. *Millennium Development Goals: A Compact among Nations to End Poverty*, New York: Oxford University Press.

Kenya National AIDS Control Council, 2006. Assessment of the Socioeconomic Impact of HIV and AIDS on Key Sectors in Kenya. Nairobi.

Kioko, U. and Enos H.N., 2004. *Funding the Fight against HIV/AIDS: Budgeting for HIV/AIDS in Developing Countries,* Guthrie, T and Hickey, A (eds), Cape Town: Idasa.

Ministry of Finance, 2003. *Development Estimates, 2003/2004,* Nairobi: Government Printer.

Ministry of Finance, 2006. *The Medium-term Budget Strategy Paper, 2006/07–2008/09,* Nairobi: Government Printer.

Ministry of Health, 2001. *Background Projections, Impact Interventions and Policy,* 6th edn., National AIDS and STDs Control Programme.

Ministry of Health and National Council for Population Development, Ministry of Planning and National Development, 1998. AIDS in Kenya: Background Projections, Impact Interventions. National AIDS and STDs Control Programme.

Ministry of Health HIV/AIDS, 2005. *Prevention and Care Programme: Coordination of the Response to HIV/AIDS,* Strategic Paper Series, No. 2., Nairobi: Government Printer.

Ministry of Health and National Council for Population Development and Ministry of Planning and National Development, 1998. *AIDS in Kenya: Background Projections, Impact Interventions,* National AIDS and STDs Control Programme, Nairobi: Government Printer.

Ministry of Planning and National Development (MoPND), 2003. *Kenya Demographic Survey preliminary report,* Nairobi: Government Printer.

National AIDS Control Council (NACC), 2002a. *Financing Framework for the HIV/AIDS Strategic Plan,* March, Nairobi: Government Printer.

National AIDS Control Council (NACC), 2002b. *Report of Technical Group 5: Planning, Finance and Budgeting,* Nairobi: Government Printer.

National AIDS Control Council (NACC), 2003. *Report on the Implementation of the Kenyan National HIV/AIDS Strategic Plan,* Office of the President, Nairobi: Government Printer.

National AIDS Control Council (NACC), 2005. *The Kenyan National HIV/AIDS Strategic Plan, 2005–2010: A Call to Action.*

Over, M., 1999. "The Public Interest in a Private Disease: An Economic Perspective on the Government Role in STD and HIV Control", in K.K. Holmes et al (eds) *Sexually Transmitted Diseases,* McGraw Hill.

PRSP 2001–2004: *Kenya Macroeconomic Evolution Since Independence,* Nairobi: Government Printer.

UNDP, 2004. *Kenya Human Development Report, 2003,* UNDP.

UNICEF, 2006. *Annual Report: PEPFAR – Support for the Prevention and Control of HIV/AIDS within the Context of Maternal and Child Health (MCH) Programmes in North Eastern Province of Kenya,* UNICEF.

World Bank (WB), 1997. *Confronting AIDS: Public Priorities in a Global Epidemic: Summary,* Washington, DC: World Bank.

World Bank (WB), 1999. Intensifying Action against HIV/AIDS in Africa: Responding to a Development Crisis. Africa Region. Washington, D.C.: The World Bank.

Malawi

Gwaza, J.B. and Hamela, G.C.

Executive Summary

This report represents a synthesis of the study that was undertaken as an initiative underlined by multiple interests and ideas about the most appropriate methodology for arriving at objective conclusions about how HIV/AIDS resources in Malawi have been managed.

The specific objectives of the analysis consisted of the following:
- To quantify total allocations for HIV/AIDS interventions;
- To document the flow of funds from sources of finance through providers to beneficiaries;
- To outline and describe the distribution of total allocations and expenditure on HIV/AIDS functions/activities and by providers;

- To evaluate efficiency and equity in the allocation of resources among various functions and levels of care; and
- To make recommendations to policymakers based on the findings obtained.

The report has therefore endeavoured to highlight to what extent people have benefited from such resources, mainly sourced from the Global Fund to Fight HIV/AIDS, TB and Malaria (GFATM), of which the members are also keen to know how efficient and effective the initiatives they finance are. The report also presents the general background to HIV/AIDS in Malawi, in terms of historical trends, prevalence, the link between HIV/AIDS and poverty, and the impact of HIV/AIDS at the national and household levels. The report further acknowledges the work of the National AIDS Commission (NAC) as a national coordinating body for all multisectoral responses to HIV/AIDS activities in Malawi.

The report provides an overview of the National HIV/AIDS Policy developed by NAC, whose objectives are:

- To prevent HIV infections;
- To improve the delivery of prevention, treatment, care and support services;
- To mitigate the impact of HIV/AIDS on individuals, families and communities;
- To reduce individual and societal vulnerability to HIV/AIDS through the creation of an enabling environment.
- To strengthen the multisectoral and multidisciplinary institutional framework aimed at coordinating and implementing HIV/AIDS programmes in the country.

Further, the study revealed a decline in HIV prevalence in the semi-urban and urban areas of the country, where prevalence among antenatal clinic attendees aged 20 to 24 years decreased from about 30% in 1999 to 16% at the semi-urban sites, and from 25% to 19% at the urban sites. In contrast, the study shows that prevalence is increasing at some rural sites. However, the causal relationship between HIV/AIDS, economic performance and poverty remains ambiguous, due to the empirical evidence, which has shown that poverty can be a cause, as well as a consequence, of HIV/AIDS. Further, poverty is known to drive those in high-risk groups, such as sex workers.

Empirical evidence from their study has shown that 47% of HIV/AIDS funds were spent on public health and prevention services, ranging from MK702 million in 2002/03 to MK1.18 billion in 2003/04. MK2.91 billion (US$ equivalent) was earmarked for HIV/AIDS in 2004/05, accounting for 39% of all HIV/AIDS expenditures in that year. More HIV/AIDS resources in Malawi were managed in the public sector; with the Ministry of Health (MoH), and NAC in particular, managing 37%, 42% and 75% of total HIV/AIDS spending in 2002/03, 2003/04 and 2004/05 respectively. NAC alone accounted for 11%, 25% and 57% of total HIV/AIDS funds. HIV/AIDS allocations have risen dramatically from 2002 to date, from MK2.54 billion in 2002/03 to MK7.53 billion in 2004/05, largely due to a steep increase in donor HIV/AIDS support disbursed through the GFATM. Donor allocation as a proportion of the total HIV/AIDS contribution was particularly high at 76% in 2003/04, due to an MK1.97 billion donor purchase of antiretroviral drugs, which were utilised in both 2003/04 and 2004/05. Nonetheless, external funding is expected to increase until 2011, due to GFATM Fifth Round commitments. Other bilateral donors, such as DFID and the Canadian International Development Agency (CIDA), have also increased their expenditures and commitments.

The following are the recommendations that can be drawn from the study:

1. NAC and other key stakeholders, including the MoH, need to institute policy and initiate campaigns encouraging employers to increase their spending on HIV/AIDS-related workplace programmes in areas of condom distribution, voluntary counselling and testing (VCT), the provision of antiretrovirals, and the treatment of opportunistic infections;

2. NAC should reconsider funding priorities to ensure that the Treasury uses a fairer proportion of HIV/AIDS funds to finance health systems strengthening, in particular the treatment and care of patients with OIs, in addition to public health and the prevention and mitigation of the disease. Huge expenditures on the administration of HIV/AIDS activities must be reduced. Bureaucratic administrative channels for the disbursement and management of HIV/AIDS need to be abolished in order to reduce the administrative costs, freeing up more funds to reach those who are the real beneficiaries, particularly women. A balance is required between the need to account and to disburse efficiently.

3. The Malawi government ensures that adequate resources are made available by establishing locally driven financing services and also by making sure that resources are used effectively, equitably and efficiently.

BACKGROUND

Resources for funding HIV/AIDS initiatives are sourced from various governments, and private and international institutions. International funds have been increasingly committed by bilateral and multilateral institutions to HIV/AIDS responses in Africa, with the international focus largely falling on how the resources are being used in terms of efficiency, equity and effectiveness. Though many resources are earmarked for HIV/AIDS initiatives, the ability of the implementing organisations to absorb all of the funds has been placed under the spotlight. Evidence has shown that implementing organisations lack sufficient financial, project management and human capacity.

The national technical working group set up to undertake the assignment agreed to use a modified model of National Health Accounts (NHA) to track, among others, HIV/AIDS resources. The composition of the technical team was drawn from civil society, the government and donors, including the MoH; NAC; the Malawi Economic Justice Network (MEJN); Action Aid International Malawi; UNAIDS/Malawi; WHO/Malawi; UNDP/Malawi; Idasa; SIDA; the Office of the President and Cabinet (OPC) HIV/AIDS Unit; and the USAID-funded PHRplus. The latter provided the overall technical support in conjunction with WHO/Malawi. The CSOs within this group also agreed to undertake a special review and analysis of the raw data and the conventional NHA report in order to develop a so-called "parallel CSO report". The parallel report will be used as an advocacy tool to influence HIV/AIDS financing policy, and to promote accountability and transparency in the allocation of HIV/ AIDS resources at all levels.

SOCIOECONOMIC BACKGROUND

Malawi is a landlocked country south of the equator in the south-eastern tip of Africa. The population of Malawi was estimated to stand at 12 757 883 in 2006 (NSO Projections Report, 1999–2023). The population is largely young, with 43.6% aged between 0 to 14 years and 46.7% aged between 15 to 49 years. Between 2000 and 2004, the estimated annual population growth was 2.25% (UNFPA, 2005, State of World Population 2005). Geographically, the country is divided into three regions: the Northern, Central, and Southern regions, whose populations are 12.5%, 40.9%, and 46.6%, respectively. The major cities are Lilongwe, the capital; Blantyre; Mzuzu; and Zomba. According to the 1998 census, the population comprised 51% men and 49% women. Approximately 85% of the Malawian population live in rural areas.

The economy of Malawi, which is a member of both the SADC and Common Markets for Eastern and Southern Africa (COMESA), is predominantly agricultural, with maize being the staple crop. Agriculture accounts for 40% of GDP and 88% of export revenues. The main export products are tobacco, tea and sugar. Other contributors to the GDP in Malawi are construction (4%); distribution (11%); transport and communication (5%); financial and professional services (6.5%); private, social and community services (6.5%); and government services (4%). The economy largely depends on substantial inflows of economic assistance from the Bretton Woods Institutions (IMF and the WB) and individual donor nations. Nonetheless, the Malawi government is struggling to develop a full-scale market economy, to build alternative and cheaper international transport routes, to improve the country's infrastructure, including educational facilities, to address environmental problems and to deal with the HIV/AIDS epidemic.

Child mortality is 103 per 1 000 live births, with there being more than a million orphans, 700 000 of whom have been made orphans because of HIV/AIDS. According to the Malawi government estimates, 14.2% of the population is HIV-positive, with 90 000 deaths in 2003 resulting from AIDS. Life expectancy in Malawi is 41.75 years for men and 41.2 years for women.

GENERAL ACCESS TO HEALTH SERVICES

Malawi has a network of health facilities belonging to the government, the private sector and religious institutions. About 85% of the population lives within 10 km of a health facility. The facilities range from small dispensaries on estates and in rural areas to large hospitals in the big cities. In 2002, 843 health facilities were estimated to exist in the country, of which more than 50% were health centres, being either dispensary or maternity units.

MoH has the largest number of health facilities, accounting for 46.5% of the total number of health facilities in Malawi, followed by the Christian Health Association of Malawi (CHAM), with 19.2%. Firms form the third largest provider, accounting for 14.9%, with the private-for-profit accounting for 11.7% of the total health facilities. Though Malawi has a network of health facilities, a JICA/MoH inventory in 2002 found that only about 9% of the government and mission health facilities were capable of providing the Essential Health Package (EHP) on site (Calcon, 2003), with each district having only one or two facilities with adequate EHP capacity. The service deficits arise from the lack of health workers, supply stock-outs, and a lack of basic utilities (specifically water, electricity, telephone services and radio communication systems) (Calcon, 2003).

The Budget Process in Malawi

Formulation of a budget using the output-based MTEF involves the setting up of objectives, activities and outcomes, whereas an incremental approach involves making allocations based on the previous year's allocations. However, in practice, Malawi has continued to use the latter approach, though to a lesser extent, with a greater tendency towards employment of the output-focused budget.

The budget cycle involves the preparation, legislation and implementation of the budget and auditing. During the preparation stage, the MoF sends out guidelines to ministries and other implementing agencies for preparing the budget. The implementing agencies are then expected to prepare estimates, which are discussed and consolidated into draft budget books, which are discussed in Parliament during the Parliamentary budget sessions. The documents discussed include the output-based document, the detailed budget, the budget statement by the Minister, and the economic report. Once satisfied, Parliament then approves the budget through the Committee of Supply. The Appropriation Bill then passed by Parliament finally provides the authority to implementation agencies to start spending. The expenditures have continuously to be monitored by the implementing agencies and the National Audit Office. Thereafter, the end-of-year accounts, which are compiled by the Accountant-General, are consolidated and discussed by the Public Accounts Committee to review any issues to do with the expenditures.

The NAC and CSOs are consulted during the pre-budget discussions about the budget. However, questions on the level and depth of discussion between the government and civil society groups exist, no matter whether their input is taken on board or not. The major challenge is that, besides being consulted by the ministries, the CSOs only monitor the implementation of the budget, and are not involved in all the stages of the budget cycle. The CSOs have the capacity to analyse the macroeconomic policies and budgets, and to assess how they respond to people's needs.

The budget process is rendered sufficiently transparent through Treasury instructions, and the Public Finance Management Act. However, the enforcement of such legal instruments is inadequate. For instance, what happens to a Permanent Secretary if s/he does not exercise prudent financial management is debatable. Government does not have the legislation in place to punish offenders. However, accountability has greatly improved due to prudent fiscal management, with the legal instruments and institutional structures for enforcing such being in existence. However, the main problem is that neither the populace nor civil societies are clear about their roles in budget formulation and in making government accountable to them. Notable improvement has been registered in terms of accessibility of the budget documents to the general public. However, there is still more room for improvement. As most people do not understand the content of the documents, due to their unwieldy nature and their consisting largely of numerous figures, the documents need to become more user-friendly.

HIV/AIDS in Malawi

History and Trends

Since the first AIDS case was identified in Malawi in 1985, HIV has spread to all parts of the country, with HIV prevalence increasing sharply from 1995 to 1999. The primary mode of HIV transmission in Malawi has been unprotected heterosexual intercourse, and, therefore, as with other countries in the region, the sexually active population has been the most affected. Since 1999, the prevalence levels have remained high, ranging between 15.0% in 1999 and 14.0% in 2005, with women being more affected than men. Of the 790 000 infected adults aged 15–49 years in 2005, 58% were women. Overall, 930 000 PLWHAs were estimated to exist in Malawi in 2005.

The Malawi Demographic and Health Survey (MDHS) (2004) found the HIV prevalence to be higher among women (13%) than men (10%) in 2004, with the HIV prevalence being higher in urban areas (17%) than in rural areas (11%). HIV prevalence tends to be higher among young women (9%) aged 15–24 years, compared with young men (2%) in the same age group.

Table 4.1: National HIV/AIDS estimates, 2005	
National adult prevalence: 15–49 years	14.0%
Number of infected adults: 15–49 years	790 000
Number of infected adult women: 15–49 years	440 000
Number of infected urban adults: 15–49 years	240 000
Number of infected rural adults: 15–49 years	550 000
Number of infected children aged 14 years and less	83 000
Number infected over age 50 years	59 000
Total HIV-positive population	930 000
New AIDS cases (all ages)	96 552
Annual AIDS deaths (all ages)	86 592
Adults needing ART	137 371
Children (0–14 years) in need of ART	49 965
Source: MoH (2005a)	

HIV Prevalence Trends

HIV prevalence is declining in the periurban and urban areas of the country, with the prevalence levels among antenatal clinic attendees aged 20 to 24 years decreasing from about 30% in 1999 to 16% in the semi-urban sites,[53] and from 25% to 19% in the urban sites.[54] Some of the sites that were found to show a decline in prevalence among young women were those located in Blantyre, Mchinji, Nkhata Bay and Nsanje. NSO 2004 found that HIV prevalence was highest in the Southern Region, followed by the Northern Region. Results from the HIV sentinel sites show that prevalence is declining in most of the urban sites, though it is increasing in some rural areas.

Figure 4.1: HIV prevalence among pregnant women aged 15–24 years

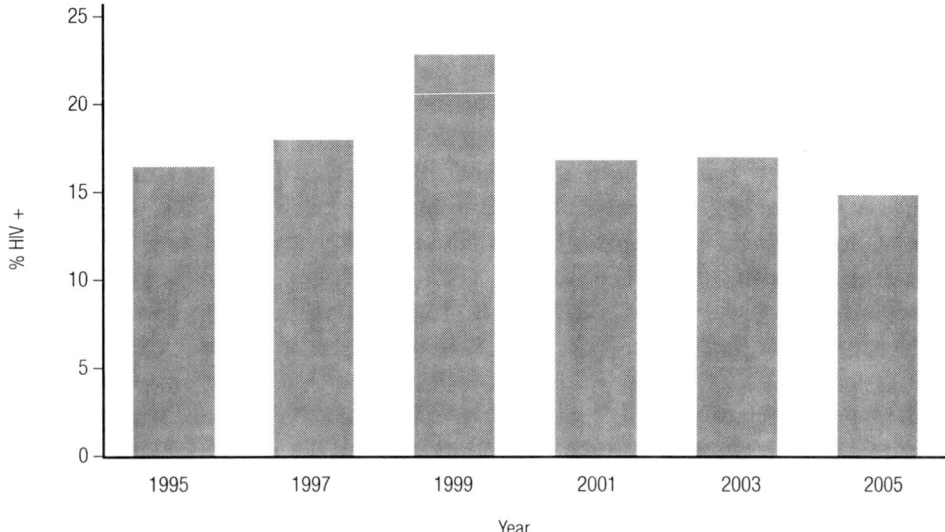

Source: NHA, 2006

HIV/AIDS and Poverty

The causal relationship between HIV/AIDS, economic performance and poverty is ambiguous, due to the empirical evidence showing that, not only can poverty cause HIV/AIDS, but that HIV/AIDS can cause poverty. In Malawi, the evidence on the link between HIV and wealth is inconclusive. Though the poverty level tends to be higher among the rural population, HIV prevalence rates tend to be higher among the urban population. The Central Region has the lowest poverty incidence and the lowest HIV prevalence. Ivaschenko and Montana (2005) also proved that the high level of poverty in the Central and South regions of Malawi is positively related to the HIV prevalence rates in the districts. The regressions showed that an increase in the share of people living below the poverty line in the district is associated with a 1% and 8% higher probability of being HIV-positive in the Central and South regions respectively.

124

Poverty is more likely to be a driving factor for the spread of HIV, especially among high-risk groups, such as prostitutes. A qualitative study of the relationship between food insecurity and HIV/AIDS showed that women in villages near Lilongwe exchanged food for sexual favours due to hunger, lack of employment opportunities, and poverty (Bryceson and Fonseca, 2005). Migrant labour is also associated with a higher risk of HIV infection, as Obare (2006) showed that those MDICP3 survey respondents whose partners usually stayed away from home were significantly more likely to be HIV positive than those whose partners usually resided at home.

Figure 4.2: Distribution of HIV/AIDS and poverty

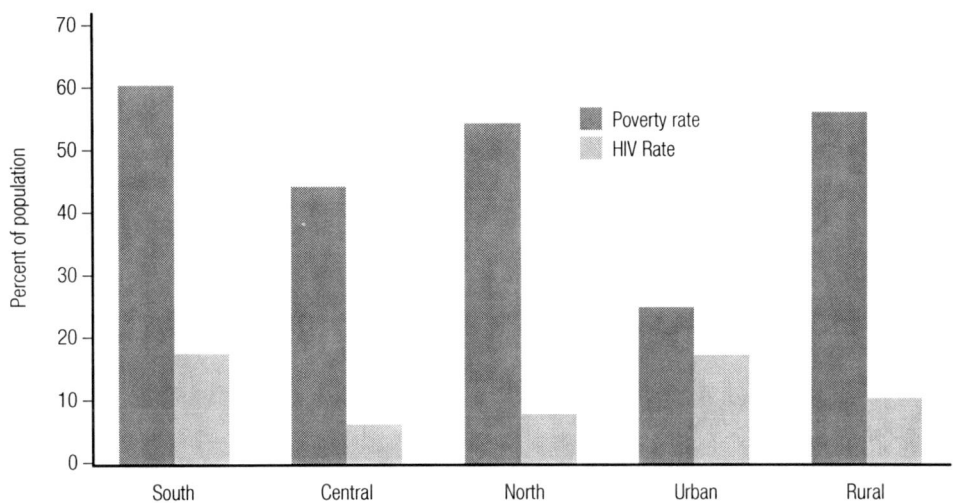

HIV/AIDS AND HOUSEHOLD ASSETS

HIV/AIDS-related illnesses are severe and devastating over several months before death. Due to the high cost of caring for such patients, households sometimes have to sell most or all of their household assets before the death of the infected person. Funeral costs are also very high, with 14% reporting losing some assets or land after the death of a household member (see Table 4.2). A larger proportion of the poor (17%) lost land after experiencing such a death than did those who were relatively more well off (13%). Conditional to experiencing such loss, the average value of lost land/assets was MK21 648 in 2006. On average, the poor who experienced the death of a PLWHA in the household lost MK15 703, while the non-poor who experienced a similar death lost an average of MK27 616. Such losses were found to amount to 24% for the poor and 22% for the non-poor of the household's total annual expenditures. The losses associated with prime-age deaths are of higher average value (more than three times) than those associated with the deaths of economically dependant household members. In households experiencing a male PLWHA death, the amount of land lost by the household was found to be almost 1.5 times as much as that lost by households that lost a female PLWHA (MK24 329 and MK16 234, respectively).

Table 4.2: Asset and land losses related to deaths in 2004/05							
	All	Household with PA death			Household with other, non-PA death		
		Non-poor	Poor	All	Non-poor	Poor	All
Percentage of households losing assets/land	9.3	12.8	16.6	14.4	8.7	5.0	7.1
Among households with any loss:							
Value of land/ assets lost (MK)	13 654	27 616	15 703	21 648	8 145	3 308	6 629
Loss (% annual household expenditure)	14.9	21.9	24.2	23.1	8.3	6.4	7.7
Source: National Statistical Office, 1HS2							

The National HIV/AIDS Response

Brief History of Malawi's Response to the HIV Epidemic

National Policy Coordination and Programme Planning

Following the emergence of the HIV/AIDS epidemic in the mid-1980s, the government of Malawi instituted strategies aimed at controlling its spread. Such strategies included the establishment of the NACP within the MoH in 1989. The Cabinet Committee on Health and HIV/AIDS was also formed to provide policy and political direction to the MoH.

In 1996, the government and its partners evaluated the national HIV/AIDS response. Some of the major findings of the evaluation included:
- Insufficient coordination of planning, implementation and M&E of activities of various agencies;
- The granting of insufficient institutional support to the NACP; and
- Over-reliance on the health sector for the national response.

To improve the multisectoral planning, implementation and coordination of HIV/AIDS activities, the government of Malawi established the NAC within the OPC in July 2001, replacing the NACP. A Board of Commissioners, comprising representatives from government, NGOs, faith-based organisations, PLWHAs, youth organisations and the private sector, oversees NAC operations. Initially, the NAC reported to the OPC through the Minister for Presidential Affairs and to the Cabinet Committee on HIV/AIDS. Currently, NAC reports to the OPC through the Principal Secretary for Nutrition (HIV/AIDS). The Board of Commissioners meets on a quarterly basis to review progress. NAC management reports to the Board of Commissioners, which is expected to meet on a monthly basis to discuss programme management issues.

NAC works closely with the Malawi HIV/AIDS Partnership Forum, founded in 2005, which advises:
- The NAC Board, and the Inter-Faith HIV/AIDS Association coordinating faith organisations;
- The Business Coalition against HIV/AIDS for the private sector; and
- The Department of Human Resource Management and Development, which coordinates the public sector responses and the umbrella bodies of the PLWHAs.

Since 1985, when the first AIDS case was identified, the country lacked an HIV policy to guide the national response. The National HIV/AIDS Policy, which was developed in 2004 through a consultative and participatory process, was launched in November of that year by the former head of state. The policy is innovative in many areas, such as HIV testing, where it is directing attention away from VCT to routine testing for all women attending antenatal clinics, the diagnostic testing of patients, and the mandatory testing for blood and organ donors.

STRATEGIC PLANS

In 1989, the Ministry of Health and Population developed a five-year Medium-term Plan (MTP-I), for the years 1989 to 1993, to guide the implementation of HIV/AIDS activities, which mainly focused on blood screening, fostering HIV/AIDS prevention through public awareness, and establishing an infrastructure for epidemiological surveillance. In 1993, a review of the MTP-I showed that much progress had been made, especially with regard to the implementation of HIV screening programmes for blood transfusions and HIV/AIDS-related awareness. However, the review noted, among other things, a lack of emphasis on the care and treatment of PLWHAs.

The second MTP (MTP-II), for the years 1994 to 1998, addressed some of the weaknesses that had been detected in the MTP-I. However, in 1996 a subsequent evaluation of the national HIV/AIDS response found that, despite a high awareness of HIV/AIDS, behaviour change had been limited and the rate of HIV incidence continued to increase. Malawi clearly needed to develop a comprehensive five-year plan to guide HIV/AIDS prevention, treatment and impact mitigation.

In response to the recommendations of the evaluation, in 1999 the National Strategic Plan (NSF) was developed through a highly participatory process involving a wide range of stakeholders in HIV/AIDS activities. The former President of Malawi launched the NSF, which covered the period 2000 to 2004, in October 1999, at which stage he also declared HIV/AIDS a national emergency. The main themes in the NSF were:
- Prevention, advocacy and behaviour change;
- Treatment, care and support;
- Sectoral mainstreaming;
- Impact mitigation; and
- Surveillance and monitoring.

The NSF also emphasised the need for the active participation of various stakeholders, including the private sector and teaching institutions, in the design, implementation, and monitoring of multisectoral and multidisciplinary HIV/AIDS interventions in the country. In 2003, the NAC developed the Strategic Management Plan (SMP), an implementation plan for the NSF covering FYs 2003/04 to 2007/08. The SMP was based on rolling annual work plans, the first of which was for FY 2004/05.

THE HIV/AIDS POLICY

Throughout the 1980s and 1990s, Malawi lacked a clear national HIV/AIDS policy for guiding the implementation of HIV/AIDS-related activities. However, after the development of the NSF, the process of developing the National AIDS Policy started in 2000 to guide the implementation of the NSF. The following areas were identified as requiring policy recommendations:
- The multisectoral approach;
- Human resources;
- HIV testing;
- Gender and HIV/AIDS;
- Sex and sexuality;
- Condom use;
- The biomedical response; and
- Legal and ethical issues.

To ensure that the policy was evidence-based, various studies were commissioned to identify issues and solicit recommendations in the eight different policy areas. In addition, a Multisectoral Policy Advisory Committee (MPAC) was formed to guide the process of policy development. The initial draft policy was presented to various community groups to develop an understanding of HIV/AIDS policy issues, to build consensus, and to seek input. Forums were conducted with parliamentarians and politicians, FBOs, youth organisations and leaders, civil society organisations, government ministries and traditional leaders, healers and birth attendants. The policy drafting team reviewed and synthesised comments from the consensus and advocacy activities for presentation to the MPAC. Based on MPAC guidance concerning the comments, a new draft of the policy was compiled and submitted to the Cabinet for approval. The National HIV/AIDS policy, which was finalised in 2004, was launched by the former president of Malawi in November 2004.

MEDIAN AGE OF SEXUAL DÉBUT

A modest increase in the median age of sexual début occurred among those aged 20 to 24 years between 2000 and 2004: from 17.1 to 17.4 years among females and from 17.7 to 18.1 years among males. Among urban young women aged 20 to 24 years, the median age at first sexual intercourse increased from 17.8 years in 2000 to 18.1 years in 2005, with the change being smaller in the rural areas (17.0 to 17.2 years).

Across the regions, the Southern region recorded a minimal increase in the median age of first sexual intercourse, compared with the significant increases made in the Northern and Central regions.

PRIMARY ABSTINENCE

Levels of primary abstinence (comprising the percentage of youth aged 15 to 19 years abstaining from sex) do not vary widely between the genders. Between 2000 and 2004, during which period abstinence among young women aged 15 to 19 years increased from 42.7% to 47.8%, a similar increase occurred among males aged 15 to 19 years from 38.9% to 47.7%. Abstinence among young women significantly increased in the urban areas and among the more educated (those with secondary or higher education). However, the proportion of those abstaining remained stable in the rural areas and among the less well educated.

Figure 4.3: Percentage of celibate youths aged 15–19 years (2000-2004)

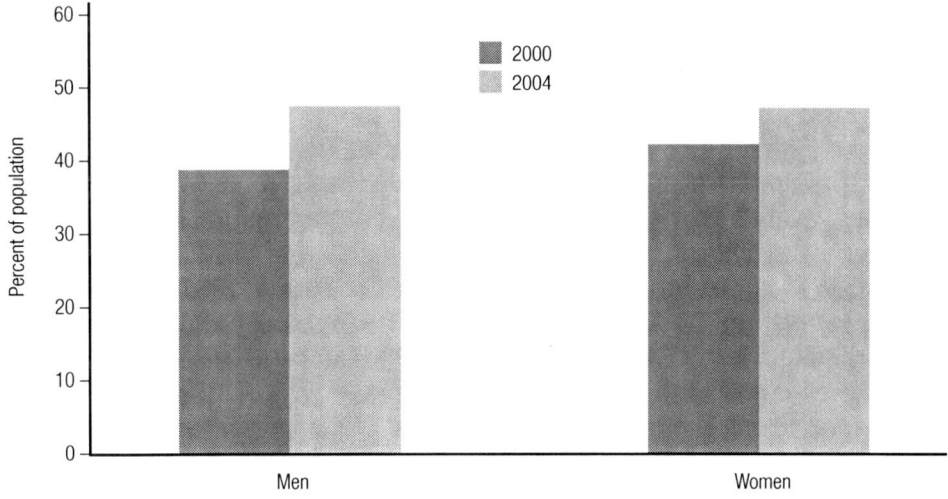

Source: UNAIDS (2006). Malawi HIV/AIDS Monitoring and Evaluation Report, 2005/06.

In 2004, the proportion of men having sex with two or more partners was highest in the Northern (19.4%) and Central (12.4%) regions, compared with the Southern region (9.5%). The practice of having sex with multiple partners was highest among men in the rural areas (12.4%) compared with those in the urban areas (9.7%). Overall, the proportion of men having sex with multiple partners decreased from 33% in 2000 to about 12% in 2004, with a dramatic decrease among male youths, from 56% in 2000 to 13% in 2004. A similar decrease occurred among female youths aged 15 to 24, from 16.4% to 1.7% over the same period.

FINANCING AND REPORTING MECHANISMS

HIV/AIDS funds originate from funding sources, which allocate the funds to the FAs, who act as intermediaries. The FAs then allocate the funds to service providers, who then implement the HIV/AIDS-directed activities. In some cases, the FA can also act as a service provider, and a FS can also be a FA. Since 2002/03, the major HIV/AIDS controller/manager has been the public sector (in particular, the MoH and NAC) at 52.2%, 42% and 75%. NAC alone accounted for 11%, 25% and 57% of the total HIV/AIDS funds.

MoH and NAC funds were received both from the MoF and donors. MoF funding to the MoH for HIV/AIDS flows through its annual allocation to the approved health budget, while donor financing to the MoH flows through their funding of the HIV/AIDS vertical programmes and the HIV/AIDS Unit at the MoH. Internationals transfer almost all their HIV/AIDS-related funding through NAC; for this reason, the role of NAC as an FA (controlling institution) for HIV/AIDS funds has increased dramatically.

The private sector, which is mainly composed of firms, CHAM, local NGOs and households, and international donors and NGOs, alternated as the second largest manager of HIV/AIDS funding during the period under review, apart from FY 2003/04, when donors were the major FAs, providing 47% of the Total HIV/AIDS Expenditure (THAE).

The latter scenario resulted from the GFATM funding the procurement of antiretroviral drugs through UNICEF, which distributed the drugs to various health care providers during both 2003/04 and 2004/05. Donor and international NGO financing and control of extensive expenditures for HIV/AIDS raises serious issues of sustainability unless in-country capacity (in particular the Central Medical Stores) for planning, budgeting and the procurement of antiretroviral drugs and drug distribution is built simultaneously. That is, the direct handling of large HIV/AIDS resources by funding agencies is commendable for the short term, but the national human and institutional capacity to gradually assume antiretroviral management responsibilities is needed in the long term.

Though not so high as in some other countries, household direct out-of-pocket spending by PLWHAs is still the major private sector FA of HIV/AIDS resources in Malawi. Such spending accounted for 28%, 29% and 35% of the total private sector spending in 2002/03, 2003/04 and 2004/05, respectively. Despite the cost of ART being highly subsidised in 2002/03 (MK2 500 per month) and antiretrovirals being made freely available since then from many different donor-funded NGOs/CBOs aiming to alleviate the financial plight of those affected and infected by HIV/AIDS, many PLWHAs continue to pay for their health care, accessing private facilities, the private wings of public hospitals, and those outpatient departments that charge user fees.

Involvement with such costs may be due to the fact that NAC funding for NGOs/CBOs is mainly spent on prevention, and public health and mitigation interventions, such as VCT, information, education and communication (IEC), sexually transmitted infections (STI), prevention, and care for orphans and vulnerable children. The funding does not cover personal needs, such as the treatment of OIs and other related health-care services, such as laboratory fees, X-rays and admissions to the private wings of public facilities. PLWHAs might also regard public services as inferior than private services, leading them to rely on private-for-profit and CHAM facilities, which charge fees. Whatever the reason for such high out-of-pocket expenditure, such spending dissuades the very poor and vulnerable from utilising needed health care and/or pushes them still further into poverty. Broadening the support needed to supply PLWHA needs would entail the provision of transport to health-care facilities and ensuring that they receive free ART and subsidised treatment of OIs from designated centres. Furthermore, employers, whose workforce is seriously affected by HIV/AIDS, need to increase the funding of their workplace programmes to ensure that PLWHAs can obtain health-care services without the latter having to pay out of their own pockets.

The government, which, at the time of going to press, was finalising the domestication of the Paris Declaration, has developed a Development Assistance Strategy (DAS). The DAS will:

- Promote national ownership by linking all development activities to the Millennium Development Goals (MDGs);
- Align donor fundings with the MDGs;
- Harmonise development partner support; and
- Manage results and mutual accountability through annual MDG reviews and Joint Country Programme Reviews.

RESOURCE MOBILISATION AND UTILISATION

Malawi has mobilised resources from multilateral and bilateral donors for managing the national response to HIV/AIDS, about two-thirds of which are channeled through NAC. In April 2004, NAC engaged a Financial Management Agency (FMA) to administer the HIV/AIDS Grants Facility, in order to facilitate the uptake of grants by implementers at all levels and to build the capacity of district assemblies to co-ordinate district-level responses. NAC engaged five international NGOs as umbrella organisations armed with clear terms of reference to mobilise district-level responses to HIV/AIDS and to coordinate district-level proposals and projects from the local CBOs, FBOs, and NGOs. The operation of this initiative has since been evaluated and the report disseminated.

The Malawi government has committed itself to contributing annually approximately US$2 million to NAC for the fight against HIV/AIDS. In addition, approximately 2% of the annual budget for each ministry/department line is expected to be allocated to HIV/AIDS interventions, while 60 to 70% of the MoH budget is dedicated to the support of HIV/AIDS-related interventions.

In the FY 2005/06, the government allocated MK210 968 487 (US$1 634 671) directly to NAC for the HIV/AIDS response, an increase from its FY 2004/05 allocation of MK108 231 900. However, such amounts are insufficient to allow the government to sustain the HIV/AIDS national response. The NHA and AIDS Accounts Survey indicated a total expenditure of MK7 527 323 449 billion on HIV/AIDS for the FY 2004/2005. Of this total, HIV/AIDS health expenditure amounted to MK6 254 069 140. The survey revealed that in FY 2005/06, the government contributed only 20% of the total HIV/AIDS funds, amounting to about MK1 505 464 690. Donors were the major financiers of HIV/AIDS programmes, accounting for 73% of the total expended on such, while private sector funding amounted to only 7%.

By end June 2006, a total of MK3.6 billion had been disbursed to various interventions, MK2.2 billion through the grants facility. Of this, MK837.9 million was disbursed to the five umbrella organisations. The NGOs constituted the largest share of the disbursed grants, accounting for MK415.5 million in the FY under discussion. Other beneficiaries of the grant disbursements in the same FY were the public sector, education and training institutions, FBOs and the private sector, the latter receiving only a very small proportion of the total amount. Until the National Health Account (NHA) report, no comprehensive data had existed on the financial resources available in Malawi by year for HIV/AIDS funding, let alone on the use of such funding by the different stakeholders concerned with this field.

SOURCES OF HIV/AIDS FUNDING IN MALAWI

HIV/AIDS allocations have risen dramatically from 2002 to date, from MK2.54 billion (US$29 million) in 2002/03 to MK7.53 billion (US$69 million) in 2004/05. Such an increase has largely been due to a steep rise in donor HIV/AIDS support through the GFATM. As already stated, donor allocation as a proportion of the total HIV/AIDS contribution was particularly high (76%) in 2003/04, due to an MK1.97 billion donor purchase of antiretroviral drugs, which were utilised during both 2003/04 and 2004/05. External funding is expected to increase until 2011 due to the GFATM Fifth Round commitments. During Phase 1, Malawi is expected to receive US$7 708 331 for OVC, amounting to a total of US$19 104 775, as well as US$65 419 162 for the reinforcement of health systems. Round 1, Phase 2 for HIV/AIDS will consume US$137 169 342 for the period 2006 to 2008. Other bilateral donors, such as DFID and CIDA, have also increased their allocations and commitments.

Most of the HIV/AIDS funds are contributed by development partners. The amount of donor support has increased through the GFATM. Of the total HIV/AIDS funding for the period under review, external financiers contributed 46% in 2002/03, 76% in 2003/04 and 80% in 2004/05. The public sector (MoF) is the second largest source of HIV/AIDS funding, contributing 26% during the period 2002 to 2005. Households contributed 7% in 2002/03, dropping to 3% in 2003/04, before increasing to 5% in 2004/05. The most likely explanation for the lower household contribution is the absence of user fees in public health facilities, in particular in the case of MoH and CHAM, who own 40% and 19% respectively of all health-care facilities in Malawi.

INSURANCE AND EMPLOYER SCHEMES

Various initiatives, such as HIV/AIDS workplace programmes, insurance contributions, and medical aid paid by employers, contributed an average of 4% of the total HIV/AIDS spending throughout the period under review. Such a contribution is very low, bearing in mind that employers are the hardest hit by HIV/AIDS in Malawi and that HIV/AIDS is threatening to disrupt their productivity, and hence the profitability of the entire economy.

GOVERNMENT

Before the disbursement of the GFATM, the government contribution in FY 2002/03 was almost comparable to the donor contribution, standing at 41% and 46% respectively. Soon after the GFATM disbursement, the government contribution fell by 22% in FY 2003/04. The reasons for such a fall are not clear. However, possibly due to the availability of GFATM funding, the government decided to shift its resources to other priority activities and let the GFATM resources suffice for the funding of most HIV/AIDS-related activities.

Figure 4.4: Financing sources for HIV/AIDS-related efforts in Malawi, 2002/03–2004/05

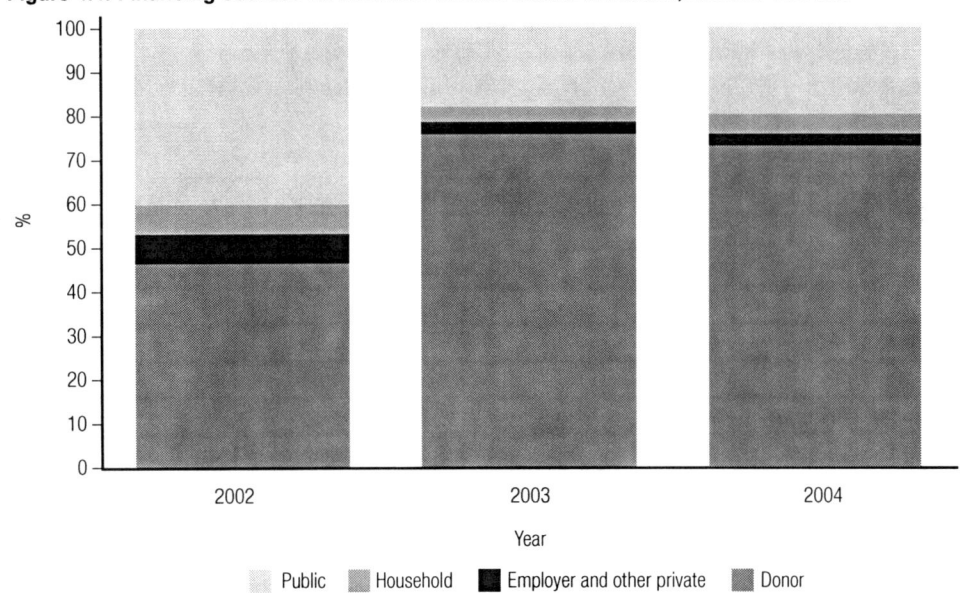

Source: NHA, 2006

Financing Agents of HIV/AIDS Funds in Malawi

Most HIV/AIDS resources in Malawi are managed by the public sector, especially by the MoH and NAC. Such FAs were responsible for 37%, 42% and 75% of the total HIV/AIDS spending in 2002/03, 2003/04 and 2004/05 respectively. NAC alone accounted for 11%, 25% and 57% of total HIV/AIDS funding.

MoH and NAC funds were received from the MoF and donors. Public funds are allocated to the MoH for HIV/AIDS-related activities through its annual health budget allocation, while donor financing of the MoH occurs through its funding of HIV/AIDS vertical programmes and the HIV/AIDS Unit within the MoH. Donors transfer almost all their HIV/AIDS-directed resources through NAC, so that the role of NAC as a controlling institution for HIV/AIDS funds has increased dramatically.

Private Sector, Non-Governmental Organisations and Households

The private sector, which is mainly composed of firms, CHAM, local NGOs and households, and international donors and NGOs alternated as the second largest managers of HIV/AIDS funding during the period under review, apart from FY 2003/04, in which year donors were the major FAs, providing 47% of the THAE.

The latter scenario resulted from the GFATM funding the procurement of antiretroviral drugs through UNICEF, which distributed the drugs to various health-care providers during both 2003/04 and 2004/05.

Table 4.3: Percentage contribution of financing agents to expenditure on HIV/AIDS, 2002/03–2004/05			
Financing agent	Year		
	2002/03	2003/04	2004/05
NAC	11.1	24.6	56.9
Public (excluding NAC)	41.0	17.6	18.5
Private	16.9	8.0	8.4
Household – out-of-pocket	6.7	3.2	4.4
Donor	24.3	46.6	11.8
Source: NHA, 2006			

When donors and international NGOs fund and manage such huge expenditures for HIV/AIDS, it raises serious issues of sustainability where inadequate capacity is not being built in the national institutions responsible for the planning, budgeting and procurement of antiretroviral drugs and their distribution. Thus, while the direct handling of large numbers of HIV/AIDS resources by funding agencies is a commendable solution in the short-term, efforts likely to build both human and institutional capacity should be made, so that the managerial responsibilities for antiretroviral procurement are smoothly transferred to the national institutions, in particular the Central Medical Stores.

Within the private sector, household direct out-of-pocket spending by PLWHAs, though not as high as in some other countries, is still the major FA of HIV/AIDS resources in Malawi, accounting for 28%, 29% and 35% of the total private sector spending in 2002/03, 2003/04 and 2004/05 respectively, despite antiretroviral provision being well subsidised in 2002/03 and freely available from 2003/04. At the time of going to press, despite antiretrovirals being freely administered by public hospitals, people were continuing to pay for their health-care needs using their own funds, when accessing the non-public sector services, central hospital private wings and paying outpatient departments. NAC funding for NGOs/CBOs is mainly designated for prevention and public health and mitigation interventions, such as VCT, IEC, STI prevention and OVCs, and not for personal treatment health needs, such as OIs.

Most public health-care services are characterised by poor working conditions, lack of drugs and dilapidated equipment, resulting in a heavy reliance on private-for-profit and CHAM facilities, which charge high fees for a better services. However the poor are prevented from accessing quality health-care goods and services by the high direct out-of-pocket expenses involved. Apart from funding prevention and mitigation intervention and providing free antiretrovirals, PLWHAs require financial support to cover transport costs to health centres, as well as to cover the costs of having to cope with OIs and other related infectious diseases. Furthermore, employers whose workforce is seriously affected by HIV need to increase funding for their workplace programmes to cover the costs of obtaining free health-care services for PLWHAs.

HIV/AIDS SERVICE PROVIDERS

HIV/AIDS service providers fund the delivery of goods and services to the population, including hospitals and health centres, providing VCT services, IEC and STI prevention services, as well as non-health HIV/AIDS services, including PLWHA support, OVC care and policy advocacy expenditures.

In order to explain the overall provider expenditure pattern, Figure 4.5 shows the expenditure trends in the period under review. There has been a steady decline in HIV/AIDS funding used by both public and private hospitals, from 59% in 2002/03, to 57% in 2003/04, to 35% in 2004/05.

Figure 4.5: Distribution of HIV/AIDS funds by provider type, 2002/03–2004/05

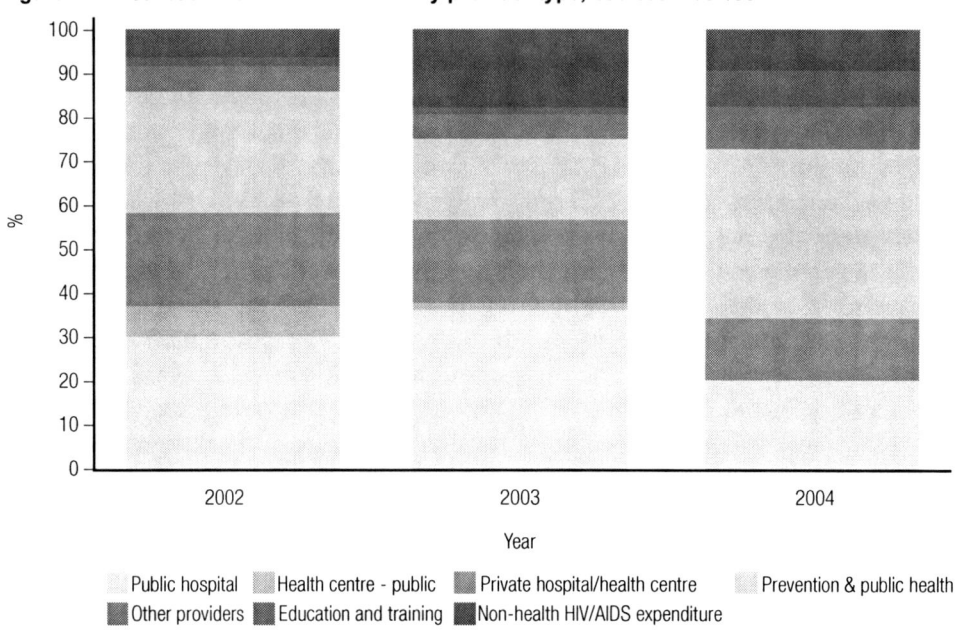

Public hospital   Health centre - public   Private hospital/health centre   Prevention & public health
Other providers   Education and training   Non-health HIV/AIDS expenditure

Source: NHA, 2006

The NHA study revealed that 47% of the HIV/AIDS funds had been spent on public health and prevention services (including IEC, PMTCT and condom distribution), increasing from MK702 million in 2002/03 to MK1.18 billion in 2003/04, with a massive MK2.91 billion being spent in 2004/05, accounting for 39% of all HIV/AIDS expenditure in that year. While health-related education and training accounted for 12%, non-health items (comprising advocacy and care for OVC) accounted for 15%. Only 12% had been spent on treatment and care at district hospitals, with nothing being spent on this area at the central hospitals.

Figure 4.6: Distribution of HIV/AIDS funds by NAC to providers, 2004/05

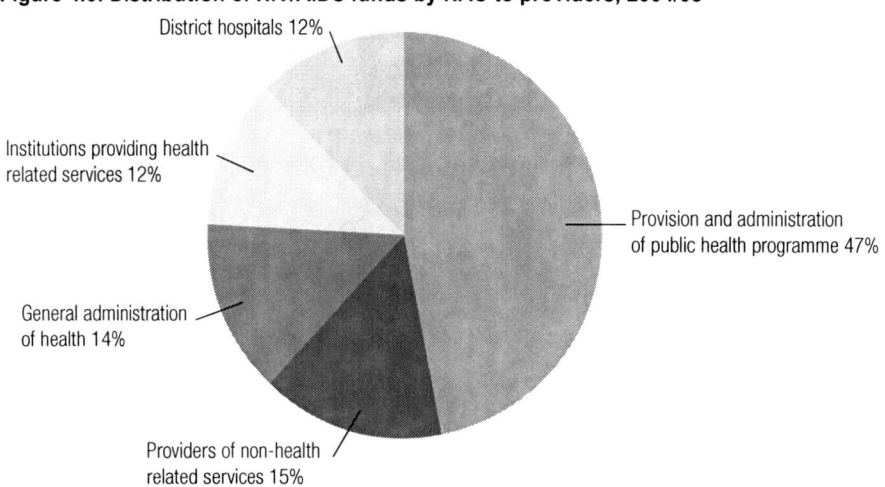

District hospitals 12%

Institutions providing health related services 12%

Provision and administration of public health programme 47%

General administration of health 14%

Providers of non-health related services 15%

Source: NHA, 2006

NAC is responsible for monitoring and documenting the impact of HIV/AIDS expenditure, and for ensuring that it targets those priority areas that can improve the lives of the most vulnerable affected by the HIV/AIDS epidemic. As noted above, despite NAC distributing substantial funding to various NGOs and CBOs, PLWHAs continue to pay high OOPE for health-care needs, thereby bringing into question the effectiveness of the funding modalities and priorities.

Though NAC is recognised as playing a key role in preventing the spread of HIV/AIDS, and in promoting an effective public health system, the sector requires strengthening to provide adequate treatment and care for all PLWHAs. The health systems should be strengthened, especially considering the additional burden that HIV/AIDS imposes on them in terms of the demand for OI-related human resources and drugs. Over 50% of bed occupancy in health facilities in Malawi is estimated to be HIV/AIDS-related. If HIV/AIDS financing continues to crowd out other diseases, inefficiencies in the health system are bound to occur.

NAC spends a great deal on general administration, including MK606 million from 2004/05 to 2005/06. The increased financial support provided by the GFATM and the recruitment of human resources should be combined with the streamlining of its functions, with maximum effort being exerted to stop the spread of HIV/AIDS and to improve the quality of life for those infected and affected by HIV/AIDS.

Figure 4.7: Distribution of PLWHA out-of-pocket funds by provider type, 2005

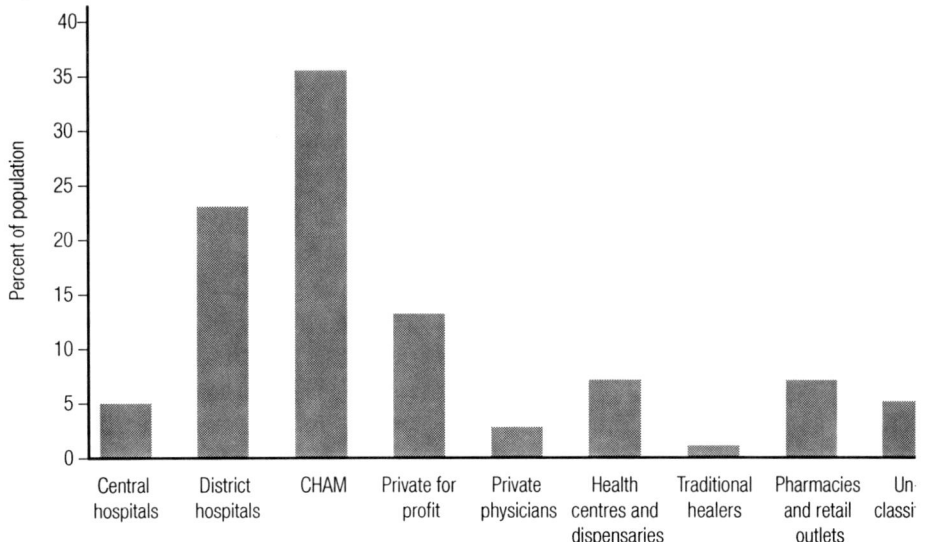

Source: NHA, 2006

The MoH's establishment of service agreements with CHAM facilities is aimed at abolishing user fees for selected services, though the implementation of such a system needs to be done both equitably and efficiently. Such agreements should only be entered into in the absence of a free use MoH facility with adequate capacity within a reasonable distance, entailing an initial targeting of priority interventions, such as: reproductive and child health, ensuring that subsidy levels are comparable between the different CHAM facilities, and avoiding over-subsidisation. A unified and comprehensive contract between the government and the CHAM facility (or any other NGO) as service provider is the best means of ensuring equity and efficiency. Such contracts would cover staff salary subventions from the MoF, the provision of drugs, and ORT-related service agreements, to help ensure greater cohesion in the financing of government and CHAM facilities. Entering into such contracts could also help avert the MoF having to pay salaries to CHAM employees, with CHAM providing additional allowances. Such a financial dispensation causes a flow of health workers away from the free-use government facilities to CHAM, leaving the public-health sector offering free services but unable to meet patient demands due to inadequate staffing. The poor have to visit an MoH facility, unstaffed by a health worker; remain without care; or pay for expensive CHAM services.

HIV/AIDS FINANCING BY FUNCTION/ACTIVITY

As the study reveals, HIV/AIDS allocations have risen dramatically from 2002 to date, from MK2.54 billion (US$29 million) in 2002/03 to MK7.53 billion (US$69 million) in 2004/05. Donor allocation, as a proportion of the total HIV/AIDS contribution, was particularly high, standing at 76% in 2003/04, due to an MK1.97 billion donor purchase of antiretroviral drugs, which were utilised during both 2003/04 and 2004/05. During the same period, external financiers contributed, of the total HIV/AIDS funds, 46% in 2002/03, 76% in 2003/04 and 73% in 2004/05. The MoF is the second largest source of HIV/AIDS funding, contributing 26% during the period 2002 to 2005. The household contribution of 7% in 2003 increased to 5% in 2004/05. The Malawi government has also allocated 2% of the annual ORT budget for each ministry/department to HIV/AIDS interventions, with 60% to 70% of the MoH budget being used to support HIV/AIDS-related interventions.

The NHA and AIDS Accounts Survey indicated a total expenditure of MK7 527 323 449 billion on HIV/AIDS, in FY 2004/2005. Of this total, HIV/AIDS health expenditure amounted to MK6 254 069 140. The survey revealed that in the same FY, the government contributed only 20% of the total HIV/AIDS funds, amounting to about MK1 505 464 690. While donors were the major financiers of HIV/AIDS programmes (73%) during the same period, private-sector funding amounted to 7%. By June 2006, NAC had MK6 751 022 840 committed funds, out of which MK4 484 206 230 had been disbursed since the inception of the grant facility, representing a disbursement rate of 66%.

Table 4.4 shows the cumulative disbursements by intervention area, with 28% of the funds disbursed for treatment, care and support mainly being used for the purchase of antiretroviral and OI drugs, and other health-related products. While 20% was disbursed to fund prevention and behavioural change activities, 24% was disbursed for mainstream activities, the majority of which focused on advocacy and prevention, resulting in 44% of disbursed funds targeting prevention programmes.

Table 4.4: Percentage distribution of total health expenditure by health-care function, 2002/03–2004/05

Health-care function	Year		
	2002/03	2003/04	2004/05
Curative	48.9	54.3	48.3
Rehabilitative	0.8	0.9	1.4
Prevention and public health	27.3	25.2	31.4
Health administration and insurance	13.8	13.0	12.4
Capital formation	0.4	0.9	0.3
Not specified by kind	8.8	5.7	6.2
Source: NHA 2006			

PROGRAMME COVERAGE

Programme coverage has significantly increased since 2001, when structures were put in place to coordinate and implement a multisectoral response to HIV/AIDS, TB and STIs. Due to the country's communication strategy, the general population tends to be well informed about HIV/AIDS, with an increasing number of people going for VCT and fewer engaging in risky sexual behaviour. Improvement in access to ART has also greatly increased the number of people going for HIV testing and counselling. In 2005, about 87 000 people died from HIV/AIDS-related illnesses, resulting in an increased number of orphans. In 2005, Malawi was estimated to have 501 963 orphans (maternal or paternal and dual) as a direct result of HIV/AIDS.

HIV TESTING

Malawi planned to have 190 operational VCT sites in FY 2005/06. By the end of the FY, 250 sites were functioning, supplied with over 1 000 counsellors, about half of whom work only part-time. The sites vary considerably in size, organisational and institutional capacity, and quality. Each district in the country has at least one site offering HIV testing. From 2001 to 2006, the number of sites offering HIV counseling and testing services has steadily increased. Almost 40% of the approximately 620 health facilities in Malawi provided counselling and testing services as of June 2005. Of the 146 sites that were offering counselling and testing services in 2005, only 70 (48%) were located in rural areas. Considering that over 85% of Malawians reside in rural areas, the provision of counselling and testing services has so far been biased towards th urban areas. The challenge for Malawi, therefore, lies in rapidly increasing counseling and testing sites in rural areas.

The number of HIV tests performed at these sites has exponentially increased annually. HIV testing has increased from 40 806 people in 2001 to about 1.9 million by mid-2007. A National HIV Testing Week has become an annual event, with about 100 000 people voluntarily going for HIV testing in 2006. The percentage of youth undergoing voluntary HIV testing increased substantially from 14% in 2005 to 22% in 2006. Despite such achievements, plans are under way to increase the number of VCT sites.

ANTIRETROVIRAL THERAPY

By the end of 2010 it is anticipated that 233 675 people will be in need of ART (UNAIDS 2006). The number of patients started on antiretroviral therapy increased from 6 414 in 2003 to 99 535 by March 2007, with a 12-month survival rate of 80%. In defined populations with good access to ART, substantial decreases in HIV/AIDS morbidity and mortality have occurred. The national ART rollout is under way in almost all districts, with referral and district health being responsible for the distribution of antiretrovirals. The government is now focusing on addressing disparities in access to antiretrovirals across different socioeconomic groups and in rural areas that are more than one kilometre away from the main roads.

CONDOM DISTRIBUTION

In Malawi, condoms are distributed using various channels, including the social marketing agencies, such as Population Services International (PSI) and *Banja la Mtsogolo* (BLM), health facilities (government, mission and private) and NGOs, either from their offices, through peer educators, or from clinics and other distribution points in the impact areas. Over 26 678 144 million condoms were distributed in 2005 and 29 million in 2006. In 2005 PSI and BLM distributed 8 852 949 and 8 328 800 condoms respectively. At least 17 181 749 socially marketed condoms were distributed to outlets in 2005. During the same period, 9 496 395 free government condoms were dispensed to end-users. More socially marketed condoms than free government condoms were distributed in the highly urbanised districts.

The government is trying to improve the dissemination of condom information, distribution and quality assurance by;

- Increasing access for those living in rural areas by employing peripheral outlets;
- Increasing access for wealthier men at acceptable sites (e.g. hotel rooms, restaurants and bars); and
- Enhancing national education campaigns to address misconceptions about condoms.

IMPACT MITIGATION

About 359 000 orphans were provided with some kind of support in FY 2005/06, exceeding a target of 120 000 orphans. The number of organisations caring for orphans and offering home-based care has also increased. By June 2006, 600 CBOs were receiving support from the NAC Grants Facility alone. At least 2 771 households have benefited from a pilot social cash-transfer scheme for Malawi, with a total of 12 686 beneficiaries, of which 36 are child-headed households and 1 819 elder-headed. In FY 2006/07 585 945 OVC received support.

Given the high prevalence of human rights abuse, especially gender-based violence, more than 3 564 victims of abuse, mostly women, were supported in the same year. NAC has also conducted sensitisation meetings on stigma and discrimination with PLWHA organisations and support groups, including the umbrella bodies, NAPHAM and Malawi Network of People Living with HIV/AIDS (MANET). Other civil rights organisations also have intensified sensitisation activities encouraging victims of crimes such as sexual assault to go for testing.

BEHAVIOUR CHANGE

The impact of the national response has been demonstrated by the positive changes made in sexual behaviour between 2000 and 2004, which has seen:
- A decrease in the proportion of men having sex with multiple partners from 33% to 12%;
- A sharp decrease in the proportion of men paying for sex from 21% to 5%;
- An increase in the proportion of male youth using condoms at last high-risk sexual encounter from 47% to 59%; and
- An increase in the age of sexual début among youth aged 15–24 years. The proportion of youth aged 15–19 years abstaining from sex increased over the four-year period from 39% to 48% among boys and from 43% to 48% among girls. Primary abstinence was found to be higher in urban areas and among youth with higher levels of education.

Successful behaviour change depends on several factors, including the type and quality of information that is provided to the population, the means by which that information is disseminated, and related socioeconomic and sociocultural factors. In order to prevent the spread of HIV, the national responses have to excel in behaviour change interventions. In Malawi, nation-wide public education has been successful in this respect. HIV/AIDS awareness was almost universal (99%) in 2004. However, levels of misconceptions were recorded as still being high among young persons aged 15–24 years. According to the 2004 Malawi Demographic Health Survey (MDHS), only 37% of young men and 25% of young women correctly identified major ways of preventing HIV and rejected major related misconceptions.

CONCLUSION

Though Malawi is receiving substantial HIV/AIDS funds from donors, the sustainability of interventions funded in this way if donors pull out is questionable. Consequently, the government should commit more resources from domestic funds.

Given that Malawi is rated among the poorest countries in the world, calls for the greater commitment of the government to the HIV/AIDS cause might appear ill advised. However, the reallocation of the available resources among the various ministries should free up a large share for HIV/AIDS and health in general. Both project and financial management by government departments and HIV/AIDS service providers has limited capacity. Donors have also contributed to the slow pace of disbursement through their strict reporting mechanisms, which delay programme implementation. While strict reporting lines are critical for accountability purposes, a balance should exist between the costs and benefits of such interventions.

REFERENCES

BLM, 2006. *2005 Annual Data*, Blantyre: Banja la Mtsogolo.

Calcon, H., 2003. *Malawi Health Facilities Inventory Survey: Final Report*, Funded by Japanese International Cooperation Agency.

Castro-Leal, F., Dayton, L., Demery, L. and Mehtra, K. "Public Spending on Health Care in Africa: Do The Poor Benefit?", *Bulletin of the World Health Organization*, 78 (1).

Data International Bangladesh, 2006. *Child Health Accounts Report.*

Eholie, S., Nolan, M., Gaumon, A. et al., 2003. "Antiretroviral Treatment Can Be Cost Saving for Industry and Lifesaving for Workers: A Case Study from Cote d'Ivoire's Private Sector".

Eichler, R., 2007. *Can "Pay for Performance" Increase Utilization by the Poor and Improve the Quality of Health Services?* Discussion Paper.

Franco, L., Mtonya, B., Mwase, T. et al, 1995. *Community Financing Experience and Options: A Study to Provide Baseline Information for Ministry of Health Decision-making.* Lilongwe:

Gwatkin, D.R., 2003. Free Government Health Services: Are They the Best Way to Reach the Poor?

Institute for Health Policy Studies and Data International, 2006. *Child Health Accounts Report: Draft*, Colombo.

International Monetary Fund, 2003. *The Impact of HIV/AIDS on the Malawian Economy*, Working Paper, Lilongwe:

Ivaschenko O and Montana L, 2005. *Using Small Area Estimation Techniques to Produce Geographic Profile of HIV/AIDS Prevalence. A Case Study of Malawi.* World Bank.

Ivaschenko and Montana, 2005. Second Integrated Household Survey.

Malawi Centre for Social Research, 2004.

Malawi Economic Justice Network, 2005. *Quality of Health Services Assessment Report*. Lilongwe.

Malawi HIV/AIDS Monitoring and Evaluation Report, 2005–2006. UNAIDS, 2006.

Malawi National TB Control Programme. *Annual Report July 2004–June 2005.* Lilongwe:

McCoy, D., Ratsma, E., and Rowson, M., 2004. *Going from Bad to Worse: Malawi's*

Maternal Mortality. Commissioned by Task Force 4 of the U.N. Millennium Project

Mills, A.J., 1991. *The Cost of the District Hospital: A Case Study from Malawi*, Washington, DC and Lilongwe: World Bank Population and Human Resources Department.

Ministry of Economic Planning and Development, 2002. *Malawi Core Welfare Indicators Questionnaire*, Lilongwe.

Ministry of Economic Planning and Development, 2002. *Poverty Reduction Strategy Paper (PRSP)*, Lilongwe.

Ministry of Education, Science, and Technology (MoEST), 2004. *Education Statistics, 2004.* Lilongwe: Ministry of Education, Science, and Technology.

Ministry of Education, Science, and Technology (MoEST), 2005. *Education Statistics, 2005.* Lilongwe: Ministry of Education, Science, and Technology.

Ministry of Education, Science, and Technology (MoEST), 2005. *Life Skills Study Report.* Lilongwe: Ministry of Education, Science, and Technology.

Ministry of Health (MoH), 1997. *Manpower Development Survey Report*, Lilongwe.

Ministry of Health (MoH), 1999. *Malawi National Health Plan: 1999–2004*, Lilongwe.

Ministry of Health (MoH), 2001. *Malawi National Health Accounts Report.* Lilongwe.

Ministry of Health (MoH), 2002a. *The Malawi Essential Health Package. Annex 3: Summary of February 2002 Dissemination Meetings*, Lilongwe:

Ministry of Health (MoH), 2002b. *National Health Facility Survey*, Lilongwe: Ministry of Health.

Ministry of Health (MoH), 2003. *Sentinel Surveillance Report, 2003.* Lilongwe: Malawi Ministry of Health.

Ministry of Health (MoH), 2004. *Programme of Work.* Lilongwe.

Ministry of Health (MoH), 2005a. *Malawi Public Expenditure Review (PER) – Health Chapter*, Lilongwe: MoH Headquarters.

Ministry of Health (MoH), 2005b. *Emergency and Obstetric Care (EmOc Survey, 2005)*, Lilongwe:

Ministry of Health (MoH), 2005c. *Sentinel Surveillance Report, 2005.* Lilongwe: Malawi Ministry of Health.

Ministry of Health (MoH), 2006a. *HMIS Bulletin: Annual Report, July 2004 to June 2005*, Lilongwe: Malawi Ministry of Health and Population.

Ministry of Health (MoH), 2006b. *Malawi Logistics System Assessment and Stock Status Report*, SLSASSR.

Ministry of Health (MoH), 2006c. *National Health Accounts and HIV/AIDS Resource Tracking Report.*

Ministry of Health (MoH), 2006d. *Report of a Country-wide Survey of HIV/AIDS services in Malawi for the year 2005.* Lilongwe: Malawi Ministry of Health and Population.

Ministry of Health (MoH), 2006e. *Report on ARV Therapy in Malawi – up to June 2006.* Lilongwe: Malawi Ministry of Health.

Ministry of Health and Population (MoH), 1995. *Health Policy Framework Paper.* Lilongwe.

Mwambaghi, F., Mtonya, B. and Manda, J., 1995. *Rural Health Unit Expenditure Study in Lilongwe District.*

Mwase, T.L., 1998. *Health Expenditure and Finance in Malawi: Do Efficiency and Equity Matter?* A study funded by WHO/Malawi and WHO/AFRO. Ministry of Health and Population.

National Health Accounts (NHA), 2006. Report.

National Statistics Office (NSO), 1998. *Population and Housing Census 1998.* Lilongwe.

National Statistics Office (NSO), 2000. *Malawi Demographic and Health Survey, 2000.* Zomba: National Statistical Office.

National Statistics Office (NSO), 2002. *Malawi Demographic and Health Survey, EdData Survey, 2002,* Zomba: National Statistical Office.

National Statistics Office (NSO), 2004. *Malawi Demographic and Health Survey, EdData Survey, 2004,* Zomba: National Statistical Office.

National Statistics Office (NSO), 2005. "Zomba, Malawi and Calverton, Maryland, USA", *Integrated Household Survey 2.* Zomba:

National Statistics Office (NSO), 2005. *Welfare Monitoring Survey.*

National Statistics Office (NSO). *Malawi Demographic and Health Survey, 2004.* Zomba: National Statistical Office.

National Statistics Office (NSO) and Measure/DHS, 2005. *Malawi Demographic and Health Survey 2004: Preliminary Report.*

Planning Unit, Ministry of Health and Population. Lilongwe.

Population, 2003.

PSI. 2005. *PSI Annual Data, 2005.* Lilongwe: Population Services International.

Statistical Office, 2002.

UNDP, 2003. *Human Development Report, Millennium Development Goals: A Compact among Nations to End Human Poverty,* New York: UNDP.

United Nations Development Programme (UNDP), 2005. *Human Development Report International Development at a Crossroads: Aid, Trade and Security in an Unequal World,* New York: UNDP.

Vision 2020, 1999. *The Vision of the Malawi Health Sector in 2020,* Lilongwe: Ministry of Health and Population, Planning Department.

WHO, 2000. *The World Health Report 2000, Health Systems: Improving Performance.* Geneva.

WHO, 2001. *Report of the Commission on Macro Economics and Health,* Geneva.

WHO, 2005. *Designing Health Financing Systems to Reduce Catastrophic Health Expenditure,* Technical Briefs for Policy Makers, No. 2, Department of Health Systems Financing.

WHO, 2006. "Are African Countries Achieving the Abuja Target of Spending 15% of Their National Budget on Health?", *WHO/NHA Policy Highlight,* No. 2/2006.

WHO, 2004. *National Health Accounts (NHA) in Eastern and Southern Africa: A Comparative Analysis.*

World Bank Poverty Net Library. World Bank Seminars, Washington:

World Bank, 2004. *Achieving the Millennium Development Goals for Malawi, 2003/04.*

World Health Organization (WHO),1994. "World Health Forum", *International Journal of Health Development,* 15 (2).

Tanzania

Kessy, F., Mashindano, O. and Kiria, I.

Executive Summary

HIV/AIDS is among the leading cross-cutting challenges to national development in Tanzania. Early cases of HIV/AIDS were reported in the 1980s in Kagera region, but by the turn of the century all administrative regions had been affected, albeit at varying rates. Institutionalised interventions addressing HIV/AIDS in Tanzania started in 1985, with the National AIDS Control Programme (NACP) being established in the same year under the MoH. In 1999, HIV/AIDS was declared a national disaster.

The Economic and Social Research Foundation (ESRF) collaborated with the Youth Action Volunteers (YAV), supported by Idasa, to undertake a study to track the expenditure on HIV/AIDS-related interventions from the source of funds to its beneficiaries, with the aim of establishing whether the allocations were, indeed, reaching the intended beneficiaries. The research employed the National AIDS Spending Assessments (NASA) tool developed by UNAIDS.

The NASA methodology was selected due to its rigour and clarity of thematic focus on resource flow. The methodology asks and answers questions on five key themes relevant to resource tracking, which are further explained below.

Based on the information available, an attempt was made to assess equity in HIV/AIDS spending in Tanzania. The National Multisectoral Strategic Framework (NMSF) emphasises that the protection of health is a basic human right for all Tanzanians, implying that resources ought to be distributed according to the needs of the different beneficiaries. HIV/AIDS prevalence rates could be a useful indicator when assessing the need for, and spatial allocation of, funds.

However, considering the diversity of socioeconomic conditions and challenges faced across the country, focusing on HIV/AIDS alone could make such a comparison unreliable. Therefore, no definite conclusions could be drawn with regard to the equity of HIV/AIDS spending, though the regression results show that urban areas tend to receive more resources than do rural areas.

The regression results also confirm that HIV/AIDS spending plays a positive role in improving health and demographic outcomes. Specifically, the analysis confirms that an increase in HIV/AIDS-related spending could help reduce the under-five mortality rate and help to reduce the number of children under 18 who are orphaned.

The share of health spending in the total budget, although not yet reaching the Abuja commitment of 15% of total government expenditure, has grown, as has the amount of spending on HIV/AIDS interventions. After becoming prioritised under the first Poverty Reduction Strategy (PRS), allocations to the health sector increased from 8.8% in 2000 to 10.6% in 2001 of the total expenditure, excluding the Consolidated Fund Services (CFS). The increase in foreign aid to the government pushed up expenditure for HIV/AIDS in 2004/05 by about 64% to TZS68.1 billion, with the total public sector and non-government expenditure also increasing to TZS80.7 billion (about US$100 million), an important target discussed in the 2003/04 PER for scaling up national HIV/AIDS interventions.

Closer scrutiny of the health spending data also shows that many donor funds and off-budget resources still are not captured by the government exchequer office.

Though NGOs were found to be significant HIV/AIDS service providers, the study identified several institutions at grassroots level that were unable to secure adequate funding for supporting interventions in areas within their vicinity. The extent of dependency on donor funding for HIV/AIDS interventions is very high, which raises concerns regarding the sustainability of interventions in the long term. The curtailing of donor financing could halt some interventions, unless local resources can be mobilised.

SOCIOECONOMIC BACKGROUND

Tanzania is the largest country in East Africa, with a total area of 945 000 square kilometres. According to the Tanzania Population and Housing Census of 2002, the country's population is estimated at 34.5 million people, of whom about 50% are youth and children, and 77% live in rural areas (URT, 2003a).

The majority of Tanzanians are poor, despite some recent achievements in social and economic growth. According to the United Nations Human Development Report of 2005, Tanzania was ranked 164 out of 177 countries surveyed (UNDP, 2005), with the overall adult literacy rate for 15 year-olds and older being 78% for males and 62% for females. Such rates are generally high, with a relatively minor gender differential.

According to the National Mortality Burden Estimates for 2001, illness and subsequent death are estimated to undermine the contribution of nearly one-third of the entire population to both individual and national development each year (URT, 2001a). Communicable diseases are the major cause of morbidity and mortality in Tanzania. According to hospital statistics, the five leading causes of death in hospitals for people (five years and above) include clinical AIDS (15.5%), non-cerebral malaria (15.3%), TB (9.9%), cerebral malaria (7.3%) and pneumonia (6.3%).

The same report further indicates that infants born in rural areas have a 30% higher probability of dying before their first birthday than do their counterparts in urban areas. Similarly, infants from the poorest quintile of mothers have a 25% higher probability of dying before the end of one year than do those in the richest quintile.

Almost all the urban areas are in close proximity to PHC facilities. According to URT (2005a), 100% of the urban population lives within five kilometers of a health centre or dispensary, compared with about 75% of the rural population. However, access to essential referral care is perhaps the single most prominent barrier to accessing health care by the poor, as they have to pay the direct health-care and transport costs involved. The difference in health service provision between rural and urban areas is a cause for concern. Most of the health centres and hospitals (private or government) providing a variety of quality health services are found in the urban areas, with most of the health-care facilities being owned by government.

Table 5.1: Percentage of births in the presence of a skilled attendant and in health facilities				
Year	% attended with a skilled attendant		% of all births at a health facility	
	Urban	Rural	Urban	Rural
1996	81.7	39.8	80.7	40.0
1999	83.3	34.7	82.8	34.5
2004	81.0	38.9	81.0	38.0
Source: National Bureau of Statistics and ORC Macro, 1997, 2000, 2005				

EMPLOYMENT

The status of employment in Tanzania reflects the economic reforms that took place in the 1990s, with the number of unemployed more than doubling over a decade, from 405 722 in 1990/91 to 912 772 in 2000/01. Agricultural occupations accounted for 73% and 79% of the total employed population in 1991/92 and 2000/01 respectively. In both urban and rural areas, more women were involved in agricultural activities than men (URT, 2002b).

The Household Budget Survey (HBS) 2000/01 shows that 44% of all Tanzanian households and over half the population living in rural areas depended on an unprotected source of drinking water. Only 40% of households had access to piped water and other protected sources, most of whom were living in the urban areas, particularly Dar es Salaam (URT, 2002a). The Tanzania HIV/AIDS Indicator Survey (THIS) 2003/2004 indicates that only about half (52%) of all households in Tanzania have access to safe water, comprising 77% of urban households and 43% of rural households (URT, 2005b).

Transport and communication systems in Tanzania are relatively better in urban areas than they are in rural areas. About 50% of the villages are inaccessible by motor vehicles, while, for some, such access is impossible during the wet seasons.[55]

The health system assumes a pyramidal pattern of referral systems made in terms of the recommendations of health planners, working upward from dispensary to consultant hospital level. The structure of health services is as follows.

VILLAGE HEALTH SERVICE/POSTS

The lowest level of health-care delivery in the country provides preventive home-based services. Usually each village health post has two village health workers, chosen by the village government from among the villagers. The workers receive only minimal training before starting to provide services.

DISPENSARY SERVICES

At the second stage of health services, the dispensary caters for from 6 000 to 10 000 people, with ward dispensaries supervising all village health posts in their wards. The dispensaries, which provide basic health care on an outpatient basis, with occasional admissions, play an important role in rural areas.

HEALTH CENTRE SERVICES

A health centre is expected to cater for 50 000 people, which corresponds to approximately the population of a single administrative division.

DISTRICT HOSPITALS

Each district is supposed to have a district general hospital. For those districts without one, the government negotiates with religious organisations to designate volunteer-run hospitals that are subsidised by the government in terms of contracts.

Regional Hospitals

Every region is supposed to have a general hospital. Regional Hospitals offer similar services to those at district level, but they have specialists in various fields and offer additional services, which are not provided at district hospitals.

Referral/Consultant Hospitals

This is the highest level of hospital services in the country. Presently there are four referral hospitals: Muhimbili National Hospital; Kilimanjaro Christian Medical Center (KCMC); Bugando Hospital; and Mbeya Hospital.

Traditional Medicine and Alternative Healing System

The health-care system in Tanzania is complimented by a well recognised traditional medicine and alternative healing system. The role of traditional and alternative health care to the people of Tanzania is significant, with 60% of the population using traditional and other forms of health care, including spiritual healing.

HIV/AIDS Epidemic in Tanzania

HIV ranks among the top impediments to a country's social and economic development as it affects all sectors of the economy. The government, in collaboration with different stakeholders, responded by committing resources, formulating policies and strategies, and by establishing specific institutions to coordinate the responses.

AIDS Cases and HIV Prevalence Rates

As stated earlier, the first cases of AIDS in the country were reported in 1983 in Kagera region in the north west of the country. Since then, the number of cases has continued to rise at a very fast rate. By 2004, there were cumulative 192 532 reported cases of AIDS in Tanzania (URT, 2005c). Figure 5.1 depicts the trend of reported AIDS cases in Tanzania from 1983–2004. In the period 1983–1986, few cases were reported to the NACP and these were not disaggregated by age.

Figure 5.1: Reported number of AIDS cases in Tanzania, 1983–2004

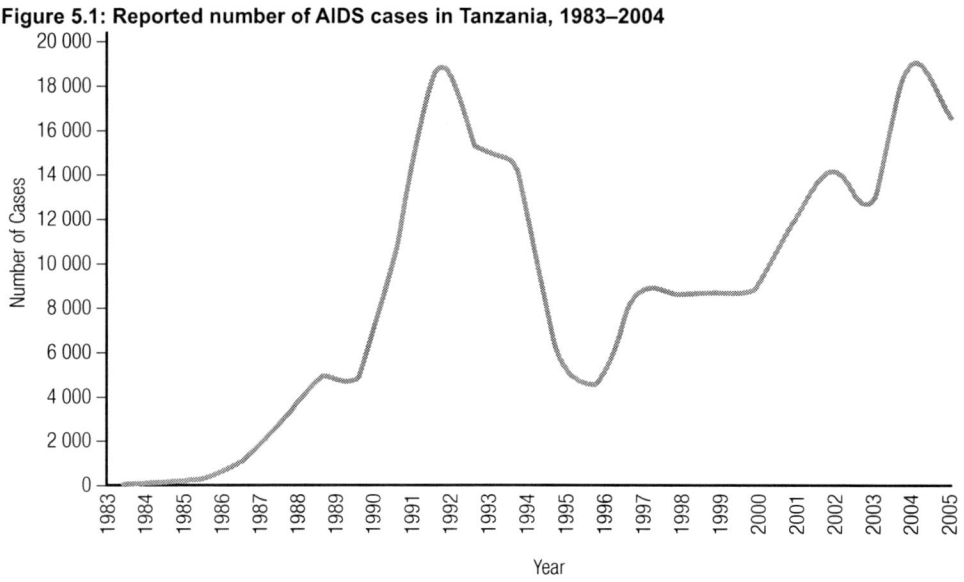

Source: URT, 2005c

HIV/AIDS prevalence varies across regions in Tanzania. THIS[56] (2003/2004) shows that 7% of Tanzania mainland adults are infected with HIV, with the prevalence being higher among women (8%) than among men (6%) (URT, 2005b). THIS further showed that HIV/AIDS prevalence was higher in urban areas (12% for women and 9.6% for men) than in rural areas (5.8% for women and 4.8% for men).

The study also revealed that Mbeya (14%) has the highest HIV prevalence, followed by Iringa and Manyara, with Kigoma having the least (2%).

Figure 5.2: Age and sex-specific distribution of reported AIDS cases in Tanzania, 2004

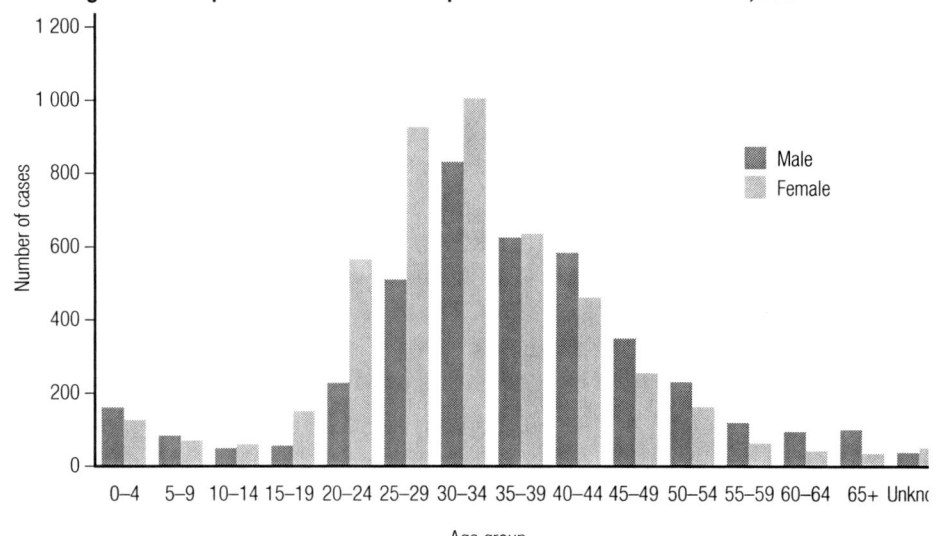

Source: URT, 2005b

In terms of the age and sex-specific cumulative case rates for 2004, females generally have a higher case rate than males (ages 15–39), though males have higher case rates, particularly for the age group 40 years and above. High case rates occur for both sexes in the age group 25–44 years.

MODE OF HIV TRANSMISSION

The predominant mode of HIV transmission has remained heterosexual contact, which accounted for 76.8% of infections in 2004, while mother–to–child transmission constituted 5.4%, and blood transfusion 0.5% (URT, 2005c).

The prevalence of HIV is related to marital status, with formally married individuals having a higher prevalence rate (18%) than other groups. Those who have never been married have a relatively low prevalence (3%), while those currently married have intermediate HIV prevalence levels of 7% among men and 8% among women. Women in polygamous unions are 10% more likely to be HIV-positive. HIV prevalence is linked to sexual risk behaviours, number of sexual partners, the age at first sex, condom use during sex, alcoholism and recent history of STIs (URT, 2005b).

LEVEL OF PUBLIC KNOWLEDGE ON HIV/AIDS

The level of knowledge of HIV/AIDS in Tanzania has remained high since 1996, with over 95% of all adults being aware of the nature of HIV/AIDS.[57] However, comprehensive knowledge on HIV/AIDS, as defined in the NBS (2005), is low.

Stigma associated with HIV/AIDS in Tanzania is said to be embedded in knowledge and beliefs about the epidemic. The 2004/2005 DHS revealed that most women and men would be willing to care at home for a relative with an HIV-related disease, and believe that an HIV-positive female teacher should be allowed to continue teaching.

About 50% of the respondents stated that they would be prepared to buy fresh food from a shopkeeper with AIDS, while 53% of women and 62% of men affirmed their belief that the HIV-positive status of a family member does not need to be kept a secret (URT, 2005b).

HIV/AIDS IMPACT ASSESSMENTS

The impact of HIV/AIDS in Tanzania is far reaching, cutting across almost all socio-economic sectors. According to URT (2003e), the epidemic has resulted in lower life expectancy, a reduction in productivity, increasing poverty, and rising infant and child mortality. In the health sector, the epidemic has added to the disease burden of Tanzanians. Especially in relation to opportunistic infections, the pandemic has exerted pressure on the already overburdened health-care system, leading to a further decline in the quality of care due to:

- The increased number of patients in health facilities, with 50% of beds being occupied by patients with HIV-related illnesses (ESRF, 2003);
- The increased workload of hospital workers in already understaffed hospitals;
- The increased expenditure involved in medical and funeral expenses on infected health-care workers;
- The deterioration of the referral systems, due to additional demand for medical care by those infected by HIV/AIDS patients;
- The staff shortage due to absenteeism and the death of HIV-infected health care workers; and
- The increased risk of HIV infection in hospital settings due to a lack of protective gear.

The country is experiencing a reversal in human development due to the epidemic. Productive sectors of the economy are experiencing a loss of skilled labour, increasing recruitment costs, sick leave costs and reduced revenues. Economic sectors such as transport, education and mining are particularly hard-hit (URT, 2003e).

A study by the Economic and Social Research Foundation (ESRF) (2003) showed the following economic and social impacts of HIV/AIDS.

IMPACT ON LABOUR SUPPLY

The epidemic has resulted in a decreased labour supply, due to increased HIV/AIDS-related mortalities and morbidities. The study revealed that the majority of PLWHAs fell in the economically active age groups (30–40 years). Results from the education sector revealed that most of the teachers who died one year prior to the survey had died of AIDS. In the private sector, companies are reported to be losing an average of six employees each a year.

IMPACT ON LABOUR PRODUCTIVITY

The loss of labour productivity has been measured by the rate of absenteeism, the total number of years of experience lost, and the amount of paid sick leave taken.

HIV/AIDS has resulted in an increased rate of absenteeism (and hence a loss of labour time), and loss of skills and experience. A study by Kessy (2004), of the impact of HIV/AIDS on agricultural performance in the Ulanga and Kilombero districts, revealed that the experience of death in the household and time taken to take care of HIV/AIDS-related problems have negatively impacted on agricultural productivity. The duration of HIV-related illness covered a total of 479 work days, equating to a loss of agricultural labour force of two farming households per month.

Further, a total of 533 work days was used to attend to and/or care for HIV-positive patients, equating to a loss of productive labour force of seven households per month.

IMPACT ON TIME ALLOCATION

HIV/AIDS was found to have affected the time allocation of infected and affected households. About 8% of the individuals interviewed at the household level indicated that they had attended to a HIV/AIDS patient in or outside their household in the 14 days prior to the survey, with the majority spending less than five hours and more than 20 hours doing so. More than 43% of women respondents spent more than 20 hours in the two weeks prior to the survey caring for HIV/AIDS patients, compared with 36% of men who did the same. Most of the respondents reported having spent at least three hours visiting an HIV/AIDS sick person in the 14 days prior to the survey. Results from the household survey further show that about 13% of the respondents reported having had to attend the funeral of a person who had died of from HIV/AIDS-related causes in the 14 days preceding the survey, with the individual amount of time spent on such activity ranging from one hour to 280 hours (ESRF, 2003).

IMPACT ON FINANCIAL RESOURCES

The medical treatment of opportunist infections affecting PLWHAs is extremely costly. Workplace findings reveal that 21% of the surveyed companies provided specific medical support (on average, about TZS11.76 million for a single company) for employees living with HIV/AIDS. Family support, terminal benefits, replacement costs, and expenditures on preventive programmes, are among other financial expenses incurred due to the epidemic. An average cost of TZS158 000 per funeral was reported at household level. Most (86%) of the surveyed companies provided funeral support for their employees. District-level data on the supply side of the education sector revealed that transport and burial costs for teachers who died of AIDS-related illness constituted a large proportion of total transport and burial costs (45–84% in 2002).

THE PLIGHT OF ORPHANS AND THE ELDERLY

The ESRF (2003) findings reveal that the number of orphans increased over the four-year period covered. The findings further suggest that the dropout rate within the orphans group is much higher than among their counterparts. Girl orphans were found to be more likely to drop out of school than boy orphans. The findings further revealed that 34% of the orphaned pupils interviewed were being taken care of by their grandparents. As a result, some orphans (15%) were forced to engage in income-generating activities during, or after, school hours.

NATIONAL RESPONSE TO HIV/AIDS

GOVERNMENT RESPONSE TO HIV/AIDS

In 1985, the NACP was created in the MoH, with the latter formulating the Short-term Plan (1985–86), and three five-year MTPs; MTP-I (1987–1991); MTP-II (1992–1996) and MTP-III (1998–2002). Initially, HIV/AIDS was perceived purely as a health problem, leading the government to focus on developing strategies to prevent, control and to mitigate the impact of the HIV/AIDS epidemic through health education and community participation. In December 1999, HIV/AIDS was declared a national disaster. In December 2000, the Tanzania Commission for AIDS (TACAIDS) was launched primarily to lead a multisectoral response against HIV. This was followed by the inauguration of a National Policy on HIV in November 2001, and the launch of an NMSF on HIV/AIDS (2003/07) in May 2003 (URT, 2003f). The NMSF provides a framework for the implementation of the National HIV/AIDS Policy.

GOVERNMENT HIV/AIDS POLICY

Tanzania's National Policy on HIV/AIDS guides and directs various multi-sectoral efforts at the HIV/AIDS response (URT, 2001b). The policy focuses on the participatory formulation of appropriate interventions. It further emphasises the protection of, and support for, vulnerable groups, and the mitigation of the social and economic impact of HIV/AIDS. The policy is based on the belief that the HIV/AIDS epidemic is a socioeconomic and cultural challenge and thus that its prevention and control greatly depends on effective community-based prevention, and care and support interventions. It also provides a framework for strengthening the capacity of institutions, communities and individuals in all sectors to curb the epidemic. The policy considers local government councils to be the foci for the coordination of public and private actors (URT, 2001b).

Objectives of the National HIV/AIDS Policy are:

- To prevent the transmission of HIV/AIDS;
- To promote HIV/AIDS testing;
- To ensure the care of PLWHAs;
- To enhance a coordinated and effective multisectoral approach towards curbing the epidemic, and to mobilise adequate financial resources for HIV/AIDS activities;
- To provide a framework to promote and coordinate multisectoral and multi-disciplinary HIV/AIDS-related research activities, and to disseminate and use the research findings;
- To create a legal framework by enacting HIV/AIDS-related legislation;
- To monitor efforts aimed at the community mobilisation of PLWHAs;
- To safeguard the rights of PLWHA in order to improve the quality of their lives and to minimise stigma;

- To provide appropriate treatment for OIs at all levels of the health-care system;
- To fight against drug and substance abuse that increases the risk of HIV transmission; and
- To prohibit misleading advertising of drugs and other products for HIV prevention, treatment and care.

The HIV/AIDS programmes delivered in Tanzania fall into the following thematic areas, as set out in the National Multi-Sectoral Strategic Framework (NMSF):

- Cross-cutting issues, comprising advocacy; fighting against stigma and discrimination; district and community responses; the mainstreaming of HIV/AIDS; HIV/AIDS and development; and poverty reduction;
- Prevention, comprising STI control and case (gender) management; condom promotion and distribution; voluntary counselling and testing; prevention of mother-to-child transmission (PMTCT); health promotion; children and youth; women and girls; men; the disabled; school-based prevention; vulnerable population groups; workplace interventions; the safety of blood products; and universal precautions; and
- Care and support, comprising medical and nursing care (treatment); psycho-social support; food and other material support; and impact mitigation.

STRUCTURES AND INSTITUTIONS FOR IMPLEMENTING GOVERNMENT PROGRAMMES

Several mechanisms and institutional arrangements have been put in place to facilitate the coordination, management, and implementation of the national HIV/AIDS programmes.

ROLES AND FUNCTION OF THE NATIONAL LEVEL

The NMSF has to be translated into a series of specific plans, programmes, projects and interventions. TACAIDS, according to URT (2001b), coordinates the multisectoral response, being responsible for:

- Formulating policy guidelines to direct the response to the HIV/AIDS epidemic and the management of its consequences on mainland Tanzania;
- Developing a strategic framework for the planning of all HIV/AIDS control programmes and activities within the overall national strategy;
- Fostering national and international linkages among all stakeholders through the proper coordination of all HIV/AIDS control programmes and activities within the overall national strategy;
- Mobilising, disbursing and monitoring resources, and ensuring their equitable distribution;
- Disseminating and sharing information on the HIV/AIDS epidemic and its consequences;

155

- Promoting HIV/AIDS-related research, information sharing and documentation;
- Promoting high-level advocacy and education on HIV/AIDS prevention and control;
- Monitoring and evaluating all continuing HIV/AIDS activities;
- Coordinating all activities related to the management of the HIV/AIDS epidemic in Tanzania;
- Facilitating efforts to find a cure, promoting access to treatment and care, and developing a vaccine;
- Protecting the human rights of people infected and affected by HIV/AIDS; and
- Advising the government on all HIV/AIDS-related matters in Tanzania.

The MoHSW, its departments and agencies and NACP are responsible for service delivery in prevention and care interventions, such as patient care, blood safety and VCT, the distribution of condoms and health-related learning materials, and research, and may influence policy-making through technical jurisdiction in the delivery of health services. Other ministries are also responsible for formulating and implementing HIV/AIDS plans, policies and activities in their respective sectors (URT, 2003e).

Roles and Functions at the Regional, District and Village Levels

At the regional level, the Regional Administrative Secretary (RAS) as well as the Regional Technical entities play an intermediate role in planning, implementing, and monitoring activities. The Regional Consultative Committee is the forum for discussing progress and other issues related to the multisectoral HIV/AIDS response at the regional level.

Local government councils are responsible for bringing together and coordinating all actors working on HIV/AIDS in the respective districts. They are foci for coordinating the public and private sector NGOs and FBOs in the planning and implementation of HIV/AIDS interventions through each Council (CMAC), Ward (WMAC) and Village Multisectoral Committee (VMAC). They also are responsible for ensuring that the councils mainstream HIV/AIDS in plans and budgets throughout the different hamlet, village, ward and council levels. All levels of local government are therefore responsible for policy making, budgeting, decision making and service delivery.

Non-State Response

The HIV/AIDS response in Tanzania has not been multisectoral. Different stakeholders, including the private sector, development partners and civil society, have responded accordingly. Different players work as sources of funds, agents, and HIV/AIDS service providers. According to the NMSF, TACAIDS should work towards holding regular consultative forums with national and international HIV/AIDS-related NGOs to discuss mechanisms through which they can participate and support the national, district and community responses (URT, 2001b).

CBOs, NGOs and FBOs, media institutions, as well as associations of PLWHAs also play a significant role in the HIV/AIDS response. Such organisations and institutions focus on different strategies, ranging from cross-cutting issues; prevention, care and treatment; and impact mitigation. Some organisations provide funds to beneficiaries either directly or through financing agents.

Over 60% of Tanzanians depend on traditional healers[58] and herbalists for treatment, illuminating the role of traditional healers in the HIV/AIDS response in the country (URT, 2003d). Traditional medicine is widely used to treat OIs. Clinical research in Tanga region has shown traditional medicine to be effective in boosting the immunity of PLWHAs. The government, by establishing the Traditional Medicine Unit at Muhimbili National Hospital, has shown that it recognises the role of traditional and alternative healing in dealing with the epidemic.

RESEARCH ACTIVITIES

The National HIV/AIDS Policy provides a framework for promoting and coordinating HIV/AIDS-related multisectoral and multidisciplinary research activities (URT, 2001b), with the coordination of research activities forming part of the NMSF. HIV/AIDS-related research has focused on ensuring the production of evidence-based information on the epidemic. The National Research and Ethics Committee for AIDS, under the leadership of TACAIDS, provides guidelines for the national research agenda, procedural aspects, the mobilisation of funds for research, and the dissemination of research findings (URT, 2003f). Research activities also form part of the non-state response to HIV/AIDS. Bilateral and multilateral organisations and development partners fund research activities.

HIV/AIDS AND THE BUDGET PROCESS IN TANZANIA

INTRODUCTION[59]

Government budgeting is a process of determining resources and their use for the attainment of national objectives. The process starts with the identification of goals and objectives that the government wants to attain in the coming financial year, guided by the medium- and long-term development plans. The main development objective of the government of Tanzania is to implement the second generation of the PRS renamed the National Strategy for Growth and Reduction of Poverty (NS-GRP), popularly known in Swahili acronym as "MKUKUTA",[60] in line with the Millennium Development Goals (MDGs).

Budget priority determination starts by assessing the availability of resources and their utilisation, which is presented in the budget guidelines. On the basis of such guidelines, the government prepares the budget by estimating revenue and expenditure needs, and allocating the available resources to different sectors. Each year the Planning Commission[61] of Tanzania provides budget guidelines to all the government ministries, departments and agencies (MDAs) and regions on projected revenues and expenditure for the following FY. Financial allocations (budget ceilings) for the MDAs are based on the expected or forecasted government revenues and the government development priorities.

Once the budget guidelines have been issued, each MDA or region prepares its budget and plans in line with the allocated budget ceiling and in accordance with the respective MDAs' priority for achieving the national development objectives, including all HIV-related objectives. The budget and MDA plans are then scrutinised by the Interministerial Technical Committee (IMTC), composed of all permanent secretaries (accounting officers of ministries). Thereafter, these plans are forwarded to the IMTC for further discussion and recommendation. Cabinet then receives and discusses the recommendations of the IMTC, and finalises the estimates, which are then presented to Parliament. In Parliament, the Finance and Economic Committee holds meetings with the government officials, studies the estimates and makes a report to the whole Parliament for discussion.

Only after the budget has been approved by Parliament does the execution of programmes start. Budget execution generally covers revenue collection and the disbursement of funds for expenditure. It also covers the monitoring and control of government operations to ensure that the budget operations are on track. Another component of the budget process is the evaluation of budget performance to identify successes and failures with respect to the prescribed goals and objectives, which occurs through the Medium-Term Expenditure Frameworks (MTEFs) and the Public Expenditure Reviews (PERs). This stage is vital in setting up new budget goals, objectives and policies. In this way, the outcome of one budget process forms the basis of the next one.

The budget process in Tanzania can be described as using both the top-down and bottom-up approach. The budget process is bottom-up in the sense that strategic action plans are prepared at each separate MDA level. The strategic action plans provide a framework for resource allocation to those activities prioritised at that particular MDA level, which are aimed at achieving the MDA targets with respect to the MKUKUTA. At the MDA's lower level, technicians prepare the first budget estimates for each priority activity, based on the budget guidelines provided by the Planning Commission. The estimates are then forwarded to the Head of Section, who then scrutinises them, makes any adjustments that are considered necessary, and forwards them upwards within the institution. Finally, the estimates are sent to the Accounting Officer, who makes a final decision regarding the estimates for the whole institution or for those MDAs concerned.

Local government authorities are required to prepare their revenue and expenditure estimates based on the subsidies that they receive from central government and on the collections from their own sources. In the preparation of such budgets, local governments are now directed to make use of the Government Finance Statistics (GFS). The use of GFS covers both the local government budget financed by own sources and the local government subsidies received from the central government budget.

The budget process can also be regarded as being top-down in the sense that the budget guidelines are issued to all MDAs by the Planning Commission. The MTP and Budget Guideline provide a guiding framework for the preparation of the medium-term expenditures for the ministries, independent departments, and executive agencies, as well as for the regions and local government authorities. The MDA plans address the Tanzania Development Vision 2025, MKUKUTA and the ruling party (*Chama cha Mapinduzi* [CCM]) election manifesto priorities. The MDAs therefore have to align their resource allocations to their priority activities in accordance with the provided budget ceilings in the budget guidelines.

In order to ensure that HIV/AIDS activities are allocated adequate funds in each sector, a "Z" code was introduced. The "Z" code denoted the MDA funding allocated to HIV activities operational for FYs 2003/04 and 2004/05. Such a system was discontinued in FY 2005/06, creating difficulty in accounting for HIV/AIDS funding to the MDAs, as the funds were grouped together with those for other activities within each MDA's budget. A specific code for HIV/AIDS funding was reintroduced in FY 2006/07, with the HIV/AIDS funds in the MDA budget being given the "A" code.

THE PARLIAMENT

The Parliament and the National Assembly jointly:
- Examine the government revenue and expenditure proposals;
- Authorise revenue collection and expenditures through the passing and enactment of the Finance and Appropriation Acts;
- Authorise supplementary revenue collection and supplementary expenditures by passing and enacting supplementary Finance and Appropriation Acts; and
- Discuss and approve the reallocation of appropriated funds between votes.

Though no specific parliamentary committee on HIV/AIDS exists, issues are frequently discussed in standing committees in Parliament. Each standing committee has an important role to play in dealing with HIV/AIDS and its linkages to specific sectoral issues, which the committee deals with as part of its normal business.

THE CABINET AND INTERMINISTERIAL TECHNICAL COMMITTEE

All ministers form part of the Cabinet, which has two main functions in the government budget process:
- The approval of government budget proposals, supplementary estimates and excess votes from all MDAs; and

- The authorisation of the minister responsible for finance to present the approved estimates to the National Assembly. The Cabinet is facilitated by the IMTC, which constitutes principal secretaries from all the ministries.

The IMTC advises and guides members of the Cabinet on budget matters and other relevant development issues.

The Role of the Public Expenditure Review Working Group

The PER working group meets biweekly, being the focus of the PER process. It develops the annual Programme of Work (PoW), supervising the implementation of specific activities. The PER process ensures that adequate resources are allocated to meet the economic growth and poverty alleviation objectives of each MKUKUTA cluster.

The role of the PER working group is to coordinate and discuss sectoral PER studies and to ensure that they address all relevant and important issues, including those to do with gender. The assumption is that PERs and MTEFs can help to improve the budget process and outcomes by clarifying policy objectives, and improving the predictability of budget allocations, the comprehensiveness of coverage, and efficiency and transparency in the use of resources, including focusing on gender issues.

The Medium-term Expenditure Framework

The MTEF comprises estimates of aggregate resources available for public expenditure consistent with the country's macroeconomic objectives and policies, and is a framework that reconciles costs with aggregate resources.

The MTEF provides the linking framework that allows expenditures to be driven by policy priorities and disciplined by budget realities. The framework links policy making to planning and budgeting, and provides a medium-term perspective on budgeting. The core of the medium-term perspective constrains choices in support of long-term development. An MTEF rests on three pillars:

- The top-down multiyear projections of resource envelope targets (what is affordable);
- The bottom-up multiyear cost estimates of sector programmes (what has to be financed, with a focus on performance); and
- The institutional (political and administrative) decision-making process to integrate the above two pillars (making the necessary trade-offs).

The Six Stages of a Comprehensive Medium-term Expenditure Framework

The comprehensive MTEF comprises six separate stages.

STAGE ONE: DEVELOPMENT OF THE MACROECONOMIC FRAMEWORK

Stage One is characterised by a macroeconomic model that projects revenues and expenditure in the medium term.

STAGE TWO: DEVELOPMENT OF SECTORAL PROGRAMMES

Stage Two is characterised by:
- Agreement on sector objectives, outputs and activities;
- The review and development of programmes and sub-programmes; and
- Programme cost estimation.

STAGE THREE: DEVELOPMENT OF THE STRATEGIC EXPENDITURE FRAMEWORK

Stage Three is characterised by:
- The analysis of inter- and intrasectoral trade-offs; and
- Consensus-building on strategic resource allocation.

STAGE FOUR: DEFINITION OF SECTORAL BUDGETS

Stage Four is characterised by the setting of medium-term sector budget ceilings.

STAGE FIVE: PREPARATION OF SECTORAL BUDGETS

Stage Five is characterised by medium-term sectoral programmes based on budget ceilings.

STAGE SIX: POLITICAL APPROVAL

Stage Six is characterised by the presentation of budget estimates to Cabinet and Parliament for approval.

MAJOR OBJECTIVES OF THE MEDIUM-TERM EXPENDITURE FRAMEWORK

The major objectives of the MTEF comprise:
- To improve macroeconomic stability through fiscal discipline;
- To improve inter- and intrasectoral resource allocation (the effective prioritisation of expenditure on the basis of the government socioeconomic programme);

- To achieve greater budgetary predictability (commitment to more credible sectoral budget ceilings);
- To achieve more efficient use of public monies (greater flexibility for line ministries, with greater accountability in managing their budgets);
- To attain greater political accountability for public expenditure outcomes (through more legitimate decision making); and
- To attain greater credibility for budgetary decision making (political restraint).

TRANSPARENCY AND PARTICIPATION IN THE BUDGET PROCESS

The report on Enhancing Aid Relationships in Tanzania (URT, 2005e) shows that transparency and participation in the budget process in Tanzania has improved considerably over the past decade. Improvements include the integration of national processes with sectors and local governments, and the public resource management process. The transparency and accountability of public financial resources has improved by rolling out the Integrated Financial Management System (IFMS) to all regions, which also has enhanced the monitoring of financial resources used by the MDAs. Stakeholder participation in policy dialogue has been broadened and is becoming more institutionalised. The sectors have been involved more explicitly and the regions have become more widely involved than in the past. However, civil society organisations are mostly involved in the ex-post budget processes. Their involvement is mainly in the PERs, which evaluate budget performance of the various MDAs in the preceding FY, and budget analysis following the presentation of the budget in Parliament. The ex-ante budget process activities are only undertaken by the experts within the various MDAs, and are approved by Cabinet and Parliament. The ex-ante budget processes can be seen to allow for limited participation by civil society.

STRENGTHS AND WEAKNESSES IN THE BUDGET PROCESS

According to the URT Report on Enhancing Aid Relationships in Tanzania (2005e), the budget has yet to function as a strategic policy and resource-allocation tool. The budget formulation process was found, so far, to be the weakest link in the policy–budget–service delivery chain. The implementation of critical MDA activities is crucial for realising the MDA's general strategic objectives, especially, in this context, those specific to HIV/AIDS. Furthermore, the budget estimated in terms of the MDA strategic plans is often larger than the available funds provided in the budget guidelines, which hampers implementation of those activities stipulated in the MDAs' strategic action plans, hindering the realisation of the MDAs' targeted outputs and activity outcomes.

HIV/AIDS FINANCIAL AND REPORTING MECHANISMS IN TANZANIA

HIV/AIDS financing and reporting mechanisms in Tanzania are dictated by the source of funds and whether the recipient organisation is a government MDA or a CSO. The financing and reporting mechanisms by the government MDAs is provided for in the rules and regulations governing government financing, while those for the NGOs are determined by the NGOs' own established rules and regulations, in line with the laws of the government of Tanzania, as well as in terms of donor conditions.

GOVERNMENT FINANCIAL AND REPORTING MECHANISMS

Government financing and finance management is regulated by the Exchequer and Audit Ordinance of 1961 and provisions set out in Chapter 7 of the Constitution. The provisions outline the financial orders on which the financial regulations and administrative procedures are based. While the financial orders are issued by the Accountant-General's Office (AGO), financial procedures are issued by the central ministries. The Controller and Auditor-General are empowered to ensure adherence to the set laws and regulations that govern public financial management, including the auditing of all government revenue and spending, and periodically present audit reports to Parliament through the Minister for Finance or the Parliamentary Accounts Committee.

The Exchequer and Audit Ordinance of 1961 requires that all money raised or received by the territory, including donor funds, be paid into the Exchequer account. The disbursement of funds is initiated by the MoF on advice from the Planning Commission, in response to a release warrant issued by the Accountant General. However, due to the poor communication within and between government departments and donors, the system is usually bypassed through disbursements being allocated directly to projects (D-funds), as well as through the opening of special accounts. This challenge, however, is being addressed through the Tanzania Aid Strategy. Government financing of the different MDAs is done through account codes. The Commissioner for Budget circulates a list of the Parliament-approved accounting codes to all MDAs. The funds approved in the government budget are therefore issued from the Exchequer to the MDAs in accordance with the amount of money budgeted for each accounting or activity code.

Government financial accounting is done by each MDA under the supervision and direction of the Accountant-General in the MoF. The MDAs prepare monthly and quarterly statements of expenditure (SOEs) and revenue receipts, and forward them to the Treasury and Controller and Auditor General (CAG). Within four months of the end of the FY, each accounting officer is required to prepare and submit appropriation accounts, annual accounts and statements to the CAG and Treasury, as prescribed under the Exchequer and Audit Ordinance No. 21 of 1961.

The government has established an IFMS, through which financial transfers to the MDAs and management are coordinated. Intergovernmental fiscal transfers are also managed within the same IFMS. The subventions supplied to the local government councils are provided to the local government to support the social service sectors, such as education and health. Funds are transferred on a quarterly basis.

As HIV/AIDS is a cross-cutting issue, and government allocation for HIV/AIDS in the different ministries is disbursed to the votes/activities within the ministries that are deemed to play a greater role in HIV/AIDS awareness raising and prevention in the country. The NACP, which administratively is established within the Department of Preventive Services of the MoH, receives funding from the government and donors (i.e. USAID, the World Bank and WHO).

At the national level, funds are disbursed by the MoF to the vote-holders accounts of each MDA on a quarterly basis. The accounting officers in each MDA then disburse the received funds for the respective activities identified in the budget estimates.

Table 5.2: Financial reports generated		
Name of report	Generated from	Reports
Expenditure Flash Report	Monthly/IFMS	Expenditure on a monthly and cumulative basis
Commitment Control Flash Report	Monthly/IFMS	Commitments on a monthly and cumulative basis
Exchequer Release	Quarterly/IFMS	All transfers from the basket account to Exchequer
Undistributed Exchequer	Quarterly/IFMS	Unallocated amounts
Quarterly Performance Report	Quarterly/IFMS	Actual and cumulative expenditures against budget
Output Monitoring Report	Quarterly/IFMS	Actual and cumulative expenditures against budget
Receipts and payment accounts	Annually/IFMS	Deposits into the basket and transfers to Exchequer

MANAGEMENT OF DONOR FUNDS FOR HIV/AIDS

MANAGEMENT OF DONOR FUNDS FOR HIV/AIDS IN THE GOVERNMENT

The External Finance Division of the Treasury is responsible for the mobilisation of all aid resources, based on the advice received from the Office of the President, Planning and Privatisation, which scrutinises and approves requests from line ministries. The legal aspects of agreements are scrutinised by the Attorney-General's Chambers. Over the last few decades, Tanzania has had to face the challenge of uncoordinated external aid.

From 2002, the government of Tanzania launched a framework for managing foreign aid resources known as the TAS, an action plan for harmonising procedures, including the channeling of donor project funds through the Exchequer system. An OECD–DAC harmonisation group has been formed to support the implementation of the TAS, which is coordinated by the MoF in close collaboration with sector ministries, local governments, civil society, and DAC. Harmonisation efforts are now focused on four areas:

- The link between the PRS and the budget requires strengthening. The outputs of the PER need to be informed by the PRS process itself. As a result, the focus should be on strengthening the link between the PER and the PRS annual reviews and the end-of-cycle revisions.
- An agreement must be reached on a common performance assessment framework for the Poverty Reduction Strategy Credit (PRSC) and Poverty Reduction Budget Support (PRBS).
- Establishing Sector Working Groups (SWGs) in all priority sectors would help to harmonise processes at sectoral level, ensuring that sector processes complement macro processes and are sequenced to merge smoothly.
- Country/portfolio annual review processes should be linked to existing in-country review processes.

In mid-2004, a Joint Assistance Strategy (JAS), based on the government's PRS and other programmes, was initiated by the Government of Tanzania, DFID and the World Bank. The JAS should combine the features of traditional country assistance strategies/programmes with the principles of "aid effectiveness". A (joint) procurement, financial management and disbursement assessment is being undertaken by a group of donors/partners with the intention of multidonor pooling through government systems for a sector-wide approach (SWAp) in terms of the Health Sector Development Programme (HSDP).

Other efforts to manage donor funds include the PER/MTEF process, involving all key stakeholders, which is now the established framework for donor–government policy dialogue. PERs have been prepared annually since 1997/98, usually comprising joint products of the government, the donor community, the European Commission and countries such as Denmark, Norway, Sweden and the UK, as well as multilateral organisations, such as UNDP and the WB. In addition, annual evaluation of fiscal performance is undertaken jointly between the WB and bilateral donors. Technical aspects, such as auditing and accounting requirements and modes of disbursements, are the major challenges often encountered in the coordination and management of donor funds.

MANAGEMENT OF DONOR FUNDS FOR HIV/AIDS IN CIVIL SOCIETY ORGANISATIONS

Civil society organisations receive funds to support HIV/AIDS activities from various sources, both internal and external. The internal sources include fundraising from charities comprising individuals, organisations and the private sector. Donor funds are channeled to local CSOs in four ways:

- Directly to the CSOs;
- Through the Rapid Fund Envelope (RFE), which was established in 2002 by TACAIDS and eight donor partners (CIDA; the Embassy of Finland; Ireland Aid; the Royal Danish Embassy; the Royal Netherlands Embassy; the Royal Norwegian Embassy; the Swiss Agency for Development and Cooperation; and USAID), whose aim it is to enable CSOs and partnerships to implement short-term HIV/AIDS projects that contribute to the long-term national strategy;

- Through other international NGOs (e.g. funds from PEPFAR which go through such international US-based NGOs as PACT, Family Health International (FHI), CARE International and Plan International); and
- Through the Exchequer (e.g. GFATM). (See Figure 5.3 for the flow of HIV funds from different sources.)

The reporting mechanisms on the status of fund utilisation depend on regulations stipulated in the Memorandum of Understanding or on a contract between the sources of funds/FA and the service provider. For funds that are provided through the RFE, CSOs are required to provide audited reports on the status of the utilisation of the funds to the RFE coordinating institution, of which copies are sent to the local governments in the areas in which the CSOs are located, as well as to TACAIDS. However, no strict sanctions are imposed on non-reporting CSOs. How the CSOs utilise the funds allocated for HIV/AIDS has been far from transparent, mainly due to the lack of mechanisms to ensure the transparent evaluation of the utilisation of funds and the implementation of CSO activities. This critical challenge needs to be addressed if effective accountability is to be ensured among CSOs.

Figure 5.3: HIV/AIDS financial flow map

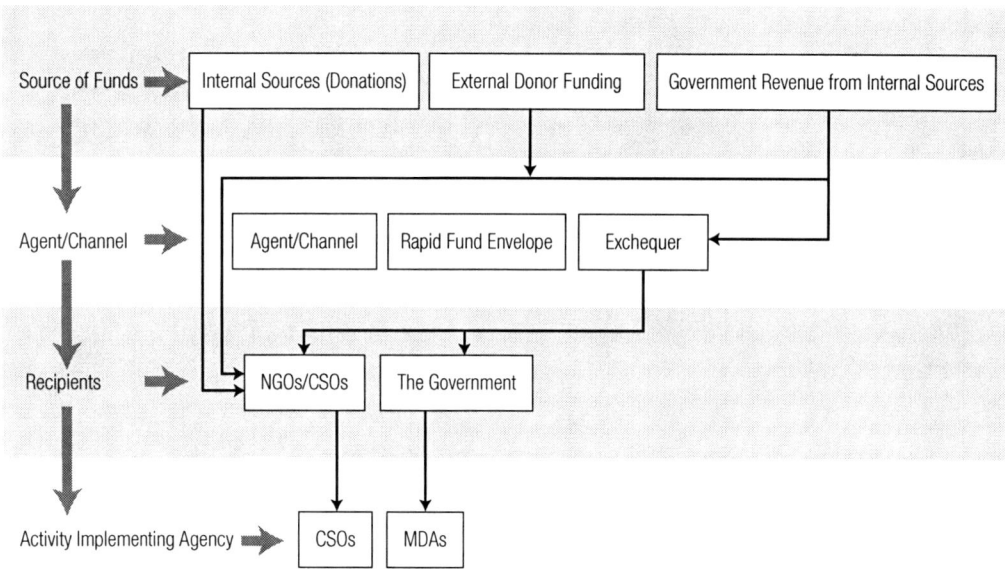

TOTAL GOVERNMENT HEALTH EXPENDITURE IN TANZANIA

Following the classification used in the 2005 Health Sector PER (URT, 2005e), health-sector expenditure is either on- or off-budget. On-budget expenditure includes:

- The recurrent and development spending at MoH headquarters;
- The allocations by the Prime Minister's Office, Regional Administration and Local Government (PMO–RALG) to regional curative and preventive sub-

votes, as well as to local government subvotes for curative and preventive health centres and dispensaries;

- The central PMO–RALG development budget related to PHC rehabilitation; and
- The contribution from the AGO to the National Health Insurance Fund (NHIF) made on behalf of public servants.

Off-budget expenditure includes the use of cost-sharing revenues by public-sector hospitals and the Community Health Fund (CHF), as well as the external funding of projects captured within the MoF external finance database.

TRENDS IN HEALTH-SECTOR SPENDING

The health sector was prioritised under the first PRS, with allocations to the sector being increased from 8.8% in 2000 to 10.6% in 2001 of the total expenditure, excluding CFS.[62] Such a trend remained constant in 2003 and 2004. The share of the health budget has also failed to meet the Abuja target, as 15% of government resources have not been allocated for health. However, the real annual increases in the health allocations have been high, comprising 34.7% in 2002/03 and 27.8% in 2005/06. Information from the MoF also shows that health-sector spending has increased as a proportion of the GDP, from about 1.3% in 2001 to 2.2% in 2005. When off-budget resources to the MoH are considered, the share of total health spending increases from 2.5% in 2002 to 3.5% of the GDP in FY 2005 (see Figure 5.4).

On-budget health spending per capita (at current prices and in real terms) has also been low. In FY 2001, per capita spending was about US$3.7 at current prices, which, however, increased to US$7.4 in the 2005 budget.

Figure 5.4: Health sector expenditure allocations, FY 2000-2005

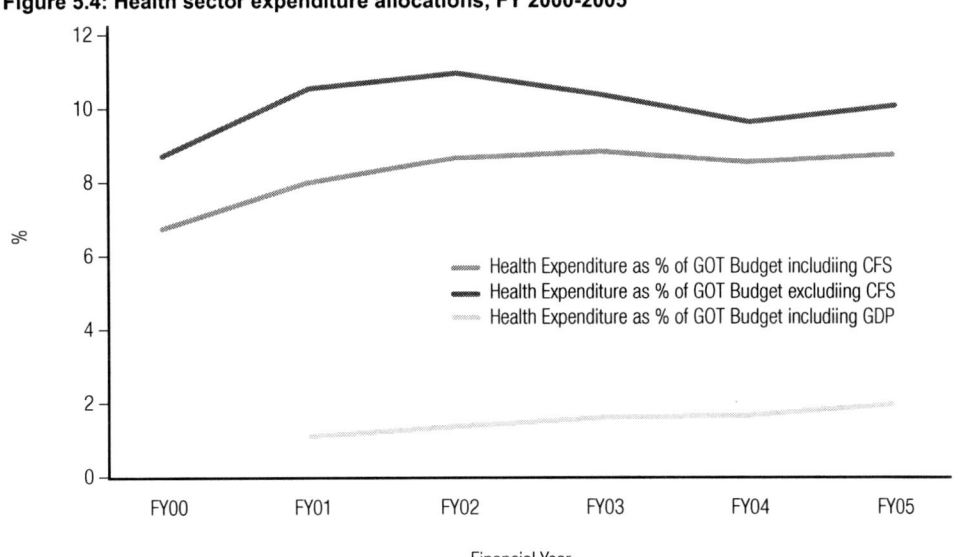

Financial Year

Source: Own calculations using data from the Health Sector 2005 PER Update

In nominal and real terms, the amount allocated to health has been increasing annually, though the growth rates have fluctuated considerably. Due to growth in the total health spending, per capita health spending increased gradually from TZS3 109 in 2001, more than doubling by FY 2005 (see Table 5.3). Such an increase is attributed to an increase in financial support from external funds for the health sector in support of the PRS. Between 2004 and 2005, disaggregated data from the MoF revealed that foreign funds earmarked for development expenditure rose from TZS59.4 billion to TZS101.9 billion as more funds were channelled through the health sector basket fund (see Figure 5.4). This led to an increase in the share of foreign financing for the health sector as a whole, from 27.3% in 2004 to 35.1%[63] in 2005.

Table 5.3: Health allocations (nominal and real), FY 2002/03-2005/06				
	2002/03 actual	2003/04 actual	2004/05 actual	2005/06 budget
Total health budget in TZS billion (current prices)	221.6	237.1	310.4	453.1
Total health budget in US$ million	237.3	236.9	288	423.2
Per capita health spending in TZS (current prices)	6 637	6 889	8 747	12 389
Per capita health spending in US$	7.11	6.88	8.12	11.57
Real allocations to health in TZS billion (real 2001 prices)	211.4	216.7	273.1	382.8
Real per capita health spending in TZS (2001 prices)	6 331	6 296	7 698	10 466
Health spending as % of GDP	2.5	2.4	2.7	3.5
Gross Domestic Product at current prices in TZS billion	8 838.10	10 062.00	11 504	12 997
Real growth of health allocations %	-0.6	22.3	36	
Inflation rate (%)	14.8	9.4	13.6	18.4
Source: Ministry of Finance data abridged from Health Sector PER update FY 2005 and own calculations				

SOURCES OF FINANCING FOR THE HEALTH SECTOR BUDGET

External funds are an important component of the health budget. However, the actual disbursement of external funds appears to be unpredictable and has fallen short of the initial budget projections in almost every year for on-budget expenditure (see Tables 5.4 and 5.5). In contrast, domestically financed health spending has each year turned out to be more than was initially budgeted for, not as a result of filling the gap in development spending caused by shortfalls in foreign funding (URT, 2005f), but due to the financing of increased recurrent expenses. There is concern, however, that scant domestic resources are set aside for development expenditure in the sector, making it highly dependent on unpredictable foreign financing.

Table 5.4: Shares of domestic and foreign funding of health budget (on-budget only), FY 2002/03-2005/06							
	2002/03		2003/04		2004/05		2005/06
	Budget	Actual	Budget	Actual	Budget	Actual	Budget
Foreign funding of health budget (%)	33.8	28.6	34.8	34.1	27.6	27.0	37.6
Domestic funding of health budget (%)	66.2	71.4	65.2	65.9	72.4	73.0	62.4
Source: Abridged from Health Sector PER Update FY 2005							

When off-budget finances are included, the picture concerning the relative shares of foreign and domestic financing of health-sector activities changes significantly. Table 5.5 shows that the actual share of foreign financing (including off-budget resources) was about 54% in FY 2002. By 2004, foreign financing of the health budget had declined to 46%, though in nominal terms it continued to grow. However, for 2005 the projections showed that about 55% of health spending would have been from foreign sources.

Table 5.5: Shares of domestic and foreign funding of health expenditure (on- and off-budget resources) as % of total health spending, FY 2002/03-2005/06							
	2002/03		2003/04		2004/05		2005/06
	Budget	Actual	Budget	Actual	Budget	Actual	Budget
Foreign funding of health spending (%)	53.2	54.0	47.9	50.3	44.6	45.9	55.3
Domestic funding of health spending (%)	46.8	46.0	52.1	49.7	54.8	54.1	44.7
Source: Abridged from Health Sector PER Update FY 2005							

THE TANZANIAN GOVERNMENT AS A SOURCE OF FUNDING FOR HIV/AIDS INITIATIVES

Table 5.6 reports the real public expenditure on HIV/AIDS from FY 2001/02 to FY 2004/05. Allocations through the Exchequer in real terms amounted to about TZS2 190.8 million in 2001/02, increasing to about TZS46 422.3 million in the 2004/05 budget. A substantial increase is also visible when other aid resources to the public sector are included.

The FY 2004/05 witnessed a sharp decline in the amount of aid for HIV/AIDS channelled through NGOs (an almost 50% decrease from FY 2003/04). While such a decline may be a result of underreporting captured on the aid database, there is also a possibility that aid to NGOs may be declining in the long run as more funds are channelled through basket funds and direct budget support (DBS) to the government.

Table 5.6: Trend in real public allocations to HIV/AIDS, FY 2001/02-2004/05				
Expenditure component	2001/02	2002/03	2003/04	2004/05
Government allocation to HIV/AIDS (US$ million) 1/	2.5	11.5	21.4	51.3
Real allocations to HIV/AIDS TZS million 1/ (in 2001 price)	2 190.8	10 521	20 334.5	46 422.3
Real growth rate of allocations to HIV/AIDS 1/	–	380.2	93.3	128.3
Total government HIV/AIDS spending including other aid to the government TZS million 2/	12 244	27 647	41 600	68 124
Total government HIV/AIDS spending including other aid to the government in current US$ million 2/	13.1	27.6	38.6	63.6
Real allocations to HIV/AIDS TZS million (2001 price) 2/	11 683.2	25 271.5	36 619.7	57 537.2
Real growth of allocations to HIV/AIDS 2/		116.3	44.9	57.1
Exchange rate TZS/US$	934	1 001	1 076	1 071
Note: 1/ Government expenditure includes only the foreign assistance captured by AGO 2/ Includes other aid to the public sector that is not directly captured by AGO Source: HIV/AIDS PER Update, 2005; URT, 2005d and author's calculations				

Expenditure on HIV/AIDS (including all aid to the public sector) has been growing. In 2001/02, the Total Public Expenditure (TPE) on HIV/AIDS was estimated at 0.8% of total government expenditure. By 2004/05, however, the figure had increased to 2.1% of the total government budget. Since some foreign assistance is not captured by the Accountant General (AG), the total expenditure reported by the AGO tends to fall short of the actual public expenditure on HIV/AIDS when other foreign assistance for HIV/AIDS is included.

Given that the health budget as a share of total expenditure is not increasing at the same proportion as the HIV/AIDS share of the health budget (see Table 5.6), the apparent crowding out of other health expenditure gives cause for concern. The response to HIV/AIDS generally requires strengthened health systems, which will only be weakened if resources are redirected to HIV/AIDS-specific responses.

Sectoral Distribution of Government Expenditure on HIV/AIDS

Based on the "Z" code (now the "A" code) information in the IFMS, the central MDAs accounted for most (about 98%) government expenditure on HIV/AIDS in FY 2004/05, with the remaining 2% financing HIV/AIDS-related activities in local government (see Table 5.7). A detailed assessment reveals that, at the central government level, the MoH, TACAIDS and the Ministry of Education and Culture accounted for nearly 90% of all HIV/AIDS-related allocations. The distribution of aid resources captured in the development budget also follows a similar pattern (see Table 5.7). Limited allocations to HIV/AIDS across various MDAs may reflect limited mainstreaming of HIV/AIDS activities in other units of the government. The HIV/AIDS PER 2005 update lists those government units that may require more funding for HIV/AIDS-related activities in future.

Table 5.7: Distribution of government expenditure for HIV/AIDS across government units (in TZS million), FY 2004/05						
Spending unit	Government domestic resources	Share (% of total)	Aid resources through AG	Share (% of total)	Aid and government resources	Share (% of total)
All MDAs	14 322	98	34 361	85	48 683	89
Regions	260	2	6 021	15	6 281	11
Total	14 582	100	40 382	100	54 964	100
Source: HIV/AIDS PER Update, 2005						

At local government level, much of the funding of HIV/AIDS activities in FY 2004/05 came from foreign sources, mainly comprising the Tanzania Multisectoral AIDS Project (TMAP) and the GFATM (Round 1). The allocation of funds for HIV/AIDS during 2004/05 shows that Dar es Salaam was the largest beneficiary of government resources from domestic revenue collection, with foreign funds being more equally distributed across the regions (see Table 5.7). On average, each region received between 3% and 6% of the total allocations for HIV/AIDS to the local governments. Mbeya region received the largest share (7%) of the total allocations to local governments, possibly due to the need to scale up HIV/AIDS mitigation activities in the regions, due to the high HIV prevalence (14%). Kigoma, Ruvuma and Rukwa received 3% each of the total resource envelope for HIV/AIDS to local governments during FY 2005.

FOREIGN/INTERNATIONAL FINANCING SOURCES FOR HIV/AIDS

With increasing HIV/AIDS prevalence rates, Tanzania continues to depend on support from its international development partners to finance its response to HIV/AIDS. Bilateral financiers include the US government, DFID, Canada, Norway, Sweden, and the European Union (EU) (see Table 5.8). The WB is currently funding TMAP, which supports the Tanzanian government's multisectoral efforts to reduce the spread of HIV/AIDS by scaling up and accelerating its national response to the HIV/AIDS epidemic, as outlined in the NMSF on HIV/AIDS. The goal of the project is to provide technical support to local government authorities (LGAs) and community groups implementing HIV/AIDS-related interventions, and to oversee the financial management of the Community Action Response Fund (CARF).

Tanzania has received funds from the GFTAM Rounds Three and Four. The WFP, which provides funding through civil society organisations for VCT programmes and for food support for those on antiretroviral treatment. While UNICEF provides funds to support activities related to the scaling up of responses to support the OVCs. UNAIDS funds HIV/AIDS prevention measures, and WHO supports VCT and activities within the NACP. As well as acting as service providers and FAs, the UN agencies spent a fair amount on programme development, support and policy development in the form of unquantified technical support. Tanzania also receives varying amounts of financial, material and technical support from the private sector for specific projects or programmes.

Table 5.8: Commitments by development partners (US$'000)				
Development partner	Before 2004	2004	2005	% in 2005
Belgium	–	213.0	213.0	0.14
CIDA	–	428.0	3 851.8	2.51
Clinton Foundation against HIV/AIDS	–		674.30	0.44
DFID	–	2 537.0	5 367.5	3.50
European Union	1 720.0	2 720.0	4 720.0	3.07
Food and Agricultural Organisation	–		232.0	0.15
Finland	410.8	91.0	88.0	0.06
France	216.0	–	–	–
Germany	12 589.4	3 096.5	2 612.1	1.70
Global Funding	–	9 674.7	9 674.7	6.30
Ireland	3 597.6	2 016.0	2 348.4	1.53
Japan/JICA	6 088.0	3 428.0	3 257.0	2.12
Netherlands Embassy	5 552.4	2 903.3	4 022.0	2.62
Norway	1 347.0	1 917.0	5009.0	3.26
Royal Danish Embassy	225	524	0	0.00
Switzerland	–	500.0	350.0	0.23
SIDA	10 712	10 594	10 273	6.69
UNAIDS	388.5	146.7	221.1	0.14
UNDP	405.0	596.0	456.0	0.30
UNFPA	3 551.0	2 650.0	873.0	0.57
UNICEF	6 066.8	5 450.0	4 449.3	2.90
USAID	–	48 750.0	81 000.0	52.75
WFP	566.0	566.0	3 850.0	2.51
World Bank	1 500.0	3 000.0	10 000.0	6.51
Total	54 935.4	101 801.1	153 542.5	100.00

Source: Christian Social Services Commission (CSSC), December 2005– 2005 Update of the partners in regard to the National Multisectoral Strategic Framework on HIV/AIDS

Structures for the Coordination and Channelling of Donor Funding

TAS, launched in June 2002, provided the framework for strengthening aid/donor co-ordination, the harmonisation of processes, partnerships, the national ownership of the development process, and the management of external resources geared towards development (URT, 2005e). TAS ensures that external resources are transparently and effectively delivered, managed and accounted for in order to achieve Tanzania's development goals.

In order to align development assistance with national priorities, URT (2004) states that the requirements are:

- Government ownership of national development agendas;
- A clear vision; and
- A strategy for development.

Tanzania's current development priorities are clearly articulated in the Vision 2025, the MTP, and the NSGRP strategy "MKUKUTA". In addition to the promotion of economic growth and poverty alleviation, HIV/AIDS is also a key priority and a cross-cutting developmental issue.

Development practitioners in Tanzania believe that, for donor funding to be effective, it has to:

- Fund national development priorities;
- Be nationally owned, predictable and integrated in the government system;
- Be delivered and managed through harmonised and rationalised processes; and
- Be complemented by capacity-building efforts.

Consequently, the TAS priority areas constitute the following:

- Increasing the predictability of aid flow;
- Integrating external funds into the government exchequer system;
- Harmonising and rationalising both government and development partner processes;
- Improving national capacities in aid coordination and external resources management; and
- Ensuring the predictability of resource flow through the formulation and adoption of the PRS paper.

Efforts have been made to move away from rigid conditionalities towards the adoption of agreed actions that are jointly adopted and monitored, and which form an integral part of the government's reform programme. The Policy Assessment Framework (PAF) of the PRBS facility and the WB PRSC were adopted in FY 2002/03. PAF sets out the agreed actions on reform, which are monitored by the development partners and the government on an annual basis. The broad assessment of progress in PAF targets provides the trigger for the release of budget support resources.

Donor funding has been integrated into the government budget system. Such integration has been facilitated through the continuing reforms of the government's public financial management system, which includes the IFMS, the PER, the MTEF, the Public Finance Act of 2001, the Procurement Act of 2001 and the Public Financial Management Reform Programme (PFMRP). The government capacity to record, monitor and control expenditures has been strengthened through the IFMS, which has been adopted and implemented in all MDAs. The IFMS has also allowed government to introduce standardised coding to facilitate the monitoring and tracking of expenditure through the budget system.

Transparency in government expenditure is also ensured through a consultative process that involves development partners and other stakeholders. The consultative processes include the PER, the MTEF and consultative group meetings. The processes have been a success in establishing an open dialogue on budgetary issues. Furthermore, confidence in the government's financial management capacity and control processes has been enhanced through the continuing implementation of the PFMRP, the Public Finance Act and the Public Procurement Act. All such efforts have contributed to the increased donor trust in the government's management of donor funds, which has encouraged them to provide direct support to the government budget, through the PRBS and PRSC facilities, and to support sector-wide basket approaches in the education and health sectors, as well as joint funding of the Poverty Monitoring System, the Legal Sector Reform Programme, and the Local Government Reform Programme.

To guide the government and development partners in moving forward on improving aid coordination and harmonisation, and in implementing the TAS, a TAS/Harmonisation Implementation Group (under the MoF), has been established, with joint membership of the government and the local Development Assistance Committee (DAC). The role of the group is to advise and oversee the implementation of TAS and harmonisation initiatives. In addition, a TAS Technical Secretariat, consisting of government and DAC representatives, has been established to support the work of the TAS/Harmonisation Implementation Group by providing technical inputs.

An Independent Monitoring Group (IMG) was established to institutionalise the process of the independent monitoring of the development partnership in Tanzania in 2002. The IMG undertakes a medium-term assessment of progress made towards the goals of the development partnership, as jointly adopted by the government and the development partners, as set out in the TAS. The group is involved in setting targets and recommending solutions to overcome any difficulties in attaining such targets.

The coordination of other international sources of HIV/AIDS channelled through the civil society is fragmented and often not transparent. Donor funds channelled to the CSOs from the bilateral and multilateral organisations are coordinated through the coordination mechanisms agreed upon by the parties in the memorandum of understanding, which are often difficult to track at national level.

Donor Priorities in Terms of HIV/AIDS Activities

Based on the Christian Social Services Commission (CSSC) analysis of funding from development partners, Table 5.9 shows, that unlike in the previous year's assessment, where the largest share was allocated for cross-cutting activities, the 2005 assessment showed that the largest share of resources committed for HIV/AIDS was channelled to care and treatment. Funds committed to care and treatment in 2005 amounted to 58.4%, compared with 16.1% in 2006, which can be explained by recent emphases on treatment, including the introduction of antiretrovirals especially by the GFATM. Among other channels, substantial amounts have been committed for care and treatment by the Clinton Foundation Against HIV/AIDS (CHAI) and GFATM. Funds committed to prevention increased from 9.1% in the 2004 assessment to 12% in 2005, which could be explained by the PEPFAR emphasis on mainly prevention activities. Nonetheless, compared with the 2004 assessment, resources for cross-cutting activities as a share of total commitments declined from 38.1% to 10.8%, with the commitment to impact mitigation accounting for 1.2%. The "other" category, which basically comprises technical support and support for administrative and logistical purposes, accounts for 3.1%.

Table 5.9: External funding in terms of specific HIV/AIDS-related thematic areas							
Code	Thematic areas	2004	2005	2006	2007	Total	%
1	Cross cutting	17 514	15 937.2	21 962.2	14 947.1	104 902.82	10.8
2	Prevention	22 352	29 515.9	31 089.0	6 680.0	116 118.50	12
3	Care and treatment	45 204	69 081.6	134 051.7	135 517.4	566 122.33	58.4
4	Impact mitigation	1 130	4 497.3	4 390.5		11 146.59	1.2
5	Others		12 439.3	17 156.1	745.0	30 340.43	3.1
6	Combined	15 159	22 275.2	30 441.0	26 505.0	140 407.30	14.5
	Total	101 359	153 746.5	239 090.5	184 394.5	969 037.97	100
Source: Christian Social Services Commission, 2005							

APPLICATION OF NATIONAL AIDS SPENDING ASSESSMENT TOOL IN TANZANIA: RESULTS FROM SELECTED DISTRICTS AND SITES

As mentioned earlier, the principle of the NASA techniques hinges on five main pillars:
- Where the money comes from (the financial sources or agents);
- Where the money goes (the service and goods providers);
- What a provider delivers (its functions in terms of prevention, treatment, etc);
- Who receives the benefits (the beneficiaries or target groups); and
- What the provider buys to deliver, meaning to produce the function (objects of expenses/budgetary items: health, medical supplies, food, etc).

SOURCE OF FUNDING

According to NASA classification, a funding agency could either be a source or an agent. At the same time, a source could also be an agent, for instance, some FBOs provide charity funds to CBOs, while, at the same time, receiving and administering funds from other sources. At the grassroots level, a total of 229 organisations were identified as sources/agents of funds, some of which are small, localised funding organisations that channel funds to local organisations and whose funds might not be captured at the national level by the MoF Exchequer system.

From the national sources, the total expenditure on HIV/AIDS interventions from the government and commitments from development partners was obtained from two sources (see Tables 10.1 and 10.2). A total of US$168 124 500 was allocated to HIV/AIDS interventions in 2004/05, both from the government (US$14 582 000) and development partner sources (US$153 542 500) for all the districts in the country, resulting in 9% government funding and 91% donor funding. Of the 16 districts under this study, the research team using the NASA data-collection tools was only able to track a total of US$19 903 180, which was transferred to the mentioned organisations in the selected districts and sites. Such funding amounts to only 12% of the HIV/AIDS funds reported at the national sources. Of the total received in the selected districts (almost US$20 million), the respondents reported they had spent US$17 602 566 (88%) on the delivery of services in the period under study. The amount reported spent was only 10.5% of the total funds reported at the national sources for the year under study.

As mentioned earlier, since the study was unable to track all the funds in the sampled districts, any discussion of the absolute numbers of what was spent might be misleading, Thus interpretation of the findings is based on the proportion of expenditures.

SERVICE PROVIDERS

Of the 189 providers sampled for the current study (see Table 2.3), the not-for-profit NGOs were found to be the leading providers of HIV/AIDS services at the grassroots level. Funds are channeled to the NGOs for the implementation of HIV/AIDS programmes and projects. The categorisation of donor support by Christian Social Services Commission (CSSC) (2005) shows that direct budget funding continues to be the key mode of support, accounting for about 88%, followed by transfers to NGOs, which account for about 8%. The RFE and in-kind both have less than 2%. On the other hand, many providers operate in the area of ancillary services, which area comprises laboratories, diagnostics centres (31.2%) and advocacy services, such as social communication (27.5%).

Table 5.10: Sampled service providers by type of service provided			
Sn.	Type of services	Number of organisations	%
1.	Advocacy	52	27.5
2.	Research and development	17	9.0
3.	Ancillary services	59	31.2
4.	Health care	37	19.6
5.	Personal health goods	10	5.3
6.	Regulation prevention and control of HIV/AIDS	14	7.4
Total		189	100.0

EXPENDITURE BY FUNCTION/AIDS SPENDING CATEGORY

The total sum reported above was spent on the interventions presented in Figure 5.5, with NASA classification referring to such interventions as "AIDS spending categories". Though many Tanzanians believe that much HIV/AIDS funding is spent on prevention programmes, which is justified by the fact that 93% of the population is not infected and needs protection, the study shows that a fairly large percentage is spent on programme development (41%). The key expenditure was followed by spending on prevention programmes and treatment and care, which consumed 24% and 22% respectively (with the findings capturing only a small proportion of funding from health facilities, including all HIV/AIDS expenditure that increases the care and treatment budget).

The study supports the findings by CSSC (2005) (www.cssc.or.tz), which show that the funds committed for care and treatment in 2005 amounted to 58.4%, compared with 16.1% in 2004 from donor funds, largely due to the recent emphasis on treatment, including the introduction of antiretrovirals. Among other channels, substantial amounts have been committed for care and treatment by the CHAI and GFATM, with 21.6% of the funds being committed for prevention, which could be attributed to PEPFAR, with a focus on prevention activities.

Figure 5.5: Sampled site proportional expenditure by NASA function, FY 2004/05

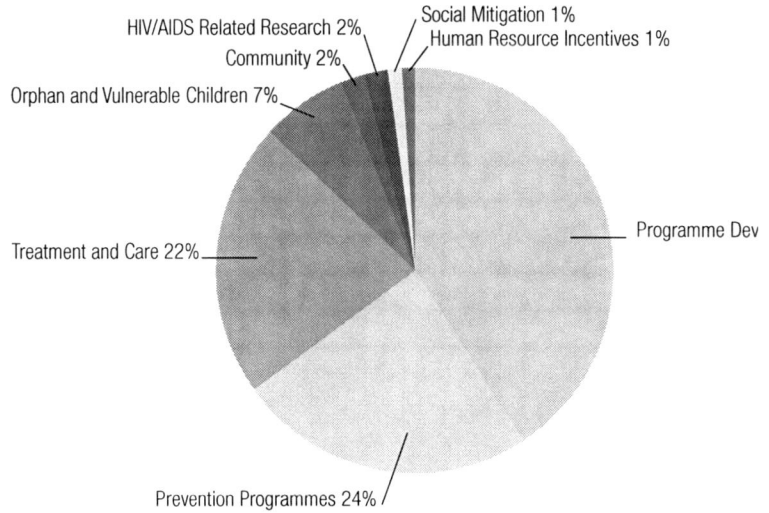

THOSE BENEFITED BY THE EXPENDITURE

Table 5.11 lists the beneficiaries of the expenditure, as reported for the sampled sites. Health-care workers benefited from 35.7% of the total funds tracked, with the next largest group consisting of the non-targeted/general population (benefiting 26.5%), followed by PLWHAs, who benefited from 25.8% of the expenditure of the total funds tracked. Only 7.2% of the tracked funds were spent on OVCs.

The expenditure on sex workers in Tanzania is low, though anecdotal evidence shows that the number of sex workers is increasing. In Tanzanian law, neither sex workers nor men who have sex with men (MSMs) are recognised, especially in the prison sector. Prisoners and prison officers were reluctant to disclose how much men-to-men sex occurs in prisons, though it is known to be common. No expenditure has been reported for prisoners and other institutionalised persons.

Table 5.11: Sampled sites reported expenditure by beneficiary group, FY 2004/05	
Beneficiary categories	% of total expenditure
People living with HIV who either have or have not been diagnosed with AIDS	25.8
Injecting drug users	0.0
Sex workers and their clients	0.1
Orphans and vulnerable children	7.2
Migrants, refugees and internally displaced persons	0.0
Prisoners and other institutionalised persons	0.0
Men and women separated from their families	0.0
Women and children affected by trafficking and violence	0.0
Youth in social risk, out of school, living in the street, members of gangs or institutionalised in centres for minors	1.2
Partners of the people living with HIV/AIDS	0.1
Children in school	0.7
Youth at school	1.5
Migrants workers, truck drivers and salespersons	0.1
Women attending reproductive health clinics	0.8
Military, police, sailors	0.0
Health-care workers	35.7
General population/ Non-targeted population	26.5
Men who have sex with other men	0.0
Special populations (unclassified)	0.2
Total	99.9

OBJECTS OF EXPENDITURE

Table 5.12 presents expenditure in terms of budgetary items, with administration (15.5%), food/meals (10.6%), health personnel (10.6%) and medical supplies (10.4%) consuming a large share of such expenditure. The total expenditure reported at this level falls short of the total expenditure cited above (US$19 903 180), because some of the respondents were unable to state their objects of expenditure.

Table 5.12: Sampled sites HIV/AIDS expenditure by object/budgetary item, FY 2004/05		
Object of expenditure	Total expenditure (US$)	% of total expenditure
Health personnel	1 864 021	10.6
Non-health personnel	423 489	2.4
Pharmaceutical products	1 016 862	5.8
Medical supplies	1 831 710	10.4
Condoms	294 522	1.7
Reagents and materials	505 712	2.9
Food/meals	1 860 608	10.6
Other materials	2 181 142	12.4
Building, remodelling and repair	562 188	3.2
Medical equipment	282 519	1.6
Non-medical equipment	208 068	1.2
Administration	2 739 554	15.5
Research and consultancy	593 130	3.4
Maintenance	108 422	0.6
Hotel and rented vehicles	515 703	2.9
Other services	1 639 032	9.3
Per diem	764 652	4.3
Monetary benefits	211 231	1.2
Total	17 602 565	100.0

EQUITY IN HIV/AIDS SPENDING IN TANZANIA

The allocation of resources for HIV/AIDS should be done equitably, with resources being distributed in accordance with the needs of different types of beneficiaries. A guiding principle of the national response initiative against the HIV/AIDS epidemic in Tanzania stated in the National Multisector Strategic Framework (NMSF) delineates that the protection of health is a basic human right of all Tanzanians. Assessing whether the allocation of HIV/AIDS resources in Tanzania reflects differential HIV/AIDS needs across regions and social groups is imperative. The findings on equity-related issues explored as follows are based on the primary data collected using NASA techniques and secondary data from government and non-governmental sources. The analysis is limited by the degree of available disaggregated data required.

Tables 5.13 and 5.14 present the HIV prevalence rates, and the proportion of expenditure by regions and districts respectively, as reported by responding organisations in the 16 districts sampled. Though the information presented in the following tables shows how much has been reported in the different regions and districts, given their socioeconomic diversity, no conclusion regarding equity issues could be drawn without further analysis. In assessing whether HIV/AIDS spending is equitable, the major determining variables are, among others:
- Allocation per specific social group (rich versus poor, women versus men, youth versus elderly);

- Allocation by geographical location (rural versus urban, depending on the population size of the location/region);
- HIV prevalence/incidence;
- HIV incidence; and
- Survival/death rates (for which data relating to the latter two variables is unavailable).

However, given the poverty prevailing generally in Tanzania, HIV allocations are also affected by other poverty-related variables.

An ordinary least square regression model with HIV/AIDS expenditure as the dependent variable and HIV/AIDS-related variables and other poverty-related variables as independent variables was applied, including:

- HIV prevalence;
- Urban/rural dummy;
- Total population;
- Population per health facility in the district;
- The number of health facilities per square kilometre;
- The percentage of the population below the poverty line;
- The percentage of households that are female headed;
- The percentage of households headed by a person 60 years of age or older;
- The percentage of children under 18 years of age whose mother and/or father has/have died; and
- The under-five mortality rate (per 1 000 live births).

(See Appendix for the summary statistics of these indicators).

Table 5.13: Share of total captured expenditure by region according to the sampled sites, FY 2004/05

Region	HIV prevalence rate	% of total expenditure	Number of organisations
Kigoma	2.0	8.88	27
Kilimanjaro	7.3	16.24	14
Dar es Salaam	10.9	37.18	50
Mbeya	13.5	10.06	13
Tabora	7.2	0.92	16
Dodoma	4.9	6.08	22
Lindi	3.6	4.43	19
Kagera	3.7	16.21	28
Total	–	100.0	189

Table 5.15 summarises the regression results, with HIV prevalence, the number of health facilities in the district, and the percentage of households headed by a person 60 years or older being strongly related to HIV/AIDS expenditure. HIV/AIDS funding is meager, being insufficient to cover the needs of the general population, or to address child-related programmes. HIV expenditure on the total/general population mainly takes the form of preventive programmes (with 93% of the population needing to be protected). However, as seen earlier, prevention interventions account for only 24% of the HIV/AIDS funds tracked. There is also a negative but significant

difference between the HIV/AIDS expenditure on the number of children under 18 who are orphaned (mother and/or father has died). This is also reflected under the funding of OVC programmes (7.2% of the tracked funds).

Table 5.14: Reported expenditure by selected districts (in US$), FY 2004/05				
Region	District	HIV prevalence rate	% of total expenditure	Number of organisations
Kigoma	Kigoma Urban	7.4	5.55	19
	Kibondo	1.4	3.53	8
Kilimanjaro	Moshi Urban	–	11.52	8
	Rombo	2.1	4.72	6
Dar es Salaam	Kinondoni	10.3	14.81	21
	Temeke	16.3	22.37	29
Mbeya	Chunya	26.5	2.01	6
	Mbeya Urban	5.6	8.05	7
Tabora	Tabora Urban	–	0.87	8
	Urambo	11.3	0.05	8
Dodoma	Dodoma Urban	4.6	3.19	11
	Kongwa	13.3	2.89	11
Lindi	Kilwa	4.7	1.74	12
	Lindi Rural	5.5	2.70	7
Kagera	Bukoba Urban	13.0	13.86	17
	Muleba	29.3	2.15	11
Total (Urban)		–	81.95	132
Total (Rural)			18.05	57
Total			100.00	189

Table 5.15: Regression results from sampled sites expenditure analysis				
Independent variables	Coefficient	Standard error	T	p>|t|
HIV prevalence	285.9642	102.8999	2.78*	0.069
Total population	-0.0079746	0.001598	-4.99*	0.015
Population per health facility	-0.055886	0.144899	-0.39	0.725
Number of health facilities per square kilometre	38 014.05	5 561.082	6.84**	0.006
% of the population below the poverty line	204.366	90.28056	2.26	0.109
% of Household that are female headed	388.3217	253.1822	1.53	0.223
% of Households headed by a person 60 or older	359.656	152.0199	2.37*	0.099
% of children under 18 who are orphaned (mother and/or father has died)	-475.6133	270.0889	-1.76	0.176
Under five mortality rate (per 1000 live births)	-48.91667	18.68618	-2.62*	0.079
Urban	2 870.034	1 449.318	1.98	0.142
Constant	-14 680.97	8 704.741	-1.69	0.190
*shows significance at 0.1 level; ** shows significance at 0.05 level				

CONCLUSION

HIV/AIDS is a serious health and socio-economic problem in Tanzania. It ranks among the top impediments to a country's social and economic development as it affects all sectors of the economy. The government, in collaboration with different stakeholders, has responded massively to the pandemic by committing resources, both human and financial, for formulating policies and strategies, and by establishing specific institutions to coordinate the response. However, there is much spending that is not captured by the AGO, and these external funds are an important contribution to the health budget. However, actual disbursement of external funds appears to be unpredictable and has fallen short of the initial budget projections almost every year. On the other hand, there is concern that very little domestic resources are set aside for development expenditure in the sector, which makes the latter highly dependent on unpredictable foreign financing.

One of the challenges to proper tracking of HIV/AIDS funds in Tanzania is the lack of a central database which shows all the players in the HIV/AIDS field and the absence of strict sanctions on non-reporting CSOs. There has also been little transparency on how CSOs utilise the funds allocated to HIV/AIDS. This is mainly due to the lack of mechanisms to enforce and ensure transparent evaluation and utilisation of funds and implementation of activities by the CSOs. This is a critical challenge that needs to be addressed if effective financial accountability is to be ensured in the country, and also because of the significant contribution made by CSOs and NGOs in the delivery of services, particularly at district level. The silence with regard to men who have sex with men, especially in prisons, has led to the failure of government to allocate resources targeting this vulnerable group. No expenditure has been reported for prisoners and other institutionalised persons. The findings showed limited expenditure that benefited women, specifically women and children affected by trafficking and violence.

REFERENCES

Economic and Social Research Foundation, 2003. *The Socio and Economic Impacts of HIV/AIDS in Tanzania: The Case of Six Districts*. Dar es Salaam: ESRF.

Haki Elimu, 2005. *Three Years of PEDP Implementation: Key Findings from Government Reviews*, July 2005. Dar es Salaam: Hakielimu.

Kessy, F., 2004. *The Impact of HIV/AIDS on Agriculture: The Case of Kilombero and Ulanga Districts*. Consultancy report submitted to the Eastern Zone Client Oriented Research and Extension Program (EZCORE).

Kessy, F., 2005. *Inventory of HIV/AIDS Service Providers in Tanzania*. Consultant Report Submitted to Swedish Cooperative Center.

National Bureau of Statistics [Tanzania] and Macro International Inc., 1997. *Tanzania Demographic and Health Survey, 1996*. Dar es Salaam; Calverton, Mld: Bureau of Statistics and Macro International.

National Bureau of Statistics (NBS) [Tanzania] and Macro International Inc., 2000.

Tanzania Reproductive and Child Health Survey, 1999. Dar es Salaam; Calverton, Ml: National Bureau of Statistics and Macro International Inc.

National Bureau of Statistics (NBS) [Tanzania] and ORC Macro, 2005. *Tanzania Demographic and Health Survey, 2004–05*. Dar es Salaam: National Bureau of Statistics and ORC Macro.

TACAIDS, 2004. *Planning, Budgeting and Monitoring Frameworks for HIV/AIDS*, A paper presented to Parliamentarians, July 2004, Dodoma.

United Nations Development Program (UNDP), 2005. *Human Development Report*, New York, Oxford: Oxford University Press.

United Republic of Tanzania (URT), 2001a. *National Mortality Burden Estimates for 2001*. National Sentinel Surveillance System, Adult Morbidity and Mortality Project. Dar es Salaam: Ministry of Health.

United Republic of Tanzania (URT), 2001b. *National Policy on HIV/AIDS*, Dar es Salaam: Prime Minister's Office.

United Republic of Tanzania (URT), 2002a. *Household Budget Survey*, Dar es Salaam: National Bureau of Statistics.

United Republic of Tanzania (URT), 2002b. *Integrated Labor Force Survey, 2000/01*, Dar es Salaam: National Bureau of Statistics, President's Office, Planning and Privatization, and Ministry of Labor, Youth Development and Sports.

United Republic of Tanzania (URT), 2002c. *Health Statistical Abstract*, Dar es Salaam: Ministry of Health.

United Republic of Tanzania (URT), 2002d. *National AIDS Control Program: HIV/ AIDS/STI Surveillance Report*, Report No. 15, Dar es Salaam: Ministry of Health.

United Republic of Tanzania (URT), 2003a. *2002 Population and Housing Census*, Dar es Salaam: National Bureau of Statistics.

United Republic of Tanzania (URT), 2003b. *Poverty and Human Development Report, 2003*, Dar es Salaam: Mkuki na Nyota Publisher.

United Republic of Tanzania (URT), 2003c. *Guide to Higher Education in Tanzania, 2003*, Dar es Salaam: Higher Education Publication Council.

United Republic of Tanzania (URT), 2003d. *National Health Policy*. Dar es Salaam: Ministry of Health.

United Republic of Tanzania (URT), 2003e. *Health Sector Strategy for HIV/AIDS (2003–2006)*, Dar es Salaam: National AIDS Control Program.

United Republic of Tanzania (URT), 2003f. *National Multi-sectoral Strategic Framework on HIV/AIDS (2003/2004)*, Dar es Salaam: Prime Minister's Office.

United Republic of Tanzania (URT), 2004. *Aid Coordination, Harmonization and Alignment in Tanzania*, Paper presented by the Ministry of Finance at the 2004 Partner Conference, 15th–17th December, 2004, Impala Hotel, Arusha.

United Republic of Tanzania (URT), 2005a. *Poverty and Human Development Report, 2005*, Dar es Salaam: Mkuki na Nyota.

United Republic of Tanzania (URT), 2005b. *Tanzania HIV/AIDS Indicator Survey, 2003–04*. Dar es Salaam: TACAIDS, National Bureau of Statistics; Calverton, Mld.: ORC Macro.

United Republic of Tanzania (URT), 2005c. *HIV/AIDS/STI Surveillance Report for January–December 2004*, No. 19, Dar es Salaam: National AIDS Control Program.

United Republic of Tanzania (URT), 2005d. *Tanzania Public Expenditure Multi-Sectoral Review: HIV/AIDS 2005 Update*, Dar es Salaam: TACAIDS and Ministry of Finance.

United Republic of Tanzania (URT), 2005e. *Enhancing Aid Relationships in Tanzania*, Report of the Independent Monitoring Group to the Government of Tanzania and Development Partners Group.

United Republic of Tanzania (URT), 2005f. *Health Sector Public Expenditure Review Update FY 05*, Dar es Salaam: Ministry of Health.

YAV, 2005. *Baseline Study on Participation of Young Persons in Governance and Management of Health Care Service in Kinondoni Municipal Council, Dar es Salaam, Tanzania*, Dar es Salaam: Youth Action Volunteers.

APPENDIX

HIV/AIDS and other poverty indicators by district									
District	HIV Prevalence	Total Population	Population per health facility	Number of health facilities per square kilometre	% of population below poverty line 2000/01	% of households that are female headed	% of households headed by a person 60 or older	% of children under 18 orphaned (mother and/or father have died	Under five mortality rate (per 1000 live births)
Kigoma Urban	7.4	144 852	12 021	0.048	27	33	13	10.2	167
Kibondo	1.4	414 764	7 013	0.014	39	33	19	6.8	136
Moshi Urban	–	144 336	7 568	0.318	18	34	8	8.4	63
Rombo	2.1	246 479	6 143	0.029	37	35	25	8.1	73
Kinondoni	10.3	1 088 867	5 162	0.384	14	28	7	12	138
Ilala	6.9	637 573	3 191	0.594	16	26	8	11	130
Temeke	16.3	771 500	6 351	0.162	29	29	8	11	134
Chunya	26.5	206 615	6 056	0.001	25	29	15	10.1	165
Mbeya Urban	5.6	266 422	6 640	0.158	12	37	10	16.2	106
Tabora Urban	–	188 808	4 273	0.029	23	33	17	9.5	123
Urambo	11.3	370 796	10 863	0.002	41	25	18	6.6	124
Dodoma Urban	4.6	324 347	5 869	0.021	27	33	16	10.8	153
Kongwa	13.3	249 760	9 209	0.007	40	31	17	7.2	195
Lindi Urban/ Kilwa	5.5	171 850	4 276	0.003	35	33	21	8.9	217
Lindi Rural	4.7	215 764	13 430	0.002	51	32	24	10.5	220
Bukoba Urban	13	81 221	7 352	0.121	11	34	10	16.3	113
Muleba	29.3	386 328	12 840	0.009	27	31	22	14.1	182
Source: URT, 2005a									

ZANZIBAR

RAMSA, N., SULTAN, O., SEHA, A. AND JUMA, S.

EXECUTIVE SUMMARY

Zanzibar, which forms part of the United Republic of Tanzania, comprises two islands – Unguja and Pemba – with an estimated population of 1 078 964[65] (RGoZ, 2002a), and covers a total surface area of 2 332 square kilometres. Zanzibar has an annual population growth rate of 3.1% and a population density of 400 people per square kilometre.

The HIV/AIDS epidemic has affected Zanzibar, with the first HIV case being reported in 1986, and the numbers having since increased to almost 4 000 cases a year to date. The Zanzibar government has embarked on ways of reducing HIV/AIDS effects together with its development partners, funding agencies, local and international NGOs, civil society organisations (CSOs), faith-based organisations (FBOs), and the citizens of Zanzibar.

The HIV/AIDS resource-tracking study aimed to review the response to the epidemic in the isles, relying on government documents, especially budget books, the first HIV/AIDS Public Expenditure Review (PER 2006/07), and other related studies. A survey conducted in 2002 showed that HIV prevalence in Zanzibar was 0.6%. Estimates using antenatal clinic data indicated HIV prevalence to be 0.87% in the age group 12-65 years by the end of 2005. Empirical evidence has shown that the number of HIV/AIDS infections in Zanzibar is increasing. The total number of cases diagnosed has increased from three in 1986 to 3 926 in 2004. Studies done in 2005 showed HIV/AIDS prevalence was 13% among substance users (SUs) and 26% among injecting drug users (IDUs).

As HIV/AIDS is both a health and a socioeconomic issue, the government has involved the Ministry of Health and Child Welfare (MoHSW) through the Zanzibar AIDS Programme (ZACP) to deal with health issues and the Zanzibar AIDS Commission (ZAC) to provide leadership of the multisectoral response. Stakeholders in the national response to HIV/AIDS include the public sector, NGOs, the private sector, CSOs, political parties and religious groups. Furthermore, the government has directed that all MDAs have a subvote in HIV/AIDS counselling. Zanzibar has both a national HIV/AIDS policy and a National Multisectoral Strategic Plan (NMSP).

The budget process in Zanzibar, which is overseen by the Ministry of Finance and Economic Affairs (MoFEA), together with the National Budget and Planning Committee (NBPC), the Sectoral Budget and Planning Committee, technical teams and revenue collection agencies, is comprehensive and includes key players and sectors in the country. The aim of such an inclusive team is to ensure that, in the planning of government expenditure, all needs of the economy are taken into consideration in the annual budget. Parliament discusses the budget plans prior to the official submission of the country's budget to ensure the fair distribution of resources to the sectors involved. The Zanzibar government has undertaken reform of the budget process, with the intention of improving financial and economic management, accountability and transparency, with a focus on PER and Medium-term Expenditure Review (MTEF) processes.

The health sector is one of the key priority areas in the Zanzibar Poverty Reduction Plan (ZPRP). The ratio of the recurrent health budget increased from 6.3% in 2002/03 to 6.9% in 2003/04 (excluding Consolidated Fund Services) as a share of the total government budget, while remaining constant at 6.6% in 2004/05 and 2005/06. The share increased to 10.7% in 2005/06 after including capital funds, thus the share of the health budget has remained substantially short of the Abuja Declaration. Health spending per capita has remained low, increasing from TZS4 323.6 in 2002/03 to TZS5 703.4 in 2004/05, but declining to TZS5 575.9 in 2005/06.

The total actual expenditure for HIV/AIDS, including government sources, donor funds through public-sector support (both on- and off-budget), the donor funding supplied directly to NGOs and international NGO expenditure, increased from TZS2 051.75 million in 2004/05 to TZS3 385.39 million in 2005/06, representing an increase of 65% in nominal terms. Regarding government revenue expenditure on HIV/AIDS, actual government expenditure increased by 69% from TZS438.52 million in 2004/05 to TZS741.1 million in 2005/06. Actual donor financing of public-sector HIV/AIDS activities increased by 54% to TZS2 001.83 million from 2004/05 to 2005/06, while total actual donor financing (including direct transfers to NGOs) increased by 63% to TZS2 629.57 million.

External funds are, therefore, an important component of both the general health and the HIV/AIDS budgets, with serious implications for planning, programme management, and the sustainability of specific programmes. Moreover, due to such dependency, delays in submitting project funding can adversely affect service delivery, and can cause inefficient spending, or "dumping", in order to expend all available funds before the end of the financial period.

Government efforts to cope with the HIV/AIDS epidemic include the increasing of budgetary allocations over time and collaborative efforts entered into with other stakeholders in controlling the spread of the virus and minimising its effects. The disbursing and reporting procedures require streamlining so as to monitor and evaluate the joint use and allocation of resources. Such gaps in the M&E systems of the different role players are seen as the main threat to the effective implementation of the proposed HIV/AIDS-related interventions.

Currently, each major donor has separate disbursement and reporting procedures, which significantly delay the implementation of HIV/AIDS-related activities. Due to the complexity of the procedures and the low recipient capacity, a substantial proportion of the available funds in each year remain unspent. Another difficulty in tracking actual expenditure arises when donors provide goods and services in kind, such as in the form of medical supplies and consultancies, without providing the recipients with any information regarding the value of such goods or services.

To assess the efficiency, effectiveness, and equity of HIV spending, PER procedure should be updated to include estimating expenditures by function, and details relating to the beneficiaries of different programmes. NASA requires that the actual expenditure is captured, and offers a comprehensive and standardised categorisation of activities, that, if adopted, would greatly enhance ZAC's ability to monitor its own expenditure, as well as that of other service providers in Zanzibar. Such categorisation would also allow for improved international comparison of efforts.

SOCIOECONOMIC CONTEXT

DEMOGRAPHIC AND GEOGRAPHICAL LOCATION

Administratively, under union arrangements, the Revolutionary Government of Zanzibar (RGoZ) maintains its own government, with its own president, cabinet, legislature and judiciary system, with full power over non-union matters.

Most of the population resides in rural areas, with agriculture as the main source of livelihood. Only 33.4% of the population lives in urban areas.

ECONOMIC GROWTH

Zanzibar has registered relatively high levels of economic growth in the last five years. The GDP of the country grew by approximately 4.0% in 2000, 8.5% in 2002, 5.9% in 2003, 6.5% in 2004 and 5.6% in 2005 (RGoZ, 2006a). In nominal terms, the GDP grew from TZS222.4 billion in 2001 to TZS286.7 billion in 2003, and TZS395.7 billion in 2005 (RGoZ, 2006a).

There was also a steady rise in per capita income from TZS236 000 in 2001 to TZS369 000 in 2005. Despite such achievements, however, the country remains among the poorest in the world, with only marginal development of its social and economic infrastructure.

The services sector continues to be the main contributor to economic growth in the isles, followed by agriculture, though its contribution to the GDP has declined from 25.4% in 2001 to 23.3% in 2005. Table 6.1 shows the GDP by activity.

Table 6.1: Gross Domestic Product by activity 2001-2005					
Sector	GDP at market prices (% shares)				
	2001	2002	2003	2004	2005
Agriculture, forestry and fishing	25.4	24.9	21.4	23.4	23.3
Industry	11.1	11.6	13.1	13.3	13.5
Services	47.9	49.3	51.8	50.4	50.7
Source: RGoZ, 2006a					

The latest Household Budget Survey (HBS) was undertaken in the isles in 2004/05. Results show that 49.1% and 13.2% of people in Zanzibar live below the basic needs poverty line and the food poverty line (head count ratios) respectively. Table 6.2 shows the poverty indicators for some key social sectors (including water, health and education).

The overall objective of the water and sanitation sector is to improve water supply and sanitation systems to both rural and urban communities. The RGoZ has empha-sised the supply of clean and safe water. About 86% of the rural and urban popula-tion has access to piped or a protected source of water, with water being available within a one kilometre radius for 91% of the population. Despite such achievements, internal regional differences are evident. Only 56.2% of the households in Miche-weni have access to a piped and protected water source, while 72.5% of households in Wete are located within one kilometre of water services.

Table 6.2: HBS national key education and health indicators, FY 2004/05			
Indicator	Total (%)	Rural (%)	Urban (%)
Percentage of adults 15 years and above with five or more years of education	66.3	55.2	82.0
Percentage of adult females 15 years and above with five or more years of education	61.9	47.9	78.0
Percentage of adults literate	75.8	65.9	89.5
Percentage of female adults literate	69.8	58.5	85.2

Percentage of households within 2 km of a primary school	88.2	82.0	98.5
Percentage of households within 5 km of a primary school	98.5	97.6	99.8
Percentage of households within km of a secondary school	93.0	89.2	99.6
Percentage of households within 5 km of a health facility	96.9	95.3	99.5
Proportion of households using piped or protected water as their source for drinking	86.2	80.5	95.9
Percentage of households within 1 km of drinking water	91.4	89.1	95.3
Source: RGoZ, 2006b			

HEALTH INDICATORS

Malaria is the leading cause of morbidity and mortality in all health facilities in Zanzibar (RGoZ, 2004a). About 50% of all outpatient attendance is due to malaria, which also accounts for 50% of the deaths of under fives. The case fatality rate ranges between 2.5% and 5%. Furthermore, between 30% and 42% of children under five years of age are anaemic, with mild and moderate anaemia. Disaggregating Demographic Health Survey (DHS) figures by district shows that Pemba North has the highest rate of moderate anaemia (51.8%) (NBS and ORC Macro, 2005). Other health problems commonly reported in hospitals comprise malnutrition, acute respiratory infections, diarrhoea, hypertension, diabetes and pneumonia. Due to the prevalence of such health conditions, life expectancy remains low (estimated to be 48 years) and maternal and child morality rates remain high in the isles. The infant mortality rate (IMR) is 90 per 1 000, with the under-five mortality rate being 114 per 1 000 live births, and the maternal mortality rate (MMR) being 377 per 100 000 live births (RGoZ, 2004a).

ACCESS TO EDUCATION

A significant proportion of adults are illiterate, with the literacy rate differing widely between rural and urban environments (see Table 6.2). Women are generally more likely to be illiterate than men, and the women in rural areas are more likely to be illiterate than women in urban areas. Almost all school-going children have been enrolled in school, as shown by the high gross enrolment ratio (GER). However, only eight out of ten school-age children are in an age-appropriate class, as indicated by the net enrolment ratio (NER) (see Table 6.2). Regionally, a high disparity exists, with Micheweni reporting a GER of 95% and an NER of 51%, while Kusini has a GER of 122% and an NER of 90% (RGoZ, 2006b).

ROADS

The total road network in Zanzibar extends 1 162 km, covering both rural and urban areas. The transport infrastructure, particularly outside the major towns, has deteriorated considerably over the years due to inadequate maintenance. Over 90% of the

Zanzibar road network is estimated to require substantial improvement. The state of the current road network is detrimental to the national economy, especially as regards access to the rural interior.

ELECTRICITY

On average, only 25.3% of households in Zanzibar are connected to electricity, with a high of 57.0% in urban areas and a low of 7.0% for the rural population. At district level, the coverage of households connected to electricity ranges from 2.4% in Micheweni to 67.6% in Mjini.

THE HEALTH-CARE SYSTEM

The overall objective of the health sector is to improve the health and well-being of the people of Zanzibar, with particular attention to women and children. Health-care services in Zanzibar are provided and managed at four levels, as illustrated in the table below.

Table 6.3: Public health-care facilities by type, location and total population served						
	Type of Facility					
District	First and second line PHF	PHCC (Cottage hospital)	General/ special hospital	Referral hospital	Total number of facilities	Population per district
Unguja Island						
Urban	7	0	2	1	10	217 945
South	9	1	0	0	10	33 520
North A	11	1	0	0	12	92 626
North B	8	0	0	0	8	56 411
Central	18	0	0	0	18	66 848
West	9	0	2	0	11	242 753
Pemba Island						
Chake Chake	11	1	1	0	13	88 661
Mkoani	14	0	1	0	15	98 782
Wete	18	0	1	0	19	109 023
Micheweni	12	1	0	0	13	88 947
Note: PHF = primary health facility						

Such level of health-service provision is supplemented by private health-care facilities. The network of health-care facilities is reportedly sufficient to place every citizen in Zanzibar within a 10 km radius of a health-care facility, and 90% of the population within 5 km walking distance of a health facility (RGoZ, 2006a).

THE HIV/AIDS EPIDEMIC IN ZANZIBAR

HIV PREVALENCE

HIV/AIDS is one of the major developmental concerns of the government of Zanzibar, as it hinders poverty alleviation efforts, undermining the improvements already made in social welfare. The population-based survey carried out in Zanzibar in 2002 revealed a prevalence rate of 0.6% in the subpopulation groups, implying that about 6 000 PLWHAs live in Zanzibar. Nearly 500 AIDS orphans have been registered with HIV/AIDS-related NGOs (RGoZ, 2004a).

A survey conducted in 2002 showed that the HIV prevalence in Zanzibar was 0.6% of the general population. Estimates using data from antenatal clinics (ZACP, 2005) indicated the HIV prevalence to be 0.87% for people between the ages of 12 and 65 years by the end of 2005. The total number of cases diagnosed increased from three in 1986 to 3 926 in 2004.

Due to the low national prevalence rates, HIV/AIDS in Zanzibar is considered a potential future threat, resulting in efforts to prevent the spread of the virus. The HIV prevalence among substance abusers and other most-at-risk-populations (MARP) is alarming, given that such groups can act as "bridging populations" for HIV/AIDS to cross over into the general population. Research has shown that the HIV epidemic in Zanzibar is concentrated in SUs, especially IDUs; both male and female sex workers and their clients; and MSM. Studies carried out in 2005 showed that the HIV prevalence was 13% among SUs and 26% among IDUs (Dahoma et al, 2005). The vulnerable groups in the population are equally affected, given the likelihood that they will engage in unsafe sex.

Currently, HIV/AIDS-related diseases in Zanzibar account for 4.02% of hospital bed occupancy, which compares with 30% in Kenya, over 50% in the Ugandan Rubaga Hospital and about 50% in the Tanzanian Muhimbili Hospital (RGoZ, 2004a).

HIV INFECTION TRENDS IN ZANZIBAR

The trends of HIV infection in Zanzibar are on the increase for some population subgroups, with the total number of HIV/AIDS cases diagnosed increasing from three in 1986 to 3 926 in 2004 (see Figure 6.1). HIV prevalence among pregnant women at antenatal clinics doubled from 0.6% in 1997 to 1% in 2002. The infection rates among voluntary counselling and testing (VCT) attendees also increased sharply from 0.6% in 2002 to 5.6% in 2003, declining to 4.3% in 2004. The HIV prevalence from the screening of donated blood doubled over a three-year period, from 0.7% in 1996 to 1.5% in 1998, declining to 0.5% in 2004.

According to the RGoZ (2005a), the young adult population is at the highest risk of infection, with females being more affected than their male counterparts (see Figure 6.1) (RGoZ, 2005a).

Figure 6.1: Cumulative frequency of HIV infection in Zanzibar, 1988–2004

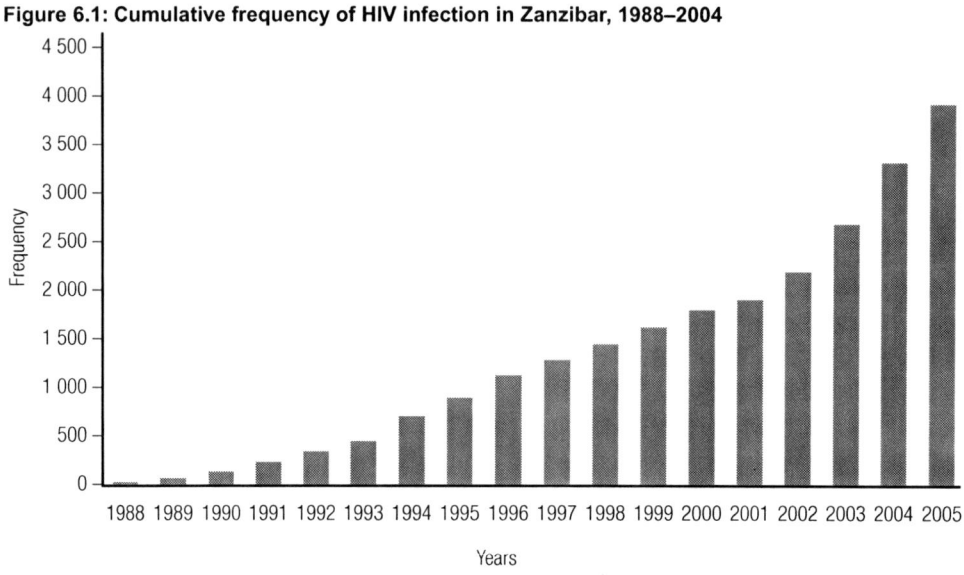

Source: RGoZ, 2005a

Primary Mode of Transmission

Unprotected sex in heterosexual relationships is the main route of HIV/AIDS transmission in Zanzibar, accounting for more than 90% of all cases. In terms of data from the ZACP, 4% of HIV/AIDS transmission is of a vertical nature, consisting of mother–to–child transmission inclusive of the breastfeeding period. HIV/AIDS transmission through the transference of body fluids and blood products in hospital settings, piercing and the use of other surgically invasive equipment account for the remaining proportions. Guidelines/directives to ensure aseptic techniques are now in use in all health facilities.

A much higher proportion of HIV-positive patients has been recorded among patients with sexually-transmitted infections (STIs) and TB, at 5.6% and 25.5% respectively. The high HIV prevalence among SUs is due to the magnitude of substance abuse in Zanzibar, particularly among the young generation, which has been increasing with time. Needle sharing among IDUs is a common phenomenon, as well as among unprotected penetrative sex, which takes place while those participating in such acts are under the influence of illicit substances. Rape and domestic violence have also been reported to result from drug abuse.

Gender and Geographical Breakdown

While the HIV prevalence in the general population is 0.6%, women show infection rates four to six times higher than that of their male counterparts (see Figure 6.2).

Gender inequalities are well-documented as influencing the high rate of HIV/ AIDS prevalence among women. Gender-related constraints caused by patriarchal

192

Figure 6.2: Trend of HIV/AIDS distribution by gender in Zanzibar, 2002–04

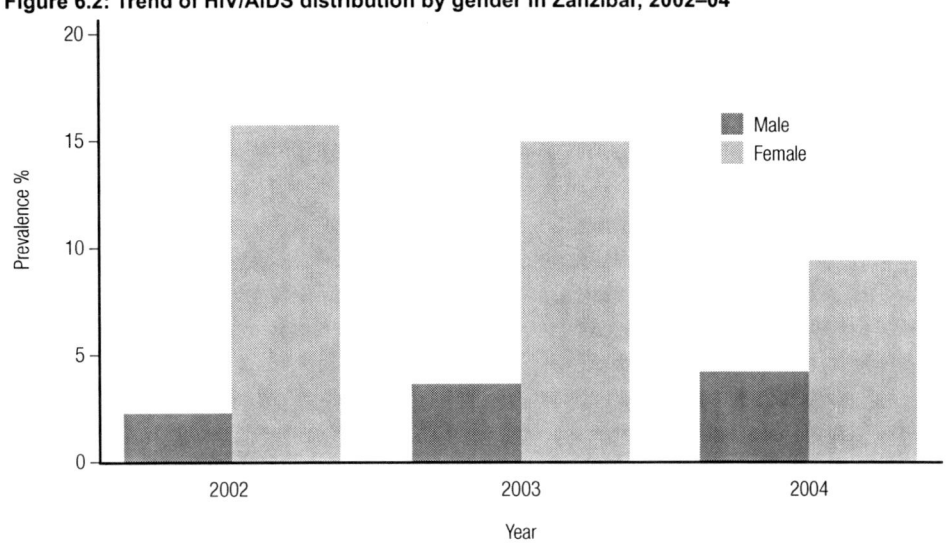

Source: RGoZ, 2005a

ideology and culture give men disproportionate power and ownership over assets and major decisions. Some of the sociocultural norms and values, policies and laws encourage an unattainable bride price, early and forced marriages, multiple partners, early sexual début among girls, high rates of teenage pregnancy and induced abortions, leading to high STI and HIV/AIDS rates (RGoZ, 2004a). Figure 6.2 shows the geographical distribution of HIV/AIDS by gender.

Overall, HIV prevalence is high in males over 45 years and females between 35 and 44. Infection rates are also high among widows and widowers (18.9%), followed by the rate among those who have been separated from matrimonial union (13.1%), while they are lowest among individuals who have never married (RGoZ, 2005a).

The highest prevalence rate in Zanzibar occurs in Chake Chake with 0.7%, with the lowest recorded in North Unguja (North B) and South Unguja (South). Table 6.4 summarises HIV prevalence by district.

Table 6.4: HIV prevalence by district, 2005[66]			
Region	District	Total population	HIV prevalence (%)
Urban West	Urban	235 413	0.2
	West	210 785	0.4
South Unguja	South	34 024	0.0
	Central	66 560	0.2
North Unguja	North A	90 834	0.2
	North B	56 650	0.0
South Pemba	Mkoani	99 354	0.1
	Chake Chake	89 236	0.7
North Pemba	Wete	109 396	0.09
	Micheweni	89 166	0.3
Total		1 081 418	0.2
Source: ZACP (2005)			

HIV/AIDS KNOWLEDGE

In Zanzibar, knowledge of HIV/AIDS is widespread among both men and women, with at least 95% of all respondents in the 2005 DHS, regardless of background, having heard of the epidemic.[67] Some 99.8% of women and 89.7% of men in Zanzibar have heard of HIV.

HIV/AIDS prevention programmes focus their messages and efforts on three important aspects of behaviour: the delaying of sexual début in young persons (abstinence); the limiting of sexual partners/staying faithful to one partner; and the use of condoms. To ascertain whether programmes have effectively communicated anti-HIV/AIDS messages, DHS 2005 asked respondents whether it was possible to reduce the chance of contracting HIV by remaining faithful to just one sexual partner, using condoms for all sexual intercourse, and abstaining from sex. Table 6.5 provides results regarding the levels of knowledge of HIV/AIDS prevention methods. Most Zanzibari women know that having only one faithful partner helps to reduce the chances of contracting HIV, with almost nine in ten women respondents in Unguja (89%) indicating that the chances of contracting HIV can be reduced by limiting sex to one uninfected partner who has no other partners. However, the knowledge that condoms can reduce the risk of contracting HIV during sexual intercourse and abstinence is low, especially among Pemba men (25.9% and 29.6% respectively). Overall, women are more knowledgeable than men regarding the three methods of prevention of transmission (see Table 6.5).

Table 6.5: Knowledge of HIV prevention methods					
	Women (%)			Men (%)		
	Using condoms	One partner	Abstinence	Using condoms	One partner	Abstinence
Unguja	66.9	89.3	88.4	43.1	78.2	85.9
Pemba	59.9	85.9	81.4	25.9	53.9	29.6
Zanzibar	64.8	88.2	86.2	37.4	70.2	67.5
Source: NBS and ORC Macro, 2005						

Comprehensive knowledge of HIV/AIDS is defined in 2005 DHS as:
- Knowing that both condom use and limiting sex partners to one uninfected partner are HIV prevention methods;
- Being aware that a healthy looking person can, nevertheless, have HIV; and
- Rejecting the two most common local misconceptions that HIV/AIDS can be transmitted through mosquito bites and by sharing food.

Both Zanzibari women and men were found likely to say that a healthy looking person can, nevertheless, be HIV-positive. Unlike with HIV prevention methods, both Zanzibari women and men are more likely than those on mainland Tanzania to say that a healthy looking person can have HIV/AIDS, and to reject the two most common misconceptions about transmission (respectively 68% and 56% for women; and 71% and 57% for men).

BEHAVIOURAL CHANGE

Changes in sexual behaviour among the high-risk groups of the population in Zanzibar have not been significant, despite the successful efforts that have been made to increase HIV awareness. Several studies show that the knowledge of specific risks in sexual practices is low among the youth and other population groups. Due to specific religious beliefs and social values and norms, the reluctance to use condoms is high. For example, a behavioural study commissioned by Africare (2001) in Zanzibar revealed that 75% of young people surveyed do not know the signs and symptoms of STIs. About 78% of the youth surveyed perceived the use of condoms to be socially unacceptable, with 65.4% of the sexually active youth surveyed reporting having not yet used a condom during sexual intercourse. A false sense of safety is prevalent among those at high risk in Zanzibar, with most youth (74%) surveyed not perceiving themselves to be at risk of contracting HIV (Africare, 2002).

STIGMA AND DISCRIMINATION

Stigma is widely reported in Zanzibar. Several of the studies cited above found unacceptable levels of stigma being practised towards PLWHAs among health-care workers and among the general population. A survey conducted by the then Ministry of Education, Culture and Sport in 2000 found that 60.5% of respondents disapproved of PLWHAs, with the Africare study concurring with such a finding. One of the respondents in this study lamented; "While I am willing to care for my blood relative infected with HIV/AIDS, my worry is that I might be infected."

DHS 2005 indicates that, while most respondents were willing to care for a family member with HIV at home (92.8%) and believed that an HIV+ female teacher should be allowed to teach (80.2%), only about half of the respondents indicated that they would buy fresh food from a shopkeeper with HIV/AIDS (46.8%), and would want the HIV-positive status of a family member to remain a secret. Only 22.1% of all respondents expressed an acceptance of all four measures of stigma.

ZANZIBAR'S NATIONAL RESPONSE TO HIV/AIDS

THE GOVERNMENT RESPONSE

Shortly after the first case of HIV/AIDS was diagnosed in 1986 in Zanzibar, the government of Zanzibar formulated a short-term plan (1987–1988) to address the situation, which was aimed at creating public awareness among, and the training of, health personnel in response to the epidemic. In 1987, the government established ZACP under the MoH. The government then came up with various five-year Mid-Term

Plans (MTPs) to strengthen the response. MTP I (1989–1991) and MTP II (1992–1996) focused on consolidating and expanding interventions made in the short-term plan, as well as on motivating behaviour change. The plans also fostered safety measures relating to the handling of blood and the promotion of counselling and care in the health sector. It was during the MTP II that the community started to become involved in providing HIV/AIDS-related education and counselling.

MTP III (1998–2000) provided a framework for multisectoral response. While implementing the plan it became evident that HIV/AIDS was both a health and a socioeconomic issue. In response to such a realisation, the government realised the need to legislate a special national structure into being, which would coordinate the national response. As a result, ZAC was established as an autonomous body.

THE ZANZIBAR AIDS COMMISSION

ZAC was established in September 2002 under the Chief Minister's Office (CMO) to provide national leadership of the epidemic. ZAC has three operational sections:
- Finance, administration and Human Resources;
- Policy, planning and national response; and
- Advocacy and IEC (information, education and communication).

Figure 6.3 shows the organisational structure of ZAC.

Figure 6.3: Zanzibar AIDS Commission Organisation Chart

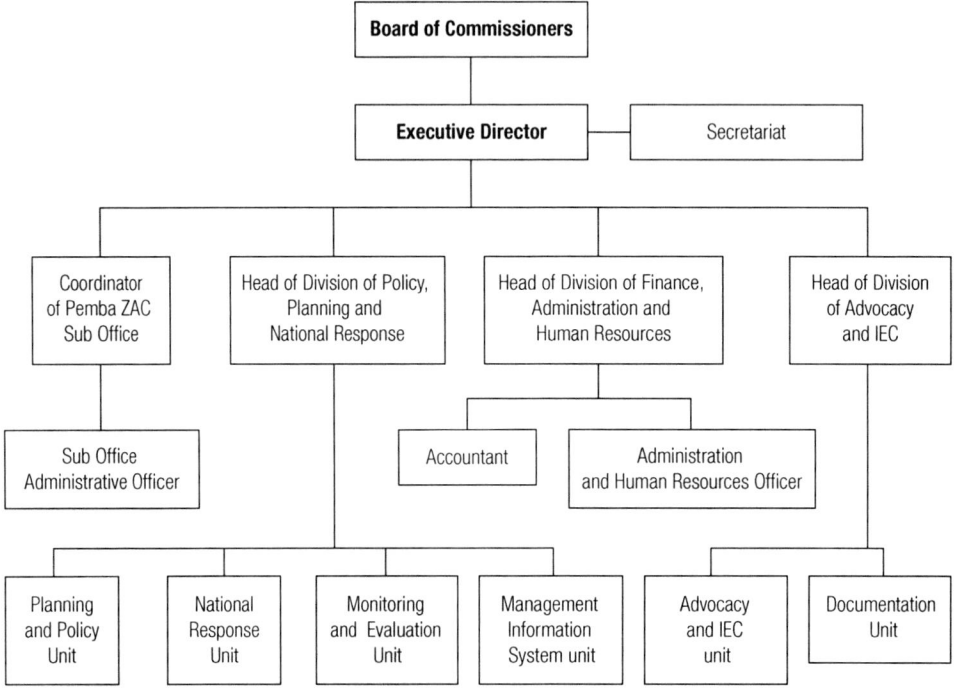

The routine operations of ZAC are mainly funded by the government, while its programmes are mainly funded by its development partners. In Zanzibar, the Commission coordinates most of the HIV/AIDS-related funds sourced from different development partners.

THE HIV/AIDS POLICY

The Zanzibar National HIV/AIDS Strategic Plan 2004/5–2008/9 (ZNSP) was developed in response to a situation and response analysis of the state of HIV/AIDS in Zanzibar undertaken in 2003. The strategic plan focuses on;
- The prevention of HIV/AIDS transmission among vulnerable groups; HIV/AIDS prevention in the workplace; and prevention, treatment, care, and support in the health sector;
- Impact mitigation; and
- Cross-cutting issues, such as coordination, advocacy, capacity-building and resource mobilisation (RGoZ, 2004b).

The strategic plan has been the main planning tool of ZAC and other organisations fighting the scourge in the isles. The latest achievement in the fight is the formulation of the national HIV/AIDS policy in Zanzibar in 2006. The overall mission of the policy is to provide a framework for the leadership and coordination of the national multisectoral response to the HIV/AIDS epidemic, leading to the reduction of HIV infections and its consequential socioeconomic impact.

The goals of the policy resonate around the prevention of new HIV infections in the population; the treatment, care and support of those who are infected; and the mitigation of the impact of HIV/AIDS on the socioeconomic status of individuals, families and communities. The policy also emphasises the enhancement of the institutional/key implementer capacity to develop/implement HIV/AIDS interventions in line with gender and human rights approaches.

COORDINATION OF THE NATIONAL RESPONSE

ZAC coordinates the HIV/AIDS response in Zanzibar through the Board of Commissioners, the ZAC secretariat and various consultative boards. At district level, coordination is undertaken by the District AIDS Coordinating Committees (DACCOMs) and the Shehia AIDS Coordinating Committees (SHACCOMs).

The various consultative boards involved with the coordination of the national response comprise:
- The quarterly meetings of the ZAC commissioners;
- The Principal Secretaries Committee on HIV/AIDS;
- The public-sector technical committee meetings;
- The consultative stakeholders meeting;
- A technical committee that involves various stakeholders from both the public and non-public sectors;

- A technical platform between various stakeholders, including UN agencies and the international NGOs; and
- Zanzibar NGO Cluster for HIV/AIDS Prevention (ZANGOC) meetings and activities.

PUBLIC-SECTOR RESPONSE

All public sectors have programmes for mainstreaming HIV/AIDS in their core functions and in the workplace. The public sector has Technical AIDS Committees (TACs) comprising representatives of members of staff and management coordinated by the HIV/AIDS focal persons. The public sector receives funds from both the government and development partners from ZAC, based on their annual work plans. They then prepare quarterly funding requests, which they submit to the Commission for consideration. Public sector focal persons meet the ZAC each quarter to review implementation. Furthermore, through a new system of M&E, the sectors are supposed to fill in the M&E forms for regular feedback and feed-forward processes. The sectors have mainstreamed their HIV/AIDS plans in their MTEF for funding from the government.

The MoHSW, through the ZACP, is mandated to coordinate the health component of HIV/AIDS at all levels. The government, through the Ministry of Regional Administration, also has the role of coordinating the community response to the epidemic via the district authorities. Generally, the public-sector response is constrained by a capacity gap in human resources, unreliable financial resources, project design and implementation, as well as M&E. At the time of writing this report, ZAC was working to address such weaknesses in order to enhance the public-sector response.

NON-STATE RESPONSE

The following table shows the HIV/AIDS non-state response in Zanzibar.

Table 6.6: Non-state response to HIV/AIDS in Zanzibar	
Partnership with development partners	Zanzibar has developed a joint programme with the United Nations system. The programme focuses on four major operational areas: • Policy and planning; • Advocacy; • Monitoring and evaluation; and • Care and treatment. The commission also has a good working relationship with its bilateral partners, mostly in the area of capacity-building and resource mobilisation. The commission has institutionalised a joint forum with the Donor Group on HIV/AIDS, which meets quarterly. The development partners are highly involved in priority setting. They are also fully involved in policy and strategic planning formulation, as well as in programme design, implementation, resource mobilisation, and monitoring and evaluation.

Civil society organisations	Civil society organisations (CSOs) have been fully involved in the fight against HIV/AIDS in Zanzibar. Currently, the 87 functional CSOs in the isles are mainly involved in the area of prevention, more specifically awareness-raising. CSOs also work in the area of support and impact mitigation and HIV testing. The NGO efforts are coordinated by an NGO umbrella organisation called ZANGOC, while the FBOs are coordinated by the Zanzibar Association of Interfaith on AIDS and Development (ZIADA). The CSO sector, through Zanzibar Against AIDS Infection and Drug Abuse (ZAIADA), has responded to the substance abuse problem, which is widespread in the isles. Nevertheless, the participation of CSOs still largely depends on the availability of funds from development partners.
Private sector response	To date, the involvement and participation of the private sector in the fight against HIV/AIDS has been limited. The private-sector response is not well coordinated, depending on the will of individual corporations. However, ZAC has supported the private sector in setting up an AIDS Business Coalition in Zanzibar (ABCZ) to coordinate and support private-sector work.
Political parties	Political parties are very influential in the lives of the people of Zanzibar, including changing the behaviour of their supporters in relation to HIV/AIDS. In spite of such an influence, however, little has been done to involve the political parties with the HIV/AIDS effort. ZAC sensitised the political party leaders on HIV issues during the political campaign running up to the 2005 general elections. As an entry point, all the political parties have included HIV messages in their election manifestos. Despite such inclusion, the parties have been silent on addressing the epidemic among their supporters, within the daily operations of the parties, including workplace interventions, as well as in the process of the political race for power.
Religious groups	As Zanzibar is predominantly Muslim, the need to involve religious leaders in the fight against HIV has become apparent. The history of the interfaith groups' response to HIV/AIDS started with the MTP III, when religious leaders started to become involved in the national response to the epidemic. The religious leaders, through open meetings and prayer sermons, helped to sensitise believers to the epidemic. The main emphasis was on prohibiting sex out of wedlock and in promoting good morals. Noting the importance of religion in the fight against HIV, ZACP and ZAC conducted sensitisation meetings to inform the religious leaders about the epidemic. In contributing to the fight, the Office of the Mufti spearheaded a publication that guides the Zanzibar Muslim community in its fight against the epidemic (Mufti's Office, 2004).

THE BUDGET PROCESS IN ZANZIBAR

The government of Zanzibar has undertaken several reforms of its budget process. Since 2000, the reforms relating to fiscal concerns have focused on public financial and budget management, being concerned with improving the management of revenue and expenditure, and with the overall objective of improving financial and economic management, accountability and transparency. Such reforms are mainly based on performance budgeting. Currently, the government has adopted the three-year MTEF budget process plan. This chapter describes the budget process in Zanzibar.

The Institutional Framework

The 1984 Zanzibar Constitution (Chapter Seven, Section One, Subsection 104(i) and Subsection 105(e)) requires the minister responsible for finance to prepare annual expenditure estimates, which s/he then tables before the House of Representatives before the beginning of a new financial year. The Principal Secretary of MoFEA, on behalf of the minister, undertakes the responsibility of preparing the expenditure estimates in collaboration with the Principal Secretaries of other line MDAs. The framework has four levels:

- The topmost level, the National Budget and Planning Committee (NBPC), which, among other functions, reviews past and current budget performance; realigns the budget framework with the national development policy; and realigns the sectoral budget estimates (recurrent/development) with the anticipated domestic and foreign resource availability;
- The Sectoral Budget and Planning Committee, which prepares budget estimates in accordance with the ceilings;
- The Technical Teams (budget drafting teams), which make proposals with regard to the national revenue portfolio (both domestic and foreign), the budget ceilings for the MDAs, and budget guidelines; and
- The revenue collection agencies.

Zanzibar has two independent tax-collection agencies, namely the Zanzibar Revenue Board (ZRB) and the Tanzania Revenue Authority (TRA). The ZRB administers the collection of domestic taxes and levies, currently administering the collection of seven different taxes, the proceeds of which are later transferred to the Zanzibar Treasury consolidated fund in an account operated by the Bank of Tanzania (BoT). The ZRB also acts as an advisor on issues pertaining to tax policies.

The TRA collects revenue on behalf of the RGoZ in the form of income tax, customs duties, excise tax and VAT on imports, which it deposits with the Treasury Consolidated Fund. In a similar role to that of the ZRB, the TRA also advises the RGoZ on tax policy. In relation to the budget process, TRA is involved in estimating revenue forecasting for the coming FY, in which capacity it takes part in the National Technical Team.

Recent Developments in the Budget Process in Zanzibar

Over the years, the budget process in Zanzibar has undergone improvements, both in its systems, as well as in their execution. The adoption of the PER process in Zanzibar[68] has also led to the introduction of the MTEF process and the undertaking of diagnostic studies in support of the implementation of the Zanzibar Poverty Reduction Plan (ZPRP). The former two processes aim to improve the linkage between policy planning and the allocation of resources, as well as to create a more consultative process for budget formulation and decision-making. By introducing the PER and MTEF, the government ensures:

- Fiscal discipline is maintained;
- Resources are allocated according to the strategic priority of government; and
- The resources are spent efficiently for their intended purposes, as explained in Table 6.7.

Table 6.7: Dimensions of public expenditure management		
Element	Underlying features	Indicators
Aggregate fiscal discipline	The budget envelope should be: • Explicit and set prior to determining the individual spending allocation; • Consistent with the broader macroeconomic framework; and • Sustainable over the medium term.	• Macroeconomic stability • Public expenditures as share of GDP • Predictability of overall resource flows
Allocative efficiency	• Consistency of expenditure allocations, both between and within sectors, with government priorities • Reallocation of resources to higher priority and more effective programmes	• Predictability of policy and programme-specific resource flows • Consistency of actual resource allocations with government policy statements • Assessment of budget formulation process and the extent to which it embraces contestable policy choices
Technical efficiency	• Achievement of continuing efficiency gains • Comparability of the efficiency of public sector operations with those of the private sector	• Benchmarking of both internal and external standards • Service delivery and unit cost data • Assessment of systems ensuring accountability
Source: Msongole and Killindo, 2003		

THE BUDGET CYCLE

The budget cycle begins with the preparation of budget guidelines for the coming FY by the National Technical Team, which takes place between November and December of each FY.

The format of the budget guidelines usually includes:

- The macroeconomic performance for the previous year, covering economic growth targets, inflation targets and capital formation;
- A review of the government finance operation for July/December;
- The macroeconomic assumptions and projections for the next FY;
- The defining of poverty reduction plan priorities for the next FY;
- Revenue estimation and projections for the next FY, including the projection of external resources (grants, loans and subsidies); and
- Expenditure estimates and projections.

The budget guidelines are then sent to the NBPC for approval. After such approval has been granted, the budget guidelines are sent to the MDAs indicating the budget ceilings and the time frames for the submission of estimates to the MoFEA. In the process of preparing the sectoral estimates, the sectoral technical teams interact with the National Technical Team for advice. Once the ZNSP has been costed, the ZAC consults the document when determining the budget allocations.

After collecting all submissions from MDAs, the MoFEA prepares comprehensive budget estimates for the whole government. After compilation, the estimates are taken through the government ratification process, first to the Principal Secretaries Committee and later to the Cabinet.

Before being taken to the House of Representatives, the budget framework and accompanying policy proposals are discussed at two outside levels. A consultative session of the three East African community governments meets to compare notes on their budget frameworks. Usually they agree on tax rates that affect the three countries and policy measures that might affect one anothers' budgets. Such a consultative meeting is usually preceded by an interstate consultation meeting between the government of Zanzibar and the government of the URT. The framework for discussion is similar to that of the three East African states.

The sessions for the House of Representatives are conducted in the following order:

- The discussion by the House Finance and Economic Committee on the national budget estimate proposal;
- The discussion of the relevant house committees to discuss proposals from sectoral ministries; and
- The full House of Representatives session to discuss and approve the budget proposals.

The major determinant for the budget comprises the previous year's baseline figures. The budget committee is mandated to determine the budget process, including the resource allocation, as well as to convene sectoral ceiling committee meetings. The committee reviews the previous year's performance in all sectors and establishes the revenue target to be collected by government institutions.

BUDGET EXECUTION

After the budget is approved and the Appropriation Bill passed, the Paymaster General requests permission from the Controller and Auditor General (CAG) for the quarterly expenditures. The revenue allocations to spending agencies are allocated monthly. The allocations are made after the monthly ceiling committee, comprising representatives from the MoF and the BoT has been held. The TRA and ZRB have set to determine the expected revenue collection level for the month.

A cash budget system is utilised in expenditure allocations, with any financing gap that accrues being covered through:

- Subventions from the URT;
- The floating of Treasury Bills; or
- Advances from the BoT.

The M&E of budget performance is currently conducted at four levels:

- A physical follow-up by officials from the budget department;

- Abstract reports submitted to the Accountant-General;
- Internal audit functions; and
- A periodic audit by the CAG.

Except for specific projects, whereby a donor may request audited accounts at any set time of the year, ZAC accounts are audited twice a year.

WEAKNESSES OF THE BUDGET PROCESS IN ZANZIBAR

The Zanzibar budget process suffers the following limitations:
1. The MDAs do not take the guidelines seriously;
2. The MDAs usually prepare their estimates disregarding provided ceilings;
3. Institutional heads do not concern themselves with budget supervision, leaving the exercise to junior staff;
4. Budgeting is regarded as an exercise purely of aligning numbers, resulting in it being left to accountants;
5. Lack of adequate resources;
6. Usually other charges and development activities receive the minimum allocation;
7. The M&E mechanism is weak;
8. The budget, particularly for development activities and HIV/AIDS, largely depends on external support; and
9. Slow disbursement of funds.

THE BUDGET PROCESS IN ZANZIBAR

The major/key player in budgeting in Zanzibar is the MoFEA which forecasts the resources to be obtained both internally and externally. ZAC, like other MDAs in Zanzibar, must plan its requirements according to the allocation assigned to it by the MoFEA. As the CMO is the parent ministry for ZAC, all submissions to MoFEA are made through the CMO.

TOTAL PUBLIC/GOVERNMENT HEALTH EXPENDITURE IN ZANZIBAR

This section presents the trends of pubic expenditure on health, as recorded in the Estimates for Recurrent and Capital Revenues and Expenditure for the Year 2005/2006 (RGoZ, 2005b). The emphasis is on general health expenditure by the MoHSW.

TRENDS IN HEALTH-SECTOR SPENDING

The ZPRP (2002/03–2004/05) underscores the importance of improving health conditions for Zanzibaris to be able to achieve increased productivity. Thus, the health sector forms one of the eight different priority sectors in ZPRP, with the others comprising agriculture, trade, tourism, education, health, housing, water and roads. The strategic cornerstone of health services for the poor under ZPRP was:

- Improved maternal and child health (MCH) and reproductive health (RH) services;
- A more efficient drug supply for the primary health centres; and
- Improved health service management (RGoZ, 2002b).

Recurrent allocations to the health sector underwent improvement, increasing from TZS4 244.2 million in 2002/03 to TZS6 108.5 million in 2005/06. In real terms, using 2001 as the base year, the amount rose from TZS4 004.4 million to TZS4 426.4 million between the two periods (see Table 6.8).

The ratio of the recurrent health budget as a share of the total government budget increased from 6.3% in 2002/03 to 6.9% in 2003/04 (excluding CFS).[69] However, the ratio remained constant at 6.6% in 2004/05 and 2005/06 (see Table 6.8). When capital funds are considered, the share increased to 10.7% in 2005/06. MoFEA-sourced information also shows that health sector spending has increased as a proportion of the GDP, from about 1.66% in 2002/03 to 1.75% in 2004/05, decreasing to 1.54% in 2005/06. Adding the capital funds allocations, the proportion increased to 2.5% in 2005/06.

The share of the health budget has, however, consistently fallen short of the Abuja Declaration of Commitment of 15% of the government budget going to health to spearhead reaching the MDGs.

Table 6.8: Allocations to MoHSW in terms of MoFEA allocations (recurrent), FY 2002/03-2005/06				
Budget Item	2002/03	2003/04	2004/05	2005/06
Total recurrent budget (TZS million)	66 978.4	70 467.6	91 460.1	91 909.0
Total recurrent health budget (TZS million)	4 244.7	4 871.5	6 011.0	6 108.5
Total health budget (US$'000)	4 487.0	4 684.2	5 509.6	5 415.3
Total share of health budget to total recurrent budget (%)	6.3	6.9	6.6	6.6
Total population (millions)	0.981	1.016	1.053	1.095
Exchange Rate (TZS to US$)	946	1 040	1 076	1 128
Per capita expenditure (US$)	4.6	4.6	5.2	4.9
Gross Domestic Product at current prices (TZS million)	256 000	286 600	344 300	395 700
Inflation	6	12	26	38
Health budget as % of GDP	1.66	1.70	1.75	1.54
Real allocations to health (TZS million) (2001 base year)	4 004.4	4 349.6	4 770.6	4 426.4
Sources: RGoZ, 2005b; RGoZ, 2006a; own calculations				

Health spending per capita (at current prices and in real terms) has been low. In nominal terms, while per capita health expenditure increased from TZS4 323.6 in 2002/03 to TZS5 703.4 in 2004/05, it declined to TZS5 575.9 in 2005/06.

Table 6.9: Capital health expenditure estimates (TZS million), 2004/05				
Category of expenditure	Government expenditure	Foreign grants	Foreign loan	Total
Immunisation and mother and child health support	34 000	674 000	0	708 000
Family planning	22 000	266 226	0	288 226
Programme for primary health care	78 000	0	6 513 300	6 591 300
Mental hospital rehabilitation	65 550	0	0	65 550
AIDS control programme	22 000	119 930	0	141 930
Total	221 550	1 060 156	6 513 300	7 795 006
Source: RGoZ, 2004c				

FUNDING FROM FOREIGN SOURCES

While recurrent expenditure has mainly been financed from government funds, capital/development expenditure has been funded by external sources. From a total of TZS7.8 billion development/capital health budget in FY 2004/05, TZS7.6 billion (equivalent to 97.4%) came from foreign sources, of which about TZS1.1 billion (equivalent to 13.6%) comprised foreign grants and TZS 6.5 billion (equivalent to 83.6%) comprised foreign loans. External funds are, therefore, an important component of the health budget. The budget dependency ratio is, therefore, very high, which does not suggest sustainability and/or stability. In 2004/05, foreign sources accounted for 97% of the capital/development expenditure, whereas in 2005/06 such sources accounted for 94%.

ALLOCATIONS TO REGIONS FROM THE MINISTRY OF FINANCE AND ECONOMIC AFFAIRS

Contrary to the Tanzania mainland, whose regions and districts receive subventions for health expenditure directly from the MoF, such levels of decentralised funding has not been achieved in the isles. No direct estimates for health in the regions appear in the budget books, partly because the MoHSW has been responsible for executing all activities relating to health provision through its several departments. Allocations for the procurement of medical supplies and services are mainly undertaken by both the preventive and curative departments.

FINANCING AND REPORTING MECHANISMS IN ZANZIBAR

Chapter Seven of the Constitution of Zanzibar 1984 sets out the financial provisions relating to RGoZ. In particular, Section 104 provides for a consolidated fund, requiring all revenue to be paid into, and all charges made out of, the fund.

Public-sector accounting and financial reporting have both been significantly strengthened by the enactment of the Financial Administration Act. The Act attempts to establish a regulatory framework to improve transparency and accountability in public-sector financial accounting and reporting, by:

- Strengthening the fiscal management of government finances;
- Making the government's monthly financial reports and individual ministry reports readily available to the general public;
- Clearly defining the form that public accounts should take; and
- Improving oversight.

The Accountant-General is responsible for preparing both monthly and annual financial statements, which are compiled on the basis of flash reports sent by the accounting officers in the line ministries. The various reporting requirements are defined below.

Table 6.10: Financial reports

Name of report	Time-frame	Coverage
Expenditure Flash Report	Monthly	Expenditure on monthly and cumulative basis
Commitment Control Flash Report	Monthly	Commitments on a monthly and cumulative basis
Exchequer Releases	Quarterly	All transfers from the basket account to the exchequer
Quarterly Performance Reports	Quarterly	Actual and cumulative expenditures against budget
Receipts and Payment Accounts	Annually	Deposits into the basket, and transfers to the exchequer

The development partners and other donors disburse their funds to the various HIV programmes largely through the MoFEA and ZAC, with a small fraction going through the MoHSW. The other funds are, however, disbursed directly to the implementing partners, particularly when it comes to the CSOs. ZAC receives funds to fight the epidemic from such bodies as the World Bank Multi-Country HIV/AIDS Programme (MAP–WB), the Global Fund to Fight HIV/AIDS, Tuberculosis and Malaria (GFATM), UNDP, UNAIDS, and Action Aid–SIPAA. The funds are either spent by the commission in undertaking routine work or disbursed to implementing partners, such as CSOs, the community, sectoral ministries and the private sector. The commission enters into agreement with subrecipients on the use of funds and reporting systems. The funds are disbursed on a quarterly basis, with no subsequent payment being undertaken before accounting for the previous expenditures. Having received reports from its subrecipients, ZAC, in turn, compiles a consolidated financial and technical report for the respective development partners.

Funds received by way of the government or ZAC from development partners and other donors are managed separately. Each partner has a separate bank account and management system to ensure transparency. Where donor funds are channelled directly to the subrecipients/implementing partners, the expenditures are also reported directly to the donor(s) concerned. Such a practice makes it difficult for the commission to track those funds and to coordinate the related activities.

Most donor HIV/AIDS funding goes to the MDAs in Zanzibar, with the CSOs receiving only 19% and 23% of captured donor funding in 2004/05 and 2005/06, respectively. Therefore, the focus is specifically on donor funds going to the MDAs. Both ZAC and ZACP receive substantial donor support and, though there is some crossover with GFATM and MAP–WB funding, they appear to act relatively independently in attracting and managing donor funds. Such independent functioning complicates tracking the available resources and actual expenditure.

Currently, each major donor has its own disbursement and reporting procedures, which cause significant delays in implementing HIV/AIDS-related activities. Due to the complexity of these procedures and the low capacity of the recipients, a substantial proportion of the funds available for each year remains unspent. Another complication arises when donors provide goods and services in kind, such as medical supplies and consultancy work, and do not provide the recipients with any information regarding the value of such goods and services. For example, ZACP has been unable to capture the value of the goods and services provided by Columbia University in 2004/05 in its accounts.

Further, some significant donors, such as PEPFAR and Columbia University, have not provided firm commitments as to the level of donor funding for a significant period of time. The global amount available under PEPFAR is voted for annually by the US Congress. Without firm funding commitments, Zanzibar is at risk of interruptions or sudden unanticipated drops in funding, which would be difficult to compensate for and could be very damaging to the national effort to fight HIV/AIDS.

TOTAL BUDGET ALLOCATIONS AND EXPENDITURE FOR HIV/AIDS IN ZANZIBAR

This section presents the trends in public expenditure on HIV/AIDS-related efforts, as recorded in the Estimates for Recurrent and Capital Revenues and Expenditure and by ZAC up to FY 2005/2006. The MoHSW, through ZACP, ZAC and HIV/AIDS-related NGOs, have been the major implementing agencies and/or institutions of HIV/AIDS programmes in the isles. According to the CSO mapping exercise completed by ZAC, approximately 87 CSOs carry out HIV/AIDS-related activities in Unguja and Pemba. However, due to HIV/AIDS being seen as a socioeconomic problem as well as a health issue, the government has issued a directive for all MDAs to have a line item for HIV/AIDS counselling. The allocations and spending analysis presented in this chapter draw heavily on the HIV/AIDS PER draft report (RGoZ, 2007).

Tables 6.11 to 6.14 (adapted from the PER, RGoZ, 2007) provide an overview of HIV/AIDS-related expenditure and financing in Zanzibar for the period June 2004 to July 2007. The analysis of actual expenditure during FY 2006/07 is omitted, due to only limited data being available.

The total actual expenditure on HIV/AIDS, including government sources, donor funding from public-sector support (both on- and off-budget), the direct donor funding of NGOs and international NGO expenditure increased from TZS2 051.75 in 2004/05 to TZS3 385.39 in 2005/06, representing an increase of 65% in nominal terms. Actual government expenditure on HIV/AIDS-related efforts increased substantially (69%) from TZS438.52 million in 2004/05 to TZS741.05 million in 2005/06. Actual donor financing of public sector HIV/AIDS activities increased by 54% to TZS2 001.83 million from 2004/05 to 2005/06, while the total actual donor financing (including direct transfers to the NGOs) increased by 63% to TZS2 629.57 million.

In 2004/05, no donor financing was captured in the government accounts, whereas in 2005/06 24% of donor financing was captured in government accounts, with 24% being accounted for by the MoHSW reporting donor financing of ZACP, with the Ministry of Agriculture, Livestock and Environment (MALE) and the Ministry of Tourism, Trade and Investment (MoTTI) reporting MAP–WB expenditure.

HIV/AIDS funding in Zanzibar is highly donor dependent, with the proportion of donor funding received by CSOs increasing from 16% in 2004/05 to 19% in 2005/06, due to the commencement of the Community AIDS Response Fund (CARF), a component of MAP–WB funding, which is expected to increase to 26% in 2007/08. The share of actual CSO expenditure is consistently higher than the budgeted share of CSO expenditure, suggesting that the CSO absorptive capacity is higher than that of the MDAs. However, neither capturing budget estimates for the CSOs in Zanzibar, nor determining the proportion of disbursed funds that was spent on the different activities and strategic beneficiaries was possible. Therefore, for most CSO funding, the actual disbursements were used as a proxy for the estimated budget and expenditure, meaning that the absorptive capacity of CSOs might have been overestimated.

FOREIGN ALLOCATIONS FOR HIV/AIDS INITIATIVES IN ZANZIBAR

Table 6.11: Donor funding of public-sector HIV/AIDS expenditure, FY 2004/05 – FY 2006/07 (in US$)				
Donor	Budget	Actual	Budget	Actual	Budget
	2004/05	2004/05	2005/06	2005/06	2006/07
SMZ	248 732 924	45 961 813	215 392 728	80 045 680	453 017 600
TMAP	1 645 619 384	395 410 464	2 558 895 120	875 137 502	2 943 034 939
Global Fund	309 875 416	231 279 009	301 622 268	232 370 085	163 282 566
UN/WHO	271 271 515	232 008 352	189 924 175	149 853 751	380 831 000
PEPFAR	126 208 000	126 208 000	537 875 000	537 875 000	–
Columbia University	11 070 000	11 070 000	50 135 488	50 135 488	461 807 500
Action Aid – SIPAA	362 481 482	300 728 131	140 010 968	117 758 771	–
CHAI	–	–	23 540 000	23 540 000	–
DFP	–	–	77 328 070	34 813 250	225 636 140
Total	2 975 258 721	1 342 665 769	4 094 723 817	2 101 529 527	4 627 609 745
Source: RGoZ, 2007				

The volatility of the major sources of donor funding is demonstrated by comparing graph 1 and graph 2. For example, Action Aid-SIPAA accounted for 22.4%

of captured funding in 2004/05, while in 2005/06 SIPAA accounted for just 5.7%. PEPFAR funding increased from 9.4% of donor funding in 2004/05 to 25.9% in 2005/06. Moreover, the budgeted funding as a proportion of the total funds differed significantly from actual funding for each of the donors involved. Such a significant difference has serious implications for planning, programme management and the sustainability of specific programmes, such as the rollout of antiretrovirals (which cannot be subjected to fluctuations and unpredictability of donor funds).

Figure 6.4: Zanzibar actual donor contribution to public-sector expenditure on HIV/AIDS activities, FY 2004/05

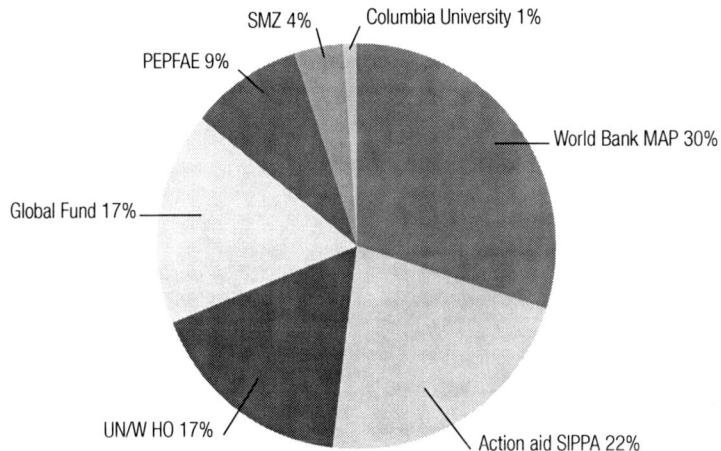

ALLOCATION OF HIV/AIDS EXPENDITURE RELATIVE TO PRIORITIES OF THE ZANZIBAR NATIONAL HIV/AIDS STRATEGIC PLAN

A costing exercise of the ZNSP was carried out by Deloitte and Touche and technical experts from Zanzibar in June 2004. Comparing the actual and budgeted expenditure against the resources identified during the costing exercise, as required for completing the ZNSP, the significant shortfall in resources is clear (see Table 6.12). Despite such a shortfall, the actual expenditure on HIV/AIDS-related activities as a proportion of the targeted amount increased from 37% in 2004/2006 to 47% in 2005/2005. For FY 2006/2007 the budgeted amount for HIV/AIDS expenditure represented 93% of the target amount identified during the costing exercise, showing a decrease in the annual resource gap. However, the cumulative gap of actual to required spending stood at TZS7 309.98 million at the time of going to press. According to the costing exercise, for Zanzibar to achieve the ZNSP, HIV/AIDS-related expenditure must equate 1.5% of the GDP.[70]

Table 6.12: Comparison of actual and budgeted expenditure to required resource level identified during ZNSP costing (TZS million), FY 2004/05-2006/07

	Budget 2004/05	Actual 2004/05	Budget 2005/06	Actual 2005/06	Budget 2006/07
Available	3 753.81	2 051.75	5 480.59	3 391.05	6 654.42
Target (ZNSP)	5 531.98	5 531.98	7 220.80	7 220.80	7 142.78
Financing gap	1 778.17	3 480.23	1 740.21	3 829.75	488.36
Available resources as % of target	68	37	76	47	93

Source: Adapted from RGoZ, 2007

The costing exercise also disaggregated the funds required to implement the ZNSP according to the thematic areas contained therein. The actual expenditure has been roughly disaggregated in order to identify the resource gap according to each thematic area and to enable commenting on the allocation of actual HIV/AIDS expenditure (see Table 6.13).

Table 6.13: Comparison of actual expenditure to required resource level identified during ZNSP costing according to thematic area (TZS million), FY 2004/05-2005/06

Thematic area	2004/05		2005/06	
	Required	Actual	Required	Actual
Prevention	1 970.41	503.37	2 951.59	1 343.18
Care and treatment	1 343.18	160.54	3 129.71	215.80
Surveillance and research	215.80	162.77	316.30	91.33
Cross-cutting issues	91.33	0.00	248.02	0.00
Institutional strengthening	771.68	902.42	575.18	1 199.40
Total	4 392.4	1 729.1	7 220.8	2 849.71

Source: RGoZ, 2007

The funds channelled to ZACP have not been included, due to the lack of information, despite the fact that ZACP routinely recorded expenditure in terms of similar thematic areas. While the selected MDAs are those which receive MAP–WB funding through ZAC, the omitted MDAs account for less than 0.5% of the budgeted HIV/AIDS expenditure, lacking any records of actual HIV/AIDS expenditure.

District and Regional Expenditure on HIV/AIDS

The government, through the Ministry of Regional Administration, coordinates the community HIV/AIDS response through DACCOMs. The DACCOMs are responsible for coordinating the community response to HIV/AIDS in the six districts in Unguja and the four districts in Pemba, as well as SHACCOM activities.

A resource-tracking exercise was undertaken by the HIV/AIDS PER team to assess the available resources and HIV/AIDS expenditure levels at the district and she- hia level in Zanzibar. As part of the exercise, three districts were visited in Unguja (Mjini, Kaskazini A and Kaskazini B) and two districts in Pemba (Mkoani and Wete). The study revealed that, apart from the funds earmarked for the commemoration of World AIDS Day, the DACCOMs had received limited or no financial support from either ZAC or the government. All DACCOMs appeared to be inactive due to a lack of resources. However, the DACCOM in Mkoani had received training from Manage- ment Sciences for Health (MSH) to build its capacity to coordinate community-based activities.

A limited number of shehia had received funding from UNAIDS as part of the District Response Initiative Programme (DRI), piloted in the districts of Mkoani and Kati (central). SHACCOMs have also received support from *Comunitá Voluntari per il Mondo* in carrying out activities and capacity-building. The national NGOs also re- ported providing support to SHACCOMs in the areas in which they operate.

In 2005/06, the level of actual expenditure at the regional level decreased by 18%, as no DRI funding was disbursed to the shehia. The DRI funding of TZS600 000 destined for eight shehia, which was originally intended for disbursal in 2004, were disbursed in 2005. In 2006, ZAC received its second disbursement of DRI funding, of which TZS24 000 000 has been made available for funding the HIV/AIDS-related ac- tivities of 12 shehia in both the Kati and Mkoani districts. The shehia plan to use the funds for peer education, capacity-building, the development of HIV/AIDS-related bylaws, community sensitisation and the support of OVC.

ABSORPTIVE CAPACITY FOR GOVERNMENT AND DONOR FUNDS

Table 6.14 provides an overview of the absorptive capacity associated with govern- ment and donor sources of funding. In 2004/05, expenditure accounted for only 18% of the budgeted government funds, while in 2005/06, expenditure increased to 36% of budgeted funds. For the total donor funding, the actual expenditure accounted for 52% and 58% of the budgeted funds for FYs 2004/05 and 2005/06 respectively. An as- sessment of this trend shows that the absorptive capacity for government funds and donor funds channeled through the public sector is very low. Though low, the ab- sorptive capacity of recipients appears to have improved over the years. The absorp- tive capacity of all MDAs is calculated by comparing the proposed annual budget of each MDA to the actual disbursements. Therefore, the shortfall in the finance MDAs request is captured relative to the funds that they had intended to spend in terms of their annual plans. For the most part, such a shortfall was caused by administrative and planning issues associated with donor funding.

Table 6.14: Overall absorptive/spending capacity for donor and government financing, FY 2004/05-2005/06		
Funding source	FY 2004/05 (%)	FY 2005/06 (%)
Government	18	36
Donor to public sector	48	52
Donor to CSOs	86	91
Total donor support	52	58
Source: Adapted from RGoZ, 2007		

For government expenditure, the low rate of absorptive capacity is due to the non-availability of government funds relative to the budgeted amount and the slow process of disbursement. A number of MDAs reported that they had been unable to undertake planned activities because required government complementary funding for MDA HIV/AIDS-related activities, which were partly donor-funded, was missing. Due to the significant level of donor funding available for HIV/AIDS-related activities, the government may be inclined to focus its limited resources on other relatively underfunded areas. Therefore, HIV/AIDS expenditure might have a lower priority than other expenditure items, with government revenue falling short of the budgeted amount by an average of about 20%, due to the government reallocating its limited resources to priority areas.

Utilisation of the Global Fund to Fight AIDS, Tuberculosis and Malaria in Zanzibar

Zanzibar has been fortunate to have received GFATM support in Rounds 1, 3, and 4 in order to enable it to address the devastating impact of the HIV/AIDS epidemic. The main focus of the GFATM project in the isles is on participatory response to HIV/AIDS for youth in Zanzibar. Response funds are managed by the Global Fund Country Coordinating Mechanism (GFCCM), which is multisectoral, consisting of representatives from various constituencies in government, civil society, private-sector organisations, development partners, religious/faith groups, members of academia, and PLWHAs. The GFCCM is chaired by the principal secretary of the CMO and co-chaired by the principal secretary of the MoHSW, with an executive committee comprised of all members of the GFCCM and three separate technical committees for HIV/AIDS, TB and malaria, each comprised of four members.

The functions and responsibilities of the GFCCM Zanzibar include the coordination, review and approval of proposals submitted by its local partners. In addition to functioning as a platform for partnership development, GFCCM is the source of coordinated information required for M&E and guidance, being the overall body responsible for programme implementation. While the executive committee meets quarterly, the technical committee meets twice quarterly.

The GFCCM is responsible for the coordination, review and approval of proposals submitted from its local partners and is a platform for partnership development. The

212

GFCCM ensures the full involvement of NGOs and CSOs in the country's proposals.

The GFATM has nine subrecipients, of which the MDA subrecipients include MoHSW, ZAC and the Mufti's Office and the CSO subrecipients include ZANGOC, the Aga-Khan Foundation, the Zanzibar Madrasa Resource Centre, ZAYADESA, the Anglican Church and the NGO Resource Centre (NGORC). Subrecipients are encouraged to request funds from, and to report to, ZAC on a quarterly basis. ZAC should request replenishments of their GFATM account every six months. However the disbursement of funds has been reported as subject to significant delays in both the first and third year of the GFATM programme.

In the third year of the programme, ZAC expected to receive funds to disburse to subrecipients in March 2006. However, due to significant delays, funds were disbursed to ZAC in mid-December. The delay was compensated for by the fact that the funds were disbursed for nine months (three-quarters) of planned activities, rather than for six months. However, the nine-month delay in disbursement must have caused significant disruption to the planned activities of subrecipients, compounded by the fact that the GFATM is the primary funding source for the majority of CSO subrecipients.

Table 6.15 compares annual subrecipient budgets with the amount that was actually disbursed by the GFATM in 2004/2005 and 2005/2006. In 2006/2007, the reported subrecipient budget equalled the amount that was disbursed by GFATM in December 2006 for nine months of activities. The final row of Table 6.15 shows the expected annual disbursements at the start of the project, with the annual budgets and actual disbursements by government and CSOs being approximately TZS650 million and TZS520 million respectively.

Table 6.15: Overview of the spending of the Global Fund funding (TZS), FY 2004/05–2005/06					
Ministry	Budget 2004/05	Actual 2004/05	Budget 2005/06	Actual 2005/06	Budget 2005/06
Mufti's Office	29 687 018	14 091 604	71 053 431	57 316 300	37 944 021
MoHSW	148 042 045	139 117 517	127 105 688	106 032 950	75 725 445
ZAC	132 146 353	78 069 888	103 463 149	69 020 836	49 613 099
CSOs	345 038 237	294 008 845	346 119 310	281 420 365	233 641 957
Total government	309 875 416	231 279 009	301 622 268	232 370 085	163 282 566
Total government and CSOs	654 913 653	525 287 854	647 741 578	513 790 450	396 924 523
Annual budget	752 640 000		459 425 000		571 375 000
Source: RGoZ, 2007					

ZAC stated that the reason for the delay in disbursements was that the initial annual reports and proposals for further funding sent by ZAC to the GFATM were incomplete. Thereafter, the subrecipient reports and funding proposals were sent back and forth between the GFATM office in Geneva and ZAC until they were agreed upon by both parties. Another reason for the negotiations taking so long is that ZAC lacks a member of staff dedicated to the coordination of the GFATM account. The subrecipients are also poorly equipped to produce suitable reports and funding proposals. Speeding up of the process would require the proposals to be well prepared and the subrecipients to produce sufficiently detailed reports. After running for almost three years, the cumulative delay in disbursement is approximately one year. Such a delay not only adversely affects service delivery, but also results in inefficient spending, or "dumping", aimed at expending funds before the end of the financial period concerned.

Table 6.16 summarises the proportion of disbursed funds that are spent by subrecipients in any given period, showing that the subrecipients were able to spend approximately 80% of the disbursed funds in both 2004/05 and 2005/06. Table 6.16 compares the amount spent in any FY relative to the available funding agreed upon at the inception of the GFATM project, with, in 2006/07, subrecipients having spent at most 69% of the available funds agreed to at the inception of the project, due to the significant delays experienced in disbursement. However, the delays have partly been compensated for by the disbursement of larger sums of funds than were agreed upon at the inception of the project for a given period of time (such as in 2005/06).

Table 6.16: Overall absorptive capacity for Global Fund financing, FY 2004/05-2006/07				
Ministry	FY 2004/05 (%)	FY 2005/06 (%)	FY 2006/07 (%)	FY 2004-2007 (%)
Mufti's Office	47	81	–	71
MoHSW	94	83	–	89
ZAC	59	67	–	62
CSOs	85	81	–	83
Total government	75	77	–	76
Total government + CSO	80	79	–	80
Annual budget	87	141	69	95
Source: RGoZ, 2007				

INTERNATIONAL NON-GOVERNMENTAL ORGANISATIONS

Table 6.17 presents details of the international NGOs that carry out HIV/AIDS activities external to, but generally in collaboration with, the government of Zanzibar. *Medicos Del Mundo* (MDM) provided significant support for the fight against HIV/AIDS, including undertaking STI testing and treatment, providing the main supply of condoms and a substantial amount of the reagents used for HIV VCT in Zanzibar.

Some international NGOs fund local NGOs to execute HIV/AIDS programmes in Zanzibar. For example, though the Zanzibar suboffice of CARE International does not directly carry out HIV/AIDS activities, CARE International Tanzania provided US$50 000 for Africare to carry out HIV/AIDS activities under the CARE TUMAINI programme in Zanzibar within one year from October 2005, in terms of which home-based care volunteers were trained and VCT kits purchased. Africare has also provided extensive support for HIV/AIDS activities in Zanzibar since 1996 in the form of the funding of activities proposed by ZANGOC and its members, which was allocated through ZANGOC to its member NGOs. In 2000, however, Africare changed its focus, channeling funds directly to seven NGOs in Zanzibar.

Table 6.17: Expenditure on HIV/AIDS efforts by international NGOs operating in Zanzibar (TZS), 2004/05-2006/07			
International NGO	Actual 2004/05	Actual 2005/06	Budget 2006/07
Africare	–	–	–
Community of Volunteers of the World	121 020 743	183 418 632	210 258 752
Aga-Khan Foundation	–	–	–
Care International	–	–	–
Save the Children	140 516 250	326 948 450	–
Medicos Del Mundo (MDM)	115 970 400	127 015 200	–
Action Aid	1 200 000	10 460 500	37 760 500
Total	378 707 393	647 842 782	248 019 252
Source: RGoZ, 2007			

The Action Aid suboffice in Zanzibar, which provided financial assistance through SIPAA support, has a limited HIV/AIDS programme in Zanzibar. Stepping Stone and Reflect (STAR), which is the main Action Aid programme, is a tool and methodology for literacy training and for facilitating HIV/AIDS committees. In 2006, Action Aid focused its STAR programme on 10 shehia in the North Unguja region and on community development officer training (under the Ministry of Labour, Youth, Women and Community Development) and regional education officer training (under the Ministry of Education and Vocational Training) at the district level. Action Aid also provides support for the Zanzibar Association of People Living with HIV/AIDS (ZAPHA+) and, in 2005, provided limited support for WAMATA.

The Aga-Khan Foundation received funding from the GFATM, via ZAC, for three projects in Zanzibar, comprising the NGORC, the Madrasa Resource Centre and the Aga-Khan VCT centre, the last of which also provides funding for its centres through recording a separate HIV/AIDS component of the funding.

Save the Children Fund has recently completed a key programme, Youth-Friendly Approaches to HIV/AIDS Education (YOFAHE), which was implemented from 2001 to 2006. The Fund has developed manuals on sexual RH, substance abuse and life skills for both health-care and education officers. Since 2005, STC has trained 300 teachers, 200 health workers and 127 peer educators in Mjini, Kati, Micheweni and Chake-Chake. Save the Children Fund has also established 11 youth-friendly information centres supplied with information, communication and technology (ICT) materials, for which sponsored youth groups write proposals and perform HIV/AIDS-related activities, as well as provided funding for local partner organisations, such as UWZ and the Zanzibar Youth Forum for HIV/AIDS-related activities.

CONCLUSION

In conclusion, the government is recognised as having exerted effort in dealing with the HIV/AIDS epidemic through nominal increases in budgetary allocations over time and its collaborative efforts with other stakeholders, such as its development partners, funding organisations, the private sector and civil society in minimising the impact of HIV/AIDS. However, many challenges to tracking HIV/AIDS expenditure by the government and key stakeholders exist. Gaps in the M&E systems of the different stakeholders threaten the effective implementation of planned HIV/AIDS interventions. The NASA framework is one positive step towards addressing some of the weaknesses observed in monitoring HIV/AIDS-related expenditure and in improving the international comparison of efforts made in this regard.

REFERENCES

Dahoma, M., Salim, A.A., Abdool, R., Othman, A.A. and Abdullah, A.S., 2005. *Prevalence of HIV, Hepatitis B and C and Syphilis Infection in Substance Users in Zanzibar, Tanzania*, Zanzibar: ZACP.

Msongole, L. and Killindo, A., 2003. *The Public Expenditure Review Process in Zanzibar*, Draft Report Submitted to MoFEA.

Mufti's Office, 2004. *HIV/AIDS Guideline for Zanzibar Muslim Community*, Zanzibar: Mufti's Office.

National Bureau of Statistics (NBS) [Tanzania] and ORC Macro, 2005. *Tanzania Demographic and Health Survey 2004–05*, Dar es Salaam: National Bureau of Statistics and ORC Macro.

Revolutionary Government of Zanzibar (RGoZ), 2002a. *Population and Housing Census*, Zanzibar: Office of the Chief Government Statistician (OCGS).

Revolutionary Government of Zanzibar (RGoZ), 2002b. *Zanzibar Poverty Reduction Plan*, Zanzibar: Ministry of Finance and Economic Affairs (MoFEA).

Revolutionary Government of Zanzibar (RGoZ), 2004a. *Zanzibar Poverty Reduction Plan – Progress Report for the Year 2003*, Zanzibar: Ministry of Finance and Economic Affairs (MoFEA).

Revolutionary Government of Zanzibar (RGoZ), 2004b. *Zanzibar National HIV/AIDS Strategic Plan 2004/5–2008/9*, Zanzibar: ZAC.

Revolutionary Government of Zanzibar (RGoZ), 2004c. *Estimates for Recurrent and Capital Revenues and Expenditure for the Year 2004/2005*, Dar es Salaam: Government Printer.

Revolutionary Government of Zanzibar (RGoZ), 2005a. *Report on Implementation of Planned Activities by the Zanzibar AIDS Control Program for the Year 2004–2005*, Zanzibar: Ministry of Health and Social Welfare.

Revolutionary Government of Zanzibar (RGoZ), 2005b. *Estimates for Recurrent and Capital Revenues and Expenditure for the Year 2005/2006*, Dar es Salaam: Government Printer.

Revolutionary Government of Zanzibar (RGoZ), 2006a. *Socio-Economic Survey 2005, Statistical Report (Preliminary Findings)*, Zanzibar: Office of the Chief Government Statistician.

Revolutionary Government of Zanzibar (RGoZ), 2006b. *Household Budget Survey: Preliminary Findings, Zanzibar*, Office of the Chief Government Statistician.

Revolutionary Government of Zanzibar (RGoZ), 2007. *Public Expenditure Review for*

HIV/AIDS: Draft Report, Zanzibar: Zanzibar AIDS Commission.

Revolutionary Government of Zanzibar (RGoZ), various. *Zanzibar HIV/AIDS Surveillance Reports, Zanzibar AIDS Control Program*, Zanzibar: Ministry of Health and Social Welfare.

Zanzibar AIDS Control Program (ZACP), 2005. *HIV Surveillance Data*.

ZAMBIA

KAMWANGA, J., CHITENGI, P. AND MALI, E.

EXECUTIVE SUMMARY

The advent of HIV/AIDS compounded an already precarious health situation in Zambia in the mid-1980s. Since the late 1980s, cooperating partners have complemented government efforts to reduce the burden of disease by allocating resources in this regard. However, the amount of resources being spent on HIV/AIDS programmes in the country is unclear. The total government health and HIV/AIDS expenditure information for purposes of this study was derived from the government budget books.

The Zambian government passed legislation that led to the establishment of the National AIDS Council (NAC) in 2002. NAC was mandated to coordinate, monitor and evaluate inputs, activities, outputs and impacts of HIV/AIDS programmes. The National HIV/AIDS/STI/TB Policy and the National HIV Intervention Strategic Plan define the country's response to the HIV epidemic. Prevention efforts are designed to help limit the spread of the virus, while mitigation efforts are intended to reduce the impact of the epidemic, with treatment and care programmes intended to support PLWHAs.

The steady increase in allocations to the health sector over the reference period entailed a steady rise in the nominal allocation from K935 million in 2002 to slightly over K1 billion in 2006. However, the real allocations were lower (after adjusting for inflation) over the reference period, having been recorded at K935 million in 2002 and K874 million by the end of 2006. Despite the discrepancy, the level of nominal per capita expenditure held steady over the years, being estimated at 93, 101, 91, 85, and 98 for the period 2002 to 2006 respectively.

In order to show the effect of the constitutional, statutory and debt-servicing budgets (CSD) on the health sector, allocations were computed both including and excluding the CSD. Health expenditure, as a proportion of the total government expenditure (TGE), remained constant over the year, being estimated at 11% over the period. However, the proportion, after discounting for CSD expenditure, increased from 10% to 17% and from 11% to 18% for 2002 and 2003 respectively. From 2004 onwards, however, the difference became smaller, thus reflecting a reduction in debt-servicing obligations.

The expenditure by target population showed that almost half of the NGOs surveyed indicated that they had spent their financial resources on the "general population", meaning that the HIV/AIDS responses were not targeted at meeting the needs of any particular social group. However, some of the organisations spent most of their HIV/AIDS resources on PLWHAs, orphans and vulnerable children, and the youth. While public funds were mostly spent on outpatient and inpatient care, the NGOs spent most of their resources on voluntary counselling and testing, programme management, human resource incentives, and workplace and IEC activities.

The government budget allocations and the Zambia National AIDS Network (ZNAN) disbursements to provinces/regions were used to show the regional variations in the allocation of HIV/AIDS funds. Based on the government expenditure on HIV/AIDS, the budgets for the Copperbelt, Southern and Eastern provinces had a strong positive relationship with their infection levels. However, a negative relationship was shown between the HIV/AIDS budget and the infection levels for Lusaka and the Central and Western provinces. Government and ZNAN resources were disbursed based on the HIV prevalence rates of the different provinces.

The steady increase in the number of partners and resources dedicated to the HIV/AIDS response has led to an increase in the collective capacity to implement prevention, treatment and care programmes, which has also resulted in coordination and administrative challenges. Tracking the resources allocated for HIV/AIDS responses and assessing whether they have been used for the intended purpose is difficult, with only the tracking of GFATM resources being relatively easy due to the centralised disbursement system.

Most of the HIV/AIDS service providers are faced with significant overlaps and duplications, and financial and programme management challenges, with the local organisations being unable to meet the stringent donor requirements. Given the already fragile health sector, the HIV/AIDS epidemic is threatening to wreak the public delivery system of activities, which is not well coordinated.

Socioeconomic Environment

Population

Zambia is a landlocked country, covering a land area of 753 000 square kilometres on the Central African interior plateau. Zambia's population is estimated to stand at 9.3 million, with a sex distribution of 51% female and 49% male, while the population density is 14 persons per square kilometre. Demographic projections (Chileshe, 2001) indicate that, at the current rate of population growth, Zambia's population will continue to grow younger on average for a long time to come. Close to 50% of the population is under the age of 15, with only about 3% over the age of 64. Zambia is one of the most urbanised countries in Sub-Saharan Africa, with about half its inhabitants living in the cities (Osei-Hwedie and Osei-Hwedie, 1992).

Socioeconomic Situation

Zambia was one of the most prosperous African nations on gaining its independence in 1964. However, external factors, such as the mid-1970s Middle East oil crisis, and bad internal economic policies, such as a rigid economic structure based on overprotectiveness, public sector dominance and import substitution, led to a precipitous economic decline that generated a severe economic crisis (Gaynor, 2005).

The economic reforms marked a dramatic departure from the populist and consumption-oriented policies of the previous United Nations Independence Party (UNIP) political regime.[71] The privatisation of state-owned mines improved the potential profitability of the mining industry. The liberalisation policies practised in the agricultural sector spurred growth over the years, which helped to boost GDP growth to 5.0% by 2004.[72] However, despite the reasonable and sustained economic growth, poverty levels have remained high, which might be due to the failure of government to redistribute income.

Health Infrastructure: Zambia Health Reforms

Rakner et al (1999) concluded that, despite the volatile economy, the combined donor and government expenditure in the health sector remained fairly steady. Paradoxically, the country experienced a steep fall in the major health indicators. The main issue confronting the country's social sector was the failure to properly and optimally allocate resources, rather than an actual lack of resources. Such inefficiencies were manifested by an excessive reliance on hospital care, and by chronic staff and supply shortages at health centres.

Furthermore, the health reforms were aimed at improving accountability. Previous MoH financial and staffing allocations reflected the prioritisation of high-technology curative care in response to political and popular pressures, rather than the official support of primary care. The reforms were aimed at redirecting attention away from the central levels to a client-focused system, in terms of which health-care providers became accountable to the local health boards.

The need to improve the coordination and participation of various actors in the health sector was underscored, with partnerships also extending to the private sector, which was expected to complement public sector service provision.

Overview of HIV/AIDS in Zambia

After the first HIV case was reported by the Ministry of Health (MoH) in 1984 (Nanyangwe, 2006), the cumulative number of cases had risen to approximately one million by 1997. HIV prevalence is higher in urban (26%) than in rural areas (16%), with the mode of transmission mainly comprising heterosexual contact. Zambian culture accepts men having multiple sex partners, which also contributes to high rates of infection.[73] Despite their increased use over the years, condoms are still only infrequently used, especially among high-risk groups,[74] such as commercial sex workers. The early commencement of sexual activity predisposes young people to the risk of infection. Circumcision, which has been noted to have a protective effect against transmission, is not widely practised in Zambia.[75]

Increasing poverty levels and the low health status of the population have also played their part in fuelling the epidemic. Women are worse affected than men, due to their low social and economic status, which enhances their susceptibility to infection.

In the latest Demographic Health Survey (DHS) (2002), the overall HIV prevalence rate for the country was about 16%. In the urban areas, the prevalence rate among 15 to 49 year-olds was more than 23%, while in the rural areas it was 11%. The overall rate is, therefore, exceedingly high, which shows that Zambia is one of the countries that has been most badly affected by HIV/AIDS. The HIV prevalence is higher in the urban regions of Lusaka and the Copperbelt provinces, where about 20% of the adults aged 15 to 49 years is HIV-positive. The rural prevalence rates are lower than the urban rates, usually ranging between 10% and 15%, compared with between 25% and 30% in the urban and periurban areas.[76]

The HIV prevalence in Lusaka remained constant at about 26% between 1990 and 1996, which could be due to a variety of reasons, including that the high HIV/AIDS incidence is offset by high mortality or that the incidence has genuinely declined (Fylkesnes, 1995).

Population-based surveys demonstrated striking differences in the age distribution of HIV prevalence, with peak prevalence rates of 50% being estimated among women aged 20 to 29 years and 42% among urban men aged 30 to 39 years (Fylkesnes et al, 1998). Young men in the age group 15 to 29 years had a much lower prevalence than did women of the same age.

Figure 7.I: HIV prevalence among Zambians aged 15-49 years, by province[77]

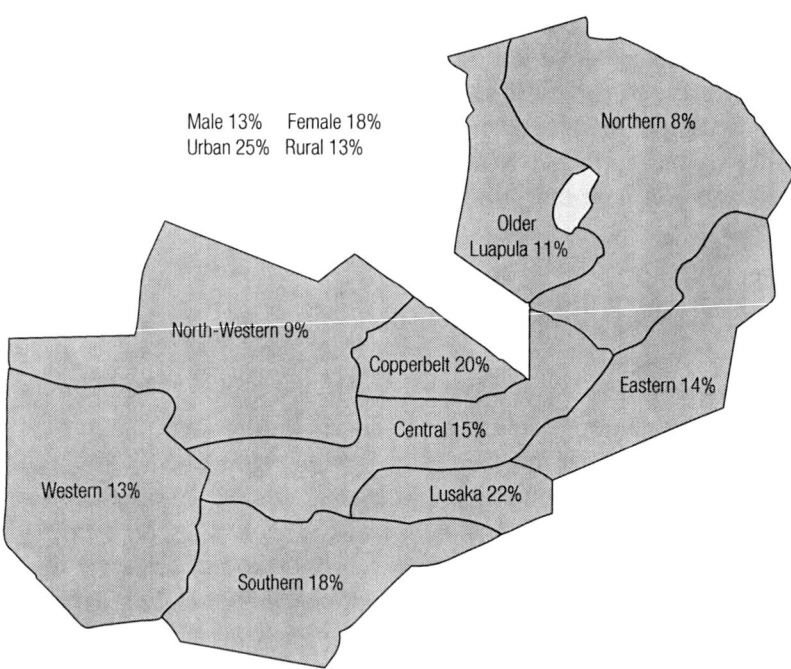

Source: Nanyangwe (2006)

According to Fylkesnes et al (1998), the infection rates among young women were higher than among young men, whereas in the upper age groups (older than 30 years), men in the urban areas were found with higher infection levels, or at comparable levels to women in the rural areas. The infection rates among men in the 15 to 19 year-old age group were relatively low in both the urban and rural populations, whereas, in the upper age groups, the rates were still high, particularly among urban men. Young women were found to be relatively more vulnerable to HIV/AIDS infection than men.

The relatively low occurrence in the 15 to 19 year-old age group shows that the rate of new infections can be reduced by widespread behaviour change.

THE NATIONAL RESPONSE TO HIV/AIDS

THE NATIONAL AIDS COUNCIL

The government passed legislation that led to the establishment of NAC in 2002, which was mandated to coordinate, monitor and evaluate inputs, activities, outputs and impacts of HIV/AIDS programmes. Subsequently, the country made a commitment and signed the UNGASS Declaration of the "Three Ones": one national AIDS coordinating agency, one strategic framework, and one monitoring and evaluation system.[78]

The specific tasks of NAC are:
- To promote the implementation of multisectoral behaviour change communication campaigns;
- To decrease the mother-to-child transmission rate by increasing access to quality PMTCT services in all districts;
- To make all blood, blood products and body parts safe for transfusion, and to promote the use of sterile syringes, blades and needles;
- To improve the quality of life of PLWHAs by encouraging positive living, good nutrition, the prevention of opportunistic infections and the avoidance of high-risk behaviour;
- To provide appropriate care, support and treatment to PLWHAs and to those affected by TB, STIs and other opportunistic infections;
- To provide improved care and support services for orphans and vulnerable children and others affected by HIV/AIDS, as well as for those at risk, such as refugees, prisoners and disabled people;
- To improve HIV/AIDS information management and decision making by developing well-coordinated databases; and
- To ensure impartial, transparent and effective programme operations by improving the coordination of the multisectoral implementation of interventions.

THE GUIDING PRINCIPLES OF THE RESPONSE

The National HIV/AIDS/STI/TB Policy (NAC Zambia, 2006) and the National HIV Intervention Strategic Plan define the country's response to the HIV/AIDS epidemic. Prevention efforts are designed to help stem further spreading of the virus, while mitigation efforts are intended to address the impact of the epidemic. Treatment and care programmes are intended to support PLWHAs. The response to HIV/AIDS is guided by the following underlying principles:
1. An appropriate legal framework, national coordination, an advocacy framework and a multisectoral approach to the HIV/AIDS epidemic are essential.
2. Information, education and communication (IEC) is needed to ensure behaviour change aimed at prevention and control.

3. Treatment, care and support are required to minimise the epidemic's impact.
4. Respecting the human rights and dignity of all people, regardless of their HIV status, and the elimination of stigma and discrimination against PLWHAs is necessary.
5. Gender mainstreaming should be regarded as a central element in the prevention of infection.
6. A supportive social and economic environment at all levels of society should enhance the responses of individuals, families and communities.

Figure 7.2: Structures and institutions for implementing government HIV/AIDS programmes

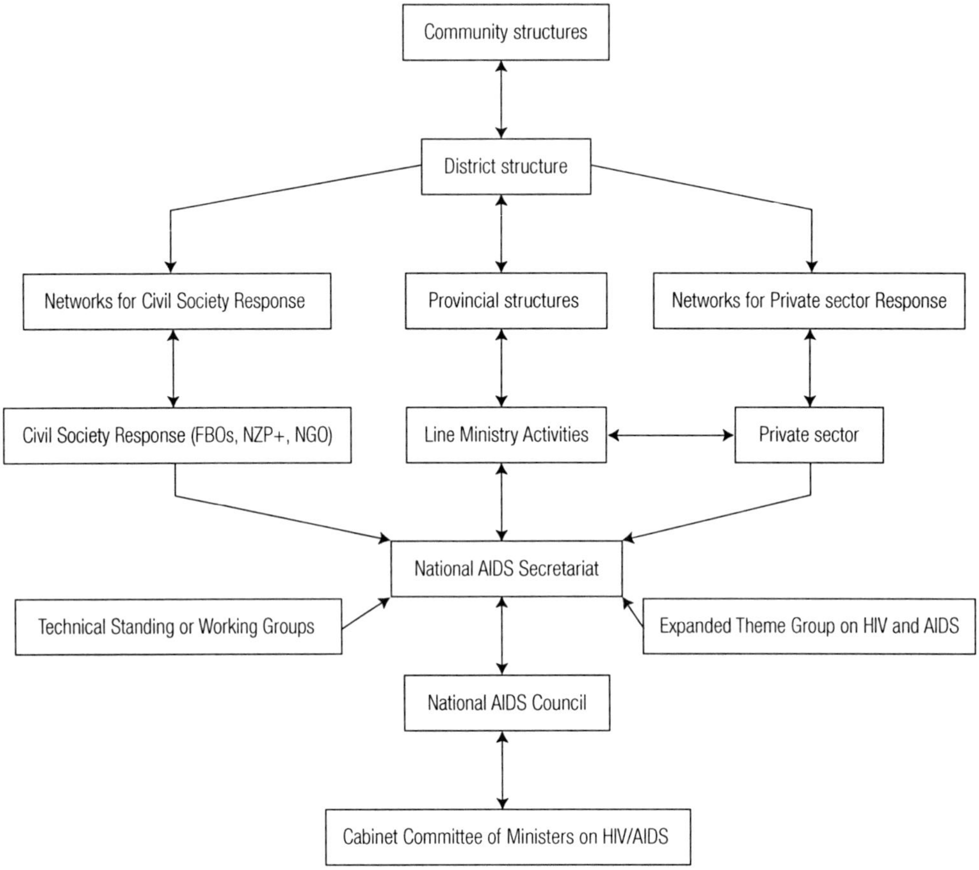

Source: NAC Zambia

INTERGOVERNMENTAL RELATIONSHIPS

NAC has substructures at provincial and district levels. At the provincial level, the NAC substructures comprise a subgroup of the Provincial Development Coordinating Committee (PDCC), known as the Provincial AIDS Task Force (PATF). At the district level, NAC is represented by a unit of the District Development Coordinating

Committee (DDCC), which is referred to as the District AIDS Task Force (DATF). Such structures are designed to enhance the multisectoral approach of the national response to HIV/AIDS, as members are drawn from state and non-state stakeholders.

BILATERAL AND MULTILATERAL PARTNERS

Multilateral and bilateral partners provide both financial and technical assistance in support of the implementation of the National Strategic Plan. International organisations also work with the government and NAC to develop strategies for addressing HIV/AIDS prevention, mitigation, and treatment and care activities through the expanded theme group. The Zambian government and some donors (Denmark, the DFID, Ireland, Norway and Sweden) contribute to the NAC basket fund referred to as the Joint Financing Arrangement (JFA).

THE NATIONAL BUDGET AND HIV/AIDS FINANCING PROCESSES

THE BUDGET PROCESS

In Zambia, the Ministry of Finance and National Planning (MoFNP) is responsible for preparing the budget. The Minister of Finance lays before the National Assembly within three months of the commencement of each financial year (FY), estimates of the revenues and expenditure of the Republic of Zambia for the relevant FY. The estimates and corresponding approved amounts are included in the Appropriation Bill after the approval of the estimates of expenditure (Mudenda et al, 2005).

The minister is also empowered to raise revenue for the Republic. The authority to charge taxes and to spend revenue is provided for in the Constitution of 1996, which stipulates, according to Article 114(1) of Chapter 687, that no tax shall be imposed or altered except by or under an Act of Parliament.[79]

The budget process starts with a call for circulars from ministries, provinces and districts in May/June, to which all the units make submissions in July/August. The budget team undertakes the aggregation and analysis of expenditure and revenue around September/October. By November, the budget is finalised, after which the draft budget is discussed in December, in readiness for the budget day in January. Figure 7.3 illustrates the budget cycle.

Figure 7.3: Flow diagram of the budget cycle

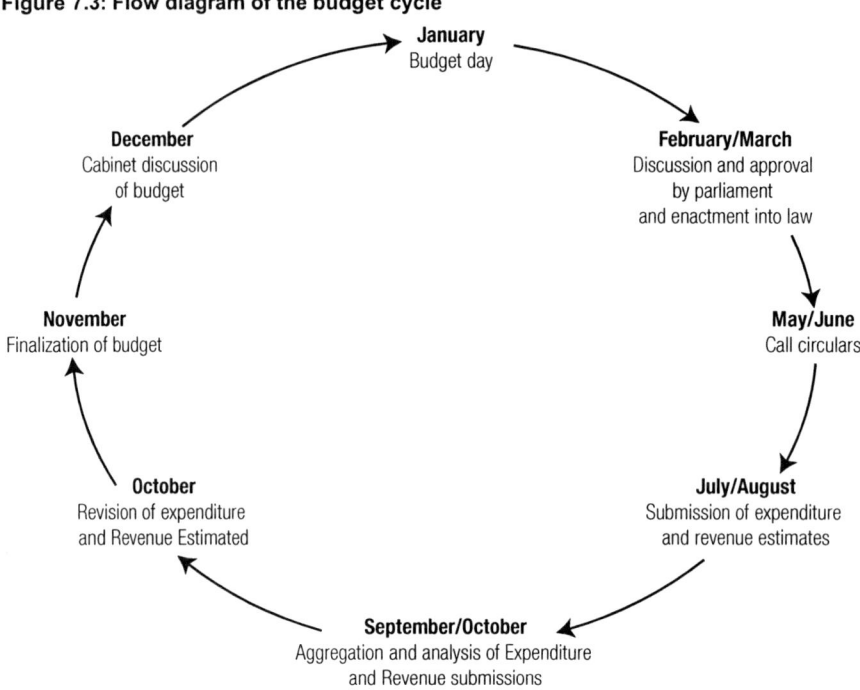

Sources: *Ministry of Finance and National Planning; NAC Zambia, 2006*

THE HIV/AIDS FINANCE PROCESS

Other than the allocations from the national budget, other sources of finance for HIV/AIDS activities in Zambia include:
- The World Bank/Zambia National Response to HIV/AIDS (ZANARA);
- The GFATM;
- The UNDP Multisectoral Response Initiative;
- The Joint Facility Arrangement; and
- The President's Emergency Plan for AIDS Relief (PEPFAR).

The information on the government HIV/AIDS allocations is obtained from the budget books, which are produced annually. The public resources include the funds sourced from local taxes and the budget support from the WB through ZANARA. Each ministry has an HIV/AIDS budget line, which shows the allocated amounts. Part of the WB funds is allocated to an umbrella organisation, (Community Response to AIDS (CRAIDS),[80] which provides financial and technical support to CBOs and disburses funds directly to the communities concerned.

The first agreement for GFTAM was signed in 2003,[81] of which the four principal recipients (financing agents) in Zambia are:
- The Churches Health Association of Zambia (CHAZ);
- The ZNAN; MoFNP; and
- NAC.

Each of the principal recipients provides funds directly to various local organisations.

The major recipients of funding from PEPFAR, which was established in 2003 in support of the national response,[82] are:

- Support to the HIV/AIDS Response in Zambia (SHARe);
- The Health Services and Systems Programme (HSSP);
- The Health Communication Project (HCP);
- Reaching HIV/AIDS-Affected People with Integrated Development and Support (RAPIDS);
- Zambian Prevention, Control and Treatment (ZPCT); and
- The Society for Family Health (SFH).

The Joint Financing Arrangement is an arrangement that brings together several donors in support of the coordination activities of NAC and the government. The five donors who form part of the JFA comprise:

- The Royal Netherlands Embassy;
- The Embassies of Sweden, Ireland and Norway; and
- The Department for International Development (United Kingdom) (DFID).

The UNDP multisectoral response to HIV/AIDS was instituted in 2003 in reaction to the capacity challenges set local government officials. The project objective is to build the capacity and skills of government officials to coordinate HIV/AIDS activities at provincial and district levels, as well as to support the M&E needs of the NAC technical working groups.

Figure 7.4: Flow of HIV/AIDS funds

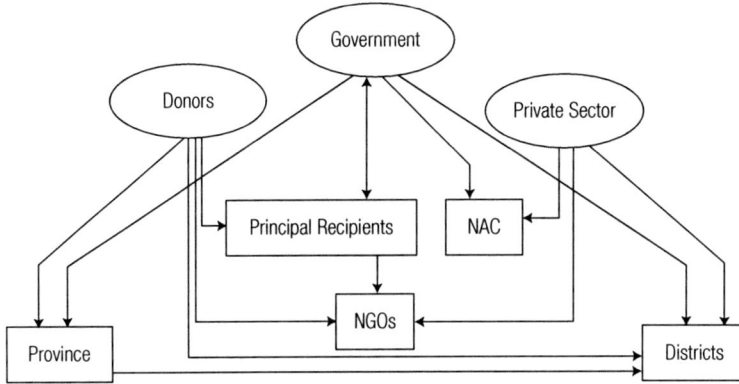

Source: NAC Zambia, 2006a

Figure 7.5: Institutional arrangements for the disbursement of the GFTAM

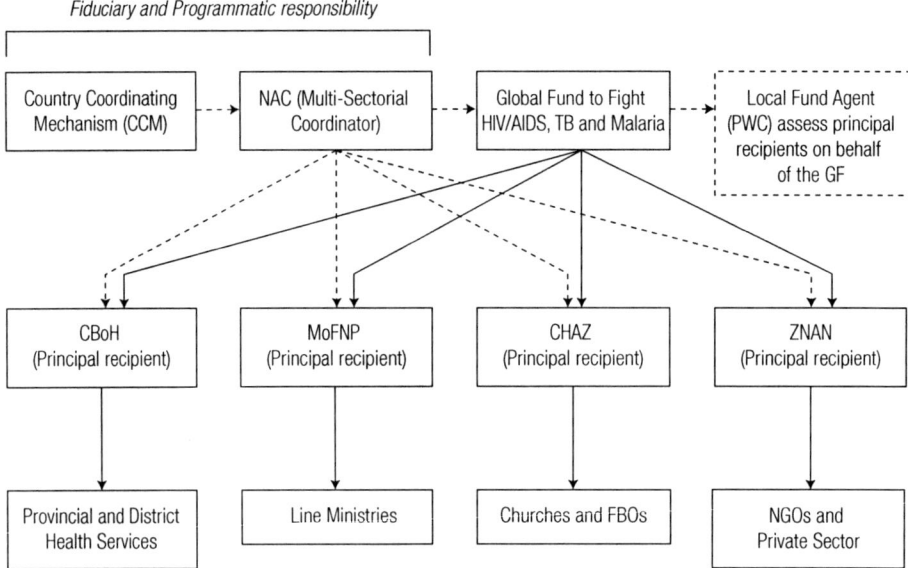

Sources: Global Fund www.theglobalfund.org/en/about/structures; NAC Zambia, 2006a

Total Public (Government) Health Expenditure

The government budgetary allocations to the health sector have steadily increased from 2002 to 2006, (Ministry of Finance and National Planning, various years), with the nominal budgetary allocations rising steadily from K935 million in 2002 to slightly over K1 billion in 2006. The real allocations (after adjusting for inflation and taking 2002 as the base year) amounted to K935 million in 2002 and K874 million by the end of 2006. While there was an increase in the absolute level of allocations, the level of nominal per capita allocations held steady over the years, being estimated at K93, K101, K91, K85 and K98 for the five years concerned, due to the rising population.

Table 7.1: Estimations of total government (public) health expenditure*					
	2002	2003	2004	2005	2006
Total health expenditure (kwacha) (TGHE)	935 044 753.00	1 033 280 147	956 663 006	918 203 246	1 085 819 257
Total health expenditure (US$)	233 761.1883	258 320.0368	239 165.7515	229 550.8115	271 454.8143
Per capita health expenditure (kwacha)	90.02519073	97.05677832	87.66835996	82.0916292	94.70955238
Per capita health expenditure (US$)	0.021434569	0.023108757	0.020873419	0.019545626	0.022549893
Per capita health expenditure (real kwacha)	93.5044753	79.954203	63.18360782	69.07866613	79.46094971
Real allocations to the health sector (kwacha)	935 044 753	815 532 870.6	663 427 882.1	739 141 727.6	874 070 446.8
Total govt expenditure (-CS)	5 255 413 343.00	5 696 818 873.00	7 561 185 385.00	7 954 823 370.00	8 751 858 586.00
Total govt expenditure (+CS)	6 126 413 343	6 931 510 010	9 036 305 385	9 779 025 370	10 236 578 586
Inflation[83]	26.7	17.2	17.5	16.8	15
Total Public Health Expenditure (TPHE)[84]					
Recurrent (MoH)	4 852 084 679	5 244 617 789	7 528 105 415	7 936 478 679	8 750 463 591
Capital	403 328 664	452 201 084	33 079 970	18 344 691	1 394 995
Medical levy			3736995	1095101	
Other foreign funds	277 597 780	27 371 689	211 715 312	114 024 940	1 271 845 111
Total Public Health Allocations	5 533 011 123	5 724 190 562	7 776 637 692	8 069 943 411	10 023 703 697
*Expenditure in '000					
Sources: Ministry of Finance and National Planning, National Budget estimates/expenditure, various years; Ministry of Health, Budgets, various years					

229

Figure 7.6: Public allocation to HIV/AIDS efforts undertaken in Zambia (Kwacha billion), 2002–06

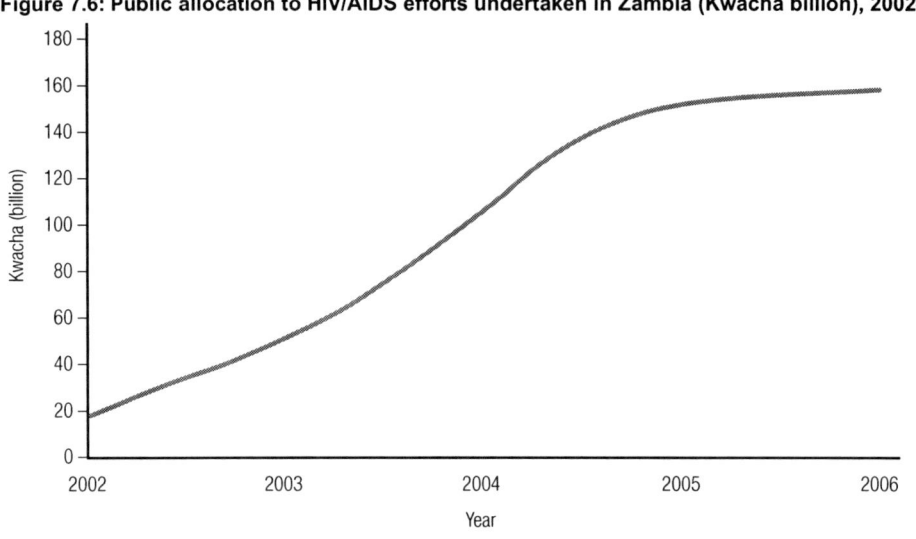

Sources: MoFNP Review of Estimates of Revenue and Expenditure Reports, 2002–2006; NAC Reports

COMPOSITION OF EXPENDITURE ON HIV/AIDS

The data given in Table 7.3 shows estimates of the total expenditure on HIV/AIDS in terms of source of funding and function of expenditure in five districts. The data for estimating total public expenditure were extrapolated from the 2002 HIV/AIDS National Health Accounts subanalysis,[85] while data for other sources of funding were based on the primary data collected from the NGOs in the five study districts. An examination of the NGO expenditure patterns[86] shows that the VCT and programme management components were the highest, followed by expenditures on incentives, workplace and IEC activities, respectively.

Almost half of the NGOs surveyed indicated that they spent their money on the general population. For the identified populations, most organisations expended their financial resources on PLWHAs, OVCs and the youth.

Table 7.2: Foreign /International financing sources for HIV/AIDS (US$), 2005		
Source of funds[87]	Amount	
	Budget/Pledge (programme/ project span)	Budget allocation (2005)
Bilateral sources		
CIDA	799,637.89	159,927.58
SIDA	1,599,000.00	400,000.00
Holland	10 609 064.00	2 900 271.73
NORAD	5 600 000.00	2 200 000.00
DFID	27 429 257.00	6 477 144.25
JICA	1 246 000.00	403 333.33
USAID	125 645 753.00	32 209 665.00
Subtotal	172 928 711.89	53 941 511.14
Multilateral Sources		
Global Fund[88]	56 657 498.00	18 885 832.67
World Bank/ZANARA	172 300 000.00	172 300 000.00
European Union	12 300 000.00	2 800 000.00
Subtotal	241 257 498.00	193 985 832.67
United Nations System		
UNFPA	3 434 758.00	1 125 871.71
UNDP	7 000 000.00	1 750 000.00
UNICEF	2 896 500.00	565 308.33
Subtotal	13 331 258.00	3 441 180.04
International NGOs/Agents		
Centre for Disease Control	7 694 000.00	7 694 000.60.
US Dept of Defence	2 208 125.00	2 208 125.00
Subtotal	9 902 125.00	9 902 125.60
Grand total	437 419 592.89	244 385 479.60
Sources: Deloitte and Touche, 2006; NAC, 2005, 2006		

Table 7.3: Estimates of total expenditure on HIV/AIDS by function of expenditure in five districts, 2005[89]		
Function of expenditure	Amount	Percentage
Advocacy and communication	9 422 169 200.00	11
VCT	168 768 964.00	0
Youth at risk	4 591 959 200.00	5
Programmes focused on sex workers	286 541 500.00	0
Workplace activities	4 309 971 266.00	5
Prevention and care programmes for PLWHAs	46 831 328 282.00	54
Condom social marketing	33 600 000.00	0
Prevention of mother-to-child transmission	462 047 117.00	1
Universal precautions	80 486 779.00	0
OVC programmes	4 603 070 998.00	5
Programme management	2 706 204 095.00	3
Monitoring and evaluation	50 040 722.00	0
Education and training	2 123 680 971.00	2
Monetary incentives for staff	50 040 722.00	0
Social services	5 850 000.00	0
Institutional development	70 764 700.00	0
Programmes focused on women	5 460 419.00	0
Income-generation projects	1 952 275 230.00	2
Construction of new health centre	262 203 588.00	0
Others	9 135 761 200.00	10
Total	87 152 224 951.00	100

ALLOCATION OF HIV/AIDS FUNDS BY REGION

The government budget allocations and ZNAN disbursements to provinces/regions showed regional variations in the allocation of HIV/AIDS funds. Lusaka, the Copperbelt, and the Southern and Central provinces had the highest HIV prevalence levels, while the Northern, North-Western and Luapula provinces had relatively low levels. The Copperbelt, Southern and Eastern provinces had bigger budgets, which were proportionate with their infection levels. Allocations to Lusaka, Central and Western provinces were low relative to their infection levels. In 2005, higher allocations were made to the Southern, Eastern and Northern provinces, while Lusaka and the Copperbelt provinces were allocated the least.

Figure 7.7: Allocation of HIV/AIDS funds by region

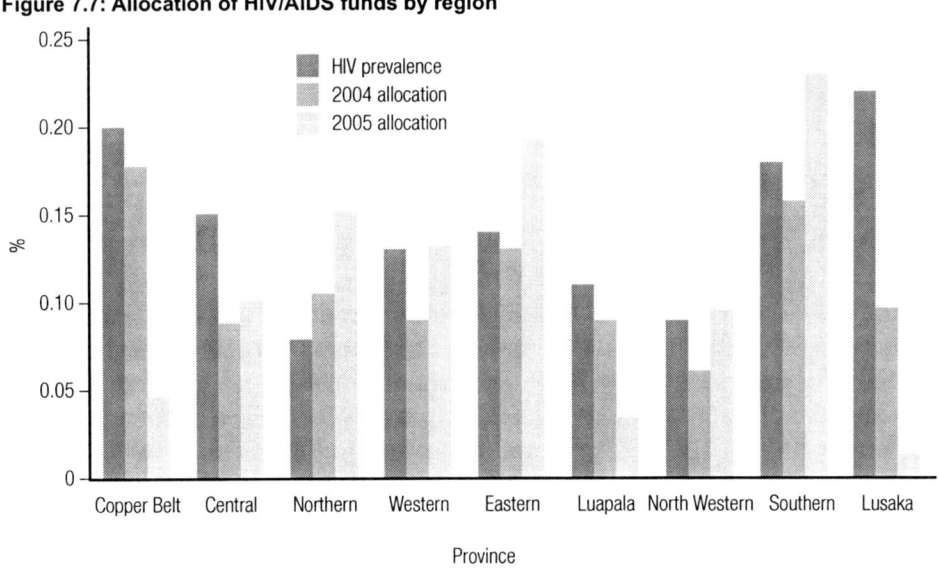

Sources: Ministry of Finance and National Planning, National Budget estimates/expenditure, various years; Ministry of Health, Budgets, 2004–2005

The data on ZNAN disbursements to the provinces were included to investigate whether they had an impact on regional budgeting differences. Thus, composite budget allocations combining public and ZNAN budgets were plotted against the provincial prevalence levels (see Figure 7.9). The findings show that the combined resources were disbursed in accordance with HIV prevalence. The three provinces with the highest prevalence Lusaka, the Copperbelt and Central also received the highest amounts, with Southern province being displaced by Eastern province.

Figure 7.8: HIV prevalence and allocation by province

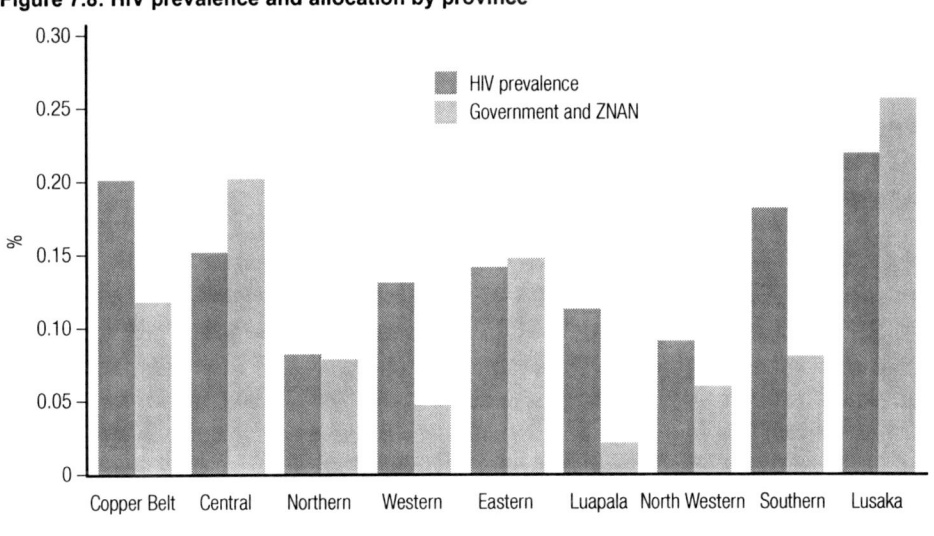

Sources: Ministry of Finance and National Planning, National Budget estimates/expenditure, various years; Ministry of Health, Budgets, 2004–2005

233

The government allocation did not reflect the prevalence levels in terms of regional differences. The addition of funds from ZNAN improved the allocation of HIV/AIDS funds, relative to the prevailing infection levels.

COORDINATION AND ADMINISTRATIVE CHALLENGES FOR HIV/AIDS ACTIVITIES – CAPTURING PEOPLE'S VOICES

Following the advent of the HIV/AIDS epidemic, the number of active partners and commensurate resources has steadily increased. This surge, while improving the collective capacity to implement prevention, treatment and care programmes, has invariably also resulted in numerous coordination and administrative challenges. Such difficulties might disrupt the delivery capacity of the public sector. The following section draws on interviews with key respondents and secondary sources to highlight such challenges.

A respondent stated:

> ...Given the scale of the HIV/AIDS problem, government resources would not be sufficient to adequately address the challenges. Hence the extra resources are welcome to the extent that they augment local efforts. For instance, without such external help, it would have been very difficult to scale up the activities, given the limited financial and technical capacity at the government's disposal. These extra resources have, for instance, led to a surge in ART services within a short period. The competence of providers has also been improved through skills upgrading.

Perverse effects have also been recorded, as stated by one of the key informants:

> .... there are challenges, when you have multiple donors and multiple financing mechanisms. We have faced challenges at the centre... at the district...and at the community level. [In response to these challenges]..the NAC has played a key role in terms of coordinating the HIV/AIDS activities...for instance through the Country Coordinating Mechanism. ...there are a number of technical working groups... At the local levels, there are the Provincial AIDS Task Forces, and District AIDS Task Forces.

> The CCM has helped in coordinating the activities. For instance, when we were allocating GFATM resources, we used the principle of comparative advantage. So CHAZ, for example, is very strong in community-based programmes, so that is where most of the resources went ....to implement such programmes. And ZNAN has another advantage in terms of community-based programmes and has funding for that. The Ministry of Health has a lot of these institutions, so it took care of all those government institutions.

While some sources of funding, such as the GF, can be relatively easily traced, given the centralised disbursement system, the many other financial sources cause tracking and auditing difficulties. Such difficulties are compounded by the lack of a uniform system, which could be used to ascertain the levels of resource inflows and utilisation patterns. The funding agencies that wanted to ascertain, in detail, how their funds were being used at a community level, were unable to retrieve such information. Due to such difficulties, the funders are becoming increasingly reluctant to release funds, even after they have been committed, resulting in the non- or late disbursement of pledged amounts. As a consequence, the subrecipients and implementers have been asked to spend the money allocated to them within a very short period in order to overcome a situation in which donors held on to their funds until they had to spend them. Upon releasing those funds, sometimes in huge amounts, they expected the implementers to utilise the funds within a short period.[90]

The coordination difficulties experienced at the central levels tended to be replicated at local implementation levels. Due to the implementers having multiple sources of funding, in some cases such agencies were unwilling to divulge their sources of funding. In the words of a key interviewee:

> ...Of course we are constrained with resources. These resources that we have at the moment are not enough. Some organisations hide information that they got funding elsewhere and with some they use the same information to get funding from different sources.

At first, implementers were allowed to undertake programmes according to their competencies, which led to multiple parallel activities. The less formally arranged interventions were, from inception, very likely to experience significant overlaps and duplications, verticality of programmes, financial tracking difficulties, and problems in understanding programme outcomes.[91] In talking about this issue, a key informant observed that:

> ...in terms of coordination, it is indirect through the National AIDS Council because the [Council] does not get data on all the activities that are taking place. Now there is another mechanism that was formed, which was made to coordinate all other activities including the World Bank. That is the UN coordinating system, the one headed by UNDP...this is a coordinating mechanism that has been....it is called the UN theme group...

Commenting still further on the coordination challenges, another respondent observed:

> ...implementation levels, such as DATFs and PATFs, are trying their best, but there are many small projects that come up that are funded directly....[and coordinating such projects in order] to ensure that there is no duplication is quite a challenge. And of course the task is probably [making] DATFS and PATFS [less effective], because these [are supposed to be for] HIV/AIDS activities, but you see there are so many donor-funded activities which are health-related, which are not directly HIV. So it might be a good idea to look at those coordinating bodies at the district level to incorporate all donor-funded programmes in order to make sure that there is synergy and no duplication.

The plethora of local HIV/AIDS activities, coupled with the varied forms of technical assistance provided by donors, strains both human and financial resources. The complexity of donor rules and regulations stretches the local organisations to such an extent that most are unable to meet the stringent requirements set. Such inability is largely due to the fact that such organisations already have other systems in place, while some donors insist on new systems being introduced.[92]

In order to address the capacity limitation experienced by coordinating HIV/AIDS activities at the local level, the UN has established local offices, which, however, are underutilised, partly because the subrecipients and implementers, instead of being obliged to report to the DATF and PATF, have to report to their donors. The public sector has been shown to be intrinsically weak, with any additional strain compounding the problem. One way in which the impact has manifested is through the movement of staff from the public to the NGO sector. Donor agencies do not, as a principle, pay salaries to volunteers or civil servants. As the salaries in the civil service are considerably lower than in the NGO sector, attracting certain skills into the civil service, which is crucial for the successful execution of projects, is extremely difficult. Even though the DATF and PATF are expected to provide technical assistance to subrecipients and implementers, they have been unable to recruit those with the requisite specialist skills.

According to CHAZ, in the words of another respondent:

> *...The fact that we still have inadequate numbers of staff is a big challenge that is yet to be solved by all these international funding arrangements. And definitely our appeal and recommendation is that in as much as these resources have come.... we feel that these initiatives should now focus more on... system-wide funding. The issues that I have articulated to you: the issue of human resources; the issue of infrastructure; the issue of transport; the issue of communication...[and] strengthening monitoring and evaluation. ...we feel that you cannot scale up an HIV/AIDS, TB or malaria programme in a vacuum... [the programmes have to] operate within a system and if that system is weak, these programmes will not succeed. So, yes, the issue of human resources is still a problem, because the numbers are small. They are not coping. We have actually done a study.... which actually shows that most of these workers have a very high burn-out.*

CONCLUSION

The absence of a central database providing details of those state and non-state actors involved in the HIV/AIDS response was, at the time of going to press, giving rise to significant overlaps and duplications, verticality of programmes, financial tracking difficulties, and challenges in tracking programme outcomes. While the efforts of DATFs and PATFs are commendable, many small projects are funded directly by donors, which makes it difficult to track their progress and to assess their impact. Given the already fragile health sector, the parallel activities, if not well coordinated, could wreak havoc on the public delivery system. The complexities of donor procedures and regulations stretch the service providers to such an extent that they end up being unable to implement the planned activities. HIV/AIDS service providers are also characterised by lack of human capacity, which compromises programme delivery.

REFERENCES

Chileshe, A., 2001. *Forestry.* Outlook Studies in Africa, Rome:

Deloitte and Touche, 2006. *Data Base for HIV/AIDS Resources in Zambia.*

Fylkesnes, K., 1995. *Updates on Patterns, Trends and Demographic: Implications of the HIV/AIDS Epidemic in Zambia,* Lusaka: National AIDS /STD/Leprosy Programme.

Fylkesnes, K., Ndhlovu, Z., Kasumba, K., Musonda, R. and Sichione, M., 1998. "Studying the Dynamics of the HIV Epidemic Population-based Data Compared to Sentinel Surveillance in Zambia", *AIDS*, 12(10).

Gaynor, C., 2005. *Structural Injustice and the MDGs: A Critical Analysis of the Zambian Experience.* Dublin.

Ministry of Finance and National Planning, Various years *National Budget Estimates, 2002–2006.*

Nanyangwe, L., 2006. *Location, Dislocation and Risk for HIV: A Case of Refugee Adolescents in Zambia, South Africa.*

National AIDS Council (NAC) (Zambia), 2005. *Second Joint Annual Programme Review of the National HIV/AIDS/STI/TB Intervention Strategic Plan (2002–2005).*

National AIDS Council (NAC) (Zambia), 2006a. *NAC Sources of Funds; National HIV/ AIDS 2005 Spending Assessment.*

National AIDS Council (NAC) (Zambia), 2006b. *The National HIV/AIDS Strategic Framework, 2006–2010.*

Mudenda, D., Ndulo, M. and Wamulume, M., 2005. "The Budgetary Processes and Economic Governance in Zambia: A Literature Review", *NEPRU* (104).

Osei-Hwedie, K. and Osei-Hwedie, B., 1992. "Reflections of Zambia's Demographic Profile and Population Policy", *Journal of Social Development in Africa*, 7(1).

Rakner, L., Walle, N. and Mulaisho, 1999. *Aid and Reform in Zambia, Country Case Study, Zambia Demographic and Health Survey, 2001–2002.*

ENDNOTES

1   http://news.bbc.co.uk/1/hi/world/africa/3503097.stm; http://www.plan.org.au/ourwork/southernafrica/malawi/733; http://www.undp.org.ls/hivaids/default.php

2   Food poverty lines measure the standard of living against which all individuals can be compared, based on the monetary value of food baskets incorporating basic minimum human nutrient requirements, such as food, water, housing, health care, and education (set at 2,250 calories per day) to be met (World Bank, 2003, p. 19). The line can also be taken to refer to the cost of obtaining the required minimum basic necessities. In 1997, the food poverty line was estimated at a K927 per month per adult equivalent for rural Kenya and K1 254 for the urban areas. Such expenditure would, on average, meet the recommended daily energy allowance per adult. Therefore, a household whose food expenditure is less than this amount is deemed to be poor (Ministry of Finance and Planning, June 2000).

3   http://www.unaids.org/en/KnowledgeCentre/HIVData/Tracking/Nasa.asp

4   Idasa previously used this methodology.

5   www.health24.com/medical/condition

6   Ethiopia, Kenya, Malawi, Tanzania, Zambia, Zanzibar

7   Foreign financiers, the governments and the private sector (including CSOs and households)

8   http://stats.oecd.org/glossary

9   http://en.wikipedia.org/wiki/Poverty_in_Africa

10   http://en.wikipedia.org/wiki/budget

11   Money can be printed when the deficit is denominated in local currency, but it has catastrophic effects on inflation.

12   http://tutor2u.net/business/accounts/incrementalbudgeting.htm

13   www.worldbank.org/publicsector/pe/mtefprocess

14   The difference lies in the different FYs, resulting in different timelines.

15   "Tanzania" refers to the mainland.

16   Though the Abuja Declaration has other clauses, this will only be used to refer to the attainment of the "15% of national budgets to the health sector".

17   As to whether the 15% should account for domestic funds only or include the foreign grants and loans allocated through the national is debatable. The current work will focus on all the funds that are disbursed through the national budget, irrespective of their origin.

18   www.thebrenthurstfoundation.org/files/Africa_Beyond_Aid/Agriculture_and_AidGames.doc -

19   www.endpoverty2015.org/files/Aideffectivenss%20-%20harmonization_25-01-05.doc -

20   http://www.uneca.org/eca_resources/Major_ECA_Websites/joint/panel.htm

21   http://www.uneca.org/eca_resources/Major_ECA_Websites/joint/panel.htm

22   http://useconomy.about.com/od/inflationfaq/f/infl_impact.htm

23   Only the local currency is affected by inflation.

24 This section only considers the situation pertaining to antiretrovirals up until 2005, since the period of study is 2004/05.

25 http://www.who.int/3by5/publications/documents/isbn9241591129/en/

26 http://www.who.int/hiv/universalaccess2010/en/index.html

27 http://data.unaids.org/publications/FactSheets03/who_fs_%20aids_treatment_nutrition_30mar05_en.htm

28 http://www.avert.org/hivcare.htm

29 http://www.aidsmap.org/en/news/A4ED06C5-E06D-4C1B-82D6-9E2D4794BB9F.asp

30 www.aidspnac.org/key-population.htm

31 Nairobi, 30 July 2004 (IRIN).

32 The endemic nature of malaria in the Ethiopian economy lies in its attacking farmers during the agricultural peak season, particularly during the harvest. The peak transmission seasons occur from September to October and, to a lesser extent, from April to May. While the former comprises the harvesting time, the latter comprises soil preparation time.

33 The framework is guided by a "Financial Calendar", which is also issued by MoFED. The objective of the Financial Calendar is to ensure that planning and budgeting are prepared, approved, appropriated and executed by adequately scheduling the tasks to be performed, the timeframe for each task and the institutions responsible for performing each task.

34 Appropriation refers to the legal authority granted to the executive by the House of Peoples Representatives to spend public funds for a stated purpose.

35 "Public body" means any organ of the federal government that has a legal mandate established by proclamation or regulation, which is partly or wholly financed by the government allocated budget, which submits its final accounts directly to the respective ministry and which is on the approved list of public bodies issued by the Prime Minister's Office.

36 The FY government's 12-month accounting period (8 July–7 July).

37 The appropriation at federal level specifies the total of the federal capital budget, the recurrent budget, the regional subsidies and the total subsidy for each region. Subsidies to regions are based on three indicators: population size (60%), the level of development hhg(25%) (with four subdevelopment indicators being considered here: the agricultural sector; the education sector; the health sector; and the water sector), and the revenue collection effort (15%).

38 "Consensus" refers to a broad understanding of the common good and the modalities of working to that end.

39 The principle of transparency is recognised by the IMF, in its "Code of Good Practices on Fiscal Transparency – Declaration of Principles" (1998). See B.H. Potter, Fiscal Transparency: The IMF Code, Paper submitted to the Second International Budget Conference entitled "Transparency and Participation in the Budget Process", Cape Town, 21–25 February 1999. Copies of the IMF transparency documents, which are now available in Arabic, Chinese, French, Portuguese, Russian and Spanish, are available at the IMF transparency web site at http://www.imf.org/external/np/fad/trans/.

40   No specific category or budget item exists for HIV/AIDS.

41   This is based on the GDP deflator, taking 1999/00 as the base year.

42   Such an amount is less than that which was allocated, which may be due to underreporting by the different regions.

43   Food poverty lines which measure the standard of living against which all individuals can be compared are based on the monetary value of food baskets that allow basic minimum human nutrient requirements such as food, water, housing, health care, and education (set at 2,250 calories per day) to be met (World Bank 2003 pp 19). The line can also be taken to refer to the cost of obtaining the required minimum basic necessities. In 1997, the food poverty line was estimated at KES927 per month per adult equivalent for rural Kenya and KES1,254 for urban areas. This is the amount of expenditure that would on average, meet the above recommended daily energy allowance per adult. Therefore, a household whose food expenditure is less than this amount is deemed to be poor (Ministry of Finance and Planning, June 2000).

44   The expected target for the MDG goals is a two-thirds reduction, between 1990 and 2015, of the under-five mortality rate, from 99/1 000 in 1990 to 33/1 000 in 2015. However, such a target is unlikely to be achieved, given that the rate has since increased to 115/1 000. The major challenge to the reduction of child mortality is the continued increase in mortality rates since the 1990s in all regions of the country. Furthermore, the inequitable access to health care services, coupled with the high cost of accessing health care, especially for the poor, remains a major obstacle to the achievement of the MDGs.

45   Poverty is more prevalent among infected and poor women than it is among men (KDHS, 2003), because a significant number of women, especially in the rural and urban slum areas, are unemployed. In such a situation, the death of a husband implies the loss of livelihood.

46   The needs assessment adopted the Futures Group model on HIV/AIDS for the estimation of resources needed for prevention and to improve the quality of care (ie care and treatment and orphan support). The model is divided into three submodels, namely, the prevention model, which calculates the cost of twelve prevention interventions contained in the HIV/AIDS Strategic Plan; care and treatment, which calculates the cost of five different care and treatment programmes; and orphan support or the mitigation of socioeconomic impact, which calculates the cost of three separate interventions to support those children orphaned by HIV/AIDS.

47   The "three ones" comprise: one agreed HIV/AIDS Action Framework, which provides the basis for the coordinated work of all partners; one National AIDS Coordinating Authority, with a broad-based multisectoral mandate; and one agreed country-level M&E system (KNASP 2005–2010).

48   The MPERs show the actual and projected expenditures for each ministry for the coming financial year.

49   The core ministries in various sectors comprise: Human Resource Development; Agriculture and Rural Development; Tourism; Trade and Industry: Public Administration; Physical Infrastructure; National Security:

Public Safety; Law and Order; and Information Technology (Republic of Kenya, 2005).

50 The per capita expenditure falls short of GoK's commitment to spend 15% of its total budget on health, as agreed to in terms of the Abuja Declaration

51 The values were taken from the approved recurrent expenditure from Treasury to the ministries during FY 2003/04 and FY 2004/05.

52 The US government contribution includes those funds channeled through CDC and PEPFAR.

53 UNAIDS (2005) AIDS epidemic update.

54 Health facilities in the three cities of Malawi.

55 See Tanzania Forum Group For Rural Transport and Development, Seminar paper on rural transport presented to Parliament under the theme: Addressing the problems of accessibility and mobility in rural areas in Tanzania, Dodoma, 14 February 2004.

56 THIS is a population-based survey showing the indicators of HIV/AIDS in Tanzania.

57 The definition used here is based on whether an individual had previously heard of HIV/AIDS. See National Bureau of Statistics (NBS) [Tanzania] and ORC Macro (2005). *Tanzania Demographic and Health Survey (DHS) 2004-05*. Dar es Salaam, Tanzania: National Bureau of Statistics and ORC Macro.

58 Traditional healers should be taken to mean herbalists who use herbs and other parts of plants to treat HIV symptoms and not witchdoctors who only pretend to be able to cure AIDS. Witchdoctors, as such, have proved a major impediment to the fight against the spread of the virus.

59 The information presented in this section was mainly drawn from the Ministry of Finance budget guidelines.

60 *Mkakati wa Kukuza Uchumi na Kuondoa Umaskini Tanzania.*

61 The Planning Commission was changed to the President's Office, Planning and Privatization (PoPP) and to the full-fledged Ministry (Ministry of Planning, Economy and Empowerment) in 2006. Further, in the same year, the Ministry of Regional Administration and Local Government was removed from the President's Office to the Prime Minister's Office.

62 CFS largely comprise debt and interest payments (both domestic and foreign), which have first claim on national resources. The GOT budget, excluding CFS, is therefore used to define the "discretionary budget" within which government has more scope to articulate its spending priorities.

63 The data contained in the Accountant General Reports differs from that held by the. For FY 2005, however, the data are very close to each other.

64 No thematic area could be identified for about 3.5 million

65 The current population projected from the 2002 Population and Housing Census (RGoZ, 2002a).

66 The Zanzibar AIDS Control Program (ZACP) and HIV Surveillance Data (2005) figures shown here might not represent the true picture of the situation, because the total number of people tested for HIV is not representative of the total population.

67 This definition is based on whether an individual has ever heard of HIV/ AIDS. See National Bureau of Statistics (NBS) [Tanzania] and ORC Macro. (2005). *Tanzania Demographic and Health Survey (DHS) 2004-05*. Dar es Salaam: National Bureau of Statistics and ORC Macro.

68 Note that the PER and MTEF processes in the Isles follow the same principles as the processes do on the Tanzania mainland.

69 The CFS largely comprises debt and interest payments (both domestic and foreign), which have first claim on national resources. The GOT budget, excluding CFS, is therefore used to define the "discretionary budget" within which the government has more scope to articulate its spending priorities.

70 The extent to which the costing exercise provides a reliable estimation of the resources required to implement ZNSP is unknown.

71 www.springerlink.com/index/D0574T3604555620.pdf

72 http://exchange.unido.org/upload/1509_Zambia%20at%20a%20glance.

73 www.who.int/hiv/HIVCP-ZMB.pdf

74 www.fhi.org/en/HIVAIDS/pub/guide

75 www.plusnews.org/indepthmain.aspx

76 www.zamstats.gov.zm

77 cfapp2.undp.org/dgo_rcar/documents/document_ZAM_445093139.ppt

78 Source: http://zambia.jhuccp.org

79 Article 115 (1) also provides that "no moneys shall be expended from the general revenues of the Republic unless: the expenditure is authorised by a warrant under the hand of the president; the expenditure is changed by the Constitution or any other law on the general revenues of the Republic; or the expenditure is received by a department of government and is made under the provisions of any law which authorises that department to retain and expend those moneys for defraying the expenses of the department". Source: www. parliament.gov.zm/index.

80 The Community Response to HIV/AIDS (CRAIDS), Project under the auspices of the World Bank. MAP was set up in provide technical and financial support to CBOs.

81 www.theglobalfund.org/programs/grantdetails

82 www.usaid.gov/zm/hiv/pepfar.htm

83 The deflators were based on the CSO annual inflation figures reflected in CSO 2006, Selected Socioeconomic indicators, Lusaka.

84 To estimate the public health expenditure, the health expenditures from all pertinent ministries, provincial and district budgets, as reflected in the annual budget books were identified and summed. The public capital expenditures appeared under the PRP for each ministry, province or district, with all such amounts being summed up to obtain an estimate of the total expenditure for the health sector.

85 The 2005 Public Estimates were derived from the 2002 HIV/AIDS subanalysis. An average growth rate of 10%, based on the 2002 to 2006 rates of change in public health expenditure, was used for the extrapolation.

86 Figure 9.2, showing the NGO expenditure function, indicates the proportion

of expenditure spent on all HIV/AIDS activities, apart from those for the general population.

87 The exact reference periods for the various donor funds are shown in the appendices. In most cases, the block-pledged/budgeted amounts were indicated by the relevant donors. In order to derive the annual figures, which were used as estimates for 2005, the block amounts were divided by the number of years covered by the programme/project. The following were the time periods for the various financiers: CIDA (2002–2007); the Netherlands (2003–2007); JICA (2000–2006); USAID (2000–2010); CDC (2004–2005); DOD (2004–2005); DFID (2003–09); Norway (2004–07); SIDA (2002–2007); World Bank (2003–2008); UNDP (2002–2006); UNFPA (2002–2006); UNICEF and WHO (1999+); the EU (2000–2007); and the Global Fund (2003–2008).

88 The four principal recipients of Global Fund resources are: the Zambia National AIDS Network (ZNAN); the Christian Health Association of Zambia (CHAZ); the Ministry of Finance and National Planning (MOFNP); and the National AIDS Council (NAC).

89 Ministry of Finance and Planning, budget estimates, various years: Ministry of Health, Budgets, various years.

90 For example, UNFPA retained possession of about Euro 200 000 of EU funds, later expecting the MOH to spend the amount retained on DHS within a fortnight; whereas, the. MOH hoped that they would have been informed about these funds earlier, enabling the Ministry to plan how to use it.

91 The National AIDS Council tried to develop a cooperating partner database that was meant to serve as a depository for all HIV/AIDS funding information in the country. Due to the joint financing mechanisms involved, the database has a major shortcoming, precluding any knowledge of the contribution made by each donor and linking of the funding to any specific geographical area.

92 For example, donor agencies have specific procurement-related regulations that must be followed. The standard procedure is to invite bids from interested parties, with only those parties satisfying certain criteria, such as bank guarantees, being shortlisted. Such regulations, however, are not universally applicable, as different rules apply to different organisations. For example, DFID indicated a willingness to use the National Tender Board, while the WB preferred to use its own system of procurement.

Printed in the United States
147449LV00003BA/5/P